COMMUNITY

HEALTH

EDUCATION

METHODS

Mon Feb 1
5-6 pm
Hp 12 52

Allen
Kaiserman

2/9
ice breaker

COMMUNITY HEALTH EDUCATION METHODS

a practical guide

THIRD EDITION

Edited by

Robert J. Bensley, Ph.D.
WESTERN MICHIGAN UNIVERSITY

Jodi Brookins-Fisher, Ph.D., CHES
CENTRAL MICHIGAN UNIVERSITY

JONES AND BARTLETT PUBLISHERS
Sudbury, Massachusetts
BOSTON   TORONTO   LONDON   SINGAPORE

World Headquarters

Jones and Bartlett Publishers
40 Tall Pine Drive
Sudbury, MA 01776
978-443-5000
info@jbpub.com
www.jbpub.com

Jones and Bartlett Publishers
Canada
6339 Ormindale Way
Mississauga, Ontario L5V 1J2
Canada

Jones and Bartlett Publishers
International
Barb House, Barb Mews
London W6 7PA
United Kingdom

Jones and Bartlett's books and products are available through most bookstores and online booksellers. To contact Jones and Bartlett Publishers directly, call 800-832-0034, fax 978-443-8000, or visit our website, www.jbpub.com.

Substantial discounts on bulk quantities of Jones and Bartlett's publications are available to corporations, professional associations, and other qualified organizations. For details and specific discount information, contact the special sales department at Jones and Bartlett via the above contact information or send an email to specialsales@jbpub.com.

Production Credits

Acquisitions Editor: Jacqueline Ann Geraci
Associate Editor: Amy L. Flagg
Editorial Assistant: Kyle Hoover
Senior Production Editor: Julie Champagne Bolduc
Production Assistant: Jessica Steele Newfell
Marketing Manager: Wendy Thayer

Marketing Associate: Meagan Norlund
Manufacturing Buyer: Therese Connell
Composition: Gryphon Publishing Services, Inc.
Cover Design: Kristin E. Ohlin
Cover Image: © Photos.com
Printing and Binding: Malloy, Inc.
Cover Printing: Malloy, Inc.

Library of Congress Cataloging-in-Publication Data
Community health education methods : a practical guide / [edited by] Robert
J. Bensley, Jodi Brookins-Fisher.—3rd. ed.
    p. ; cm.
    Includes bibliographical references and index.
    ISBN 978-0-7637-5533-1 (pbk. : alk. paper)
    1. Health education—Handbooks, manuals, etc. 2. Community health
services—Handbooks, manuals, etc. 3. Health education—Handbooks, manuals,
etc. I. Bensley, Robert J. II. Brookins-Fisher, Jodi.
    [DNLM: 1. Health Education--methods. 2. Community Health
Services—methods. 3. Health Promotion—methods. WA 590 C7355 2008]
    RA440.C66 2008
    613.071--dc22
                        2007049469

Photo Credits
p. 6, © Michael G. Smith/ShutterStock, Inc.; p. 27, © Jack Hollingsworth/PhotoDisc; p. 59, © Arne Trautmann/ShutterStock, Inc.; p. 64, © Marc Dietrich, ShutterStock, Inc.; p. 89, © PhotoLink/PhotoDisc; p. 93, © foto.fritz/ShutterStock, Inc.; p. 171, © Jack Hollingsworth/PhotoDisc; p. 202, © Ben Blankenburg/Stockphoto; p. 243, © S. Meltzer/PhotoLink/PhotoDisc; p. 245, © Jones and Bartlett Publishers; p. 283, © AbleStock; p. 286, © ArrowStudio/ShutterStock, Inc.; p. 309, © Duncan Smith/PhotoDisc; p. 345, Courtesy of the Centers for Disease Control and Prevention; p. 347, © Ryan McVay/PhotoDisc.

6048
Printed in the United States of America
12 11 10 09 08   10 9 8 7 6 5 4 3 2 1

This book is dedicated to the past and present students who have spent numerous hours and years completing professional preparation programs in community or public health education. It is through the process of studying how to become a health educator that students learn the skills necessary to be effective practitioners. May the concepts presented in this book continue this process.

CONTENTS

Welcome to the third edition of *Community Health Education Methods: A Practical Guide*. This text is designed to assist you in effectively communicating messages and affecting norms and behaviors of individuals and communities. It is a book about the methods we use as health educators—the ways in which we tell a story and empower others to seek healthy lifestyles. It explains the basic tools we need in order to communicate messages to those we are trying to serve, and it provides an understanding of the skills we need to make a difference.

This text is unique because many of the chapters are written by and for local health education practitioners. Much of the material within this text comes straight from the trenches, where real health education occurs. It is a guide designed to assist the health educator who exists on a shoestring budget and is attempting to implement the strategies that theorists and researchers have proved to be effective. It is for the overburdened practitioner who is working with multiple populations, across multiple settings, experiencing multiple problems. It is a guide to assist those on the front lines of health education in completing their mission.

This edition has been expanded in several ways, all of which are designed to provide both student and practitioner with an expanded understanding of the application of skills related to the practice of health education. New to this edition is a chapter that focuses on professionalism in health education ("Developing Professionalism as a Health Educator"). All chapters have been revised to reflect new trends in health education methods, including the impact of the Internet and technology across all methods. Although maintaining a practitioner's focus, perspectives from national leaders in health education are incorporated into existing chapters. In addition, each chapter continues to be user friendly by conforming to a common chapter format, including key terms, additional resources, and interesting "Did You Know?" facts. A series of "Community Connections" vignettes appears in each chapter, designed to provide readers with an easy-to-understand, practical application of the concepts presented in the chapters.

The text is divided into three sections, each containing chapters that center on a common theme. Section I provides an overview of models and concepts relevant across all health education methods, including the chapters "Using Theory and Ethics to Guide Method Selection and Application," "Promoting Health Education in a Multicultural Society," "Developing Professionalism as a Health Educator," and chapters introducing health communication and social marketing concepts.

Sections II and III follow a similar format that includes an introduction to the topics, steps for implementing the skill, tips and techniques for successful implementation, strategies for overcoming challenges, and expected outcomes. Section II comprises chapters that focus on health education methods designed to influence behavior at the individual level. "Facilitating Support Groups" provides guidance on how to effectively facilitate support group processes, "Selecting Presentation Methods" and "Developing Effective Presentations" direct the reader through the entire presentation process, "Developing and Selecting Print Materials" presents skills for creating materials appropriate for a target population, and "Working with the Media" identifies how to utilize existing media avenues.

Section III comprises chapters that pertain to methods utilized at the community or policy level. "Facilitating Groups" and "Building and Sustaining Coalitions" provide information on how to coordinate and maintain community group efforts, while "Using Advocacy to Affect Policy" and "Using Media Advocacy to Influence Policy" focus on skills associated with strategies to promote health-related policy change.

It is our intent that this third edition will continue to assist students and practitioners in the acquisition and delivery of health education skills.

Robert J. Bensley, Ph.D.
Western Michigan University

Jodi Brookins-Fisher, Ph.D., CHES
Central Michigan University

ACKNOWLEDGMENTS

As with any project of this magnitude, there are numerous individuals whose contributions are usually "behind the scenes" but are paramount to its success. It is in part due to their efforts that the third edition of this text has come to fruition.

First and foremost, we want to acknowledge the individual authors of this text for agreeing to contribute their experiences and knowledge related to community health education practices. Without them, this book would not exist. Their integrity, dedication, knowledge, patience, and understanding are definitely appreciated.

We also would like to acknowledge the efforts of many who had a part in creating, editing, and reviewing various parts of this text. A list of names is difficult to provide, as each individual author has sought input from their own sources during the creation of their chapters. However, it is important for us to recognize their contributions in making this a highly credible text. We would like to particularly acknowledge Jones and Bartlett Publishers for their willingness to travel this road with us.

The health educators who have shared offices with, served as mentors to, and collaborated on projects with the authors of this text deserve recognition for the roles they have played in shaping the skills and experiences of the authors. The agencies and institutions for which the authors work and the populations they serve also deserve credit for providing authors with opportunities to gain knowledge and practical experiences.

We would also like to thank Irene O'Boyle, Ph.D., CHES of Central Michigan University for updating the TestBank, PowerPoints, and Instructor's Manual. Her expertise was greatly appreciated.

Finally, we thank our families for their unwavering support during this project. Kathy, Kara, Katilee, Jack, Bekah, Paul, Max, Katie, and Ben, we thank you for your patience, support, and understanding. Your unconditional belief and hope is what keeps us going.

Michael D. Barnes, Ph.D.

Dr. Barnes is a Professor of Public Health Education within the Department of Health Science at Brigham Young University, where he also serves as Director for the Master of Public Health program. Dr. Barnes' research interests include health communication interventions and policy advocacy, for which he has garnered many publications and received notable grants and awards. His passion for the profession is constantly sparked by training and mentoring students, and by serving on national and international boards within prominent professional associations.

Loren B. Bensley, Jr., Ed.D.

Dr. Bensley is a Professor Emeritus of Central Michigan University, where he served for 33 years in the professional preparation of health educators. His interest in learning theory and its relationship to methodology had its origin during his first years of teaching in secondary school. As a university professor, his research and teaching reflected his continued interest in helping students understand learning theory and applying it to the selection of school and community health education methods. During his career, Dr. Bensley was active in professional associations at the state, national, and international levels. One of his interests was improving standards by advocating a professional code of ethics. As chair of the American Advancement for Health Education (AAHE) Committee on Ethics, he participated in the early stages of what is now the current Health Education Code of Ethics.

Robert J. Bensley, Ph.D.

Dr. Bensley is currently a Professor of Community Health Education at Western Michigan University. His research interests focus on the use of advancing technology modalities as a means of influencing behavior change, for which he has been awarded over $1,000,000 in funding as principal investigator in technology-based projects. He is the creator of www.wichealth. org, a parent–child nutrition education behavior change project that has served over 175,000 WIC participants across seven states. He is also working with the Heart and Stroke Foundation of Ontario in developing Internet-based solutions for blood pressure management and healthy weight management. Dr. Bensley received a Fulbright Senior Scholar Award in 2003 and spent six months engaging in health promotion activities associated with the University of Port Elizabeth, South Africa. Prior to entering the health education profession, Dr. Bensley was employed by IBM, where he served as a systems engineer providing technical assistance and education to educational institutions, hospitals, and local government agencies.

Jodi Brookins-Fisher, Ph.D., CHES

Dr. Brookins-Fisher is a Professor in the School of Health Sciences at Central Michigan University (CMU), where she also is currently the Undergraduate Internship Coordinator. Her research interests include the evaluation of university–community partnerships, programs for underserved populations, and sexuality education. Dr. Brookins-Fisher has been involved in several national and state professional organizations, including the local chapter of Eta Sigma Gamma. She has received CMU's Teaching Excellence Award, Registered Student Organization Advisor Award, and Outstanding Teacher Award in her department. Additionally, Dr. Brookins-Fisher has received both the Great Lakes Chapter Society for Public Health Education (SOPHE) and national Eta Sigma Gamma Distinguished Service Awards. A human rights advocate, Dr. Brookins-Fisher has been recognized for her contributions to underserved populations.

Frances Dunn Butterfoss, Ph.D., M.S.Ed.

Dr. Butterfoss is the Foundation Professor and Director of the Division of Community Health and Research in the Department of Pediatrics at Eastern Virginia Medical School (EVMS) in Norfolk, Virginia. She is the founder and board member of the Consortium for Infant and Child Health (CINCH) and Project Immunize Virginia (PIV). Dr. Butterfoss teaches in the ODU/EVMS Master of Public Health Program, directs several grants, and consults on building and maintaining effective coalitions for health promotion and disease prevention. She is an Associate Editor of Health Promotion Practice and is a past President of SOPHE. She recently published a comprehensive text on coalitions, *Coalitions and Partnerships in Community Health*.

Lori Dorfman, Dr.P.H.

Dr. Dorfman directs Berkeley Media Studies Group (BMSG), a project of the Public Health Institute. She directs BMSG's research on how public health issues appear in the media, which BMSG applies to its media advocacy with community groups and to its professional education for journalists. Her research and media advocacy cover a range of public health issues, from alcohol and tobacco to nutrition and physical activity to violence prevention. Dr. Dorfman teaches a course on mass communication and public health at the School of Public Health at the University of California, Berkeley; consults on strategic communications with foundations, public health groups, and government agencies; and is co-author of *Media Advocacy and Public Health: Power for Prevention* and *News for a Change: An Advocate's Guide to Working with the Media*.

Karen Denard Goldman, Ph.D., CHES

Dr. Goldman has been a health educator for over 20 years, enjoying a fulfilling career as a full-time academic at the graduate and undergraduate levels. As director of KDG Health Education Consulting, Dr. Goldman has provided health education and social marketing technical assistance, training, and keynote presentations for over 15 years. She currently serves on the health education faculty of Kingsborough Community College and The City University of New York (CUNY). Dr. Goldman is a Public Health Association of New York City Board member, an Associate Editor of *Health Promotion Practice*, and creator and co-author of *Health Education Tools of the Trade: Tools for Tasks That Didn't Come with the Job Description*. She has previously served as President of the national SOPHE, Coordinator of the New York State Coalition for Health Education, and Coordinator of the Professional Development Board of the National Commission for Health Education Credentialing (NCHEC). Dr. Goldman conducted the first federally funded, nationally broadcast conference on social marketing in New York City, and she has conducted social marketing orientation and training for community and public health personnel across the country.

Lynne Durrant, Ph.D.

Dr. Durrant is an Associate Professor in the Department of Health Promotion and Education and Adjunct Assistant Professor in the Department of Nutrition at the University of Utah. She was previously the Substance Abuse Prevention Director at the Community Counseling Center in Salt Lake City. Her research areas of interest include individual and group health behavior change; alcohol, tobacco, and other drugs prevention; and substance abuse prevention through community coalitions. Dr. Durrant is the Project Director for the Neighborhood Action Coalition, which has been funded through the Center for Substance Abuse Prevention and the Department of Justice continuously since 1990. She is the author of two junior high school textbooks on drug education and prevention, and she received the University of Utah's Distinguished Teaching Award in 1999.

Malcolm Goldsmith, Ph.D., CHES

Dr. Goldsmith has taught professional preparation methods and curriculum classes for over 30 years and has been involved in numerous leadership roles at the state and national levels, including coordinating a risk reduction program for the Hawaii State Health Department. Presently, he serves as Professor and Coordinator of Health Education at Southern Illinois University at Edwardsville. Dr. Goldsmith is the current Chairperson of the Board of Commissioners of NCHEC, and he also serves as Director of Chapter Development for Eta Sigma Gamma, the National Health Education Honorary. He has co-authored two books on peer health education and delivered numerous presentations to the health education profession as well as to business and industry.

Gary L. Kreps, Ph.D.

Dr. Kreps is the Eileen and Steve Mandell Professor of Health Communication at George Mason University, where he serves as Chair of the Department of Communication, Director of the Center for Health and Risk Communication, Governing Board Member for the Center for Social Science Research, and faculty affiliate of the National Center for Biodefense and Infectious Disease. Prior to his appointment at Mason, he served as founding Chief of the Health Communication and Informatics Research Branch at the National Cancer Institute (NIH), where he developed and coordinated major national research initiatives concerning risk communication, health promotion, behavior change, technology development, and information dissemination to promote effective cancer prevention and control. He also has served as the Founding Dean of the School of Communication at Hofstra University, as Executive Director of the Greenspun School of Communication at the University of Nevada, Las Vegas, and in faculty and administrative roles at Northern Illinois, Rutgers, Indiana, and Purdue Universities. Dr. Kreps' areas of expertise include health and organizational communication, health promotion, ehealth, multimedia edutainment, multicultural relations, and applied research methods.

Sue Lachenmayr, M.P.H., CHES

Ms. Lachenmayr is a past President of SOPHE and has served as chair of the national SOPHE's Advocacy Committee and as Advocacy Committee Chair and President of the New Jersey SOPHE. She is an Adjunct Professor at the University of Medicine and Dentistry of New Jersey School of Public Health and is a health education consultant, particularly in the areas of advocacy and media advocacy training at the university, state, and national levels. She was former State Public Policy Coordinator for the Alzheimer's Association State Public Policy Coalition and a member of the New Jersey Commission on Aging. Ms. Lachenmayr is co-author of *Amplifying Our Voices: Training for Public Health Advocacy* and winner of SOPHE's 2001 Program Excellence Award, as well as the author of publications and programs training health educators to be effective advocates.

Brad L. Neiger, Ph.D., CHES

Dr. Neiger is currently employed as a Professor and Chair of the Department of Health Science at Brigham Young University. His previous positions include Director of the Bureau of Health Promotion at the Utah Department of Health, Director of Health Education at FHP (managed care), and Director of Health Promotion at the Davis County Health Department (Utah). He also taught at Utah State University and currently retains adjunct faculty status at the University of Utah. Dr. Neiger has served in leadership roles in many state and national health education associations, including vice-chair of the Board of Commissioners on NCHEC. Dr. Neiger's research interests include social marketing and health communication.

Mike Perko, Ph.D., CHES, FAAHE

Dr. Perko is an Associate Professor and Chair of the Department of Health Science at the University of Alabama and serves as a mentor to students in the University of Alabama's Ph.D. program in Health Education and Promotion. Formerly chair of the Worksite Health Promotion group for the American Public Health Association (APHA), Dr. Perko has consulted and spoken extensively on worksite wellness and currently serves as Associate Editor of the Wellness Council of America's national publication, *Absolute Advantage*. The 2003 Health Educator of the Year in North Carolina, as well as an AAHE Fellow, Dr. Perko has authored two books, published more than 30 articles in professional journals, and presented more than 75 peer-reviewed papers.

Kathy Delavan Plomer, M.P.H.

Ms. Delavan Plomer has been in the field of health education in varying capacities for the last 15 years. Her experience includes work at a local health department and three nonprofit health agencies and extensive community volunteer work. During her years in health education, Ms. Delavan Plomer has seen technology change the way that information is sent, received, and processed, but recognized that the printed word is as vital as ever in getting health messages out to the public. She has helped inform health educators how to create easy-to-read, audience-centered print materials that allow everyone, regardless of reading ability, language status, or other barriers, to get the health information they need to take care of themselves and improve their lives.

Keely S. Rees, Ph.D., CHES

Dr. Rees is an Associate Professor at the University of Wisconsin La Crosse, where she teaches courses in community health foundations, women's health, grant seeking, aspects of aging, and nutrition education. Dr. Rees' research interests are exercise and health habits during and after pregnancy, nutrition for families, and worksite wellness. Dr. Rees has been a faculty co-advisor for Eta Sigma Gamma for the last seven years and served as At-Large Board Member nationally for the last three years.

Traci Rieckmann, Ph.D.

Dr. Rieckmann is a Research Assistant Professor within the Department of Public Health and Preventive Medicine at Oregon Health and Science University. Her field of focus is primarily adoption of evidence-based practices (EBPs) in substance abuse treatment services. Dr. Rieckmann is the principal investigator on an award examining the impact of a state mandate that requires the use of EBPs, a second investigation exploring state authority strategies aimed at increasing the use of EBPs, and an investigator for the NIDA Clinical Trials Network and the Network for the Improvement of Addiction Treatment. She was previously a Visiting Assistant Professor within the Department of Social and Behavioral Sciences at the University of Portland and a clinical resident in private practice. Dr. Rieckmann also has an extensive background working with adolescents in a variety of settings. She generated a gang intervention curriculum and community-based substance abuse prevention and intervention groups while working as a youth counselor and program coordinator.

Jason Rivas, M.P.A.

Mr. Rivas is the Program Manager for the eHealth Innovations Group at Western Michigan University (WMU), where his responsibility is the development and oversight of several Internet-based behavior change programs. He has extensive experience with Web design, development, and usability and is passionate about integrating innovative technology into health education. Previously, he served as an health educator for a Michigan tri-county health department and an HIV test counselor for the health center at WMU. He also has spent two years in rural Japan teaching English as a second language.

Kathleen Roe, Dr.P.H., M.P.H.

Dr. Roe is Chair of the Health Science Department and Professor of Community Health Education at San José State University in Northern California. As Founder and Director of the Community Health Studies Group, Dr. Roe has been involved in community health promotion efforts for over 25 years, including HIV prevention planning, neighborhood capacity building for health, violence prevention, breast and cervical cancer outreach, health promotion in public housing, and community support for relative caregivers. Dr. Roe is a past President of SOPHE and a former member of the Governing Council of APHA. She serves as co-editor of the Circle of Research and Practice Department of Health Promotion Practice. Dr. Roe has been acknowledged for her professional accomplishments and commitments many times, including the Northern California SOPHE's Dorothy Nyswander Award for Leadership in Health Education. In 2006, she was named a Distinguished Fellow of SOPHE.

Kevin Roe, M.P.H.

Mr. Roe is the Community Organizer at Magnet, a gay men's health and community center in San Francisco. Over the last ten years, Mr. Roe, with the Community Health Studies Group, has been involved in community health promotion efforts throughout California, including HIV prevention and health services planning processes in San Francisco, Alameda, and Santa Clara counties; Our Lives, a Photovoice project with African American non-gay–identified men who have sex with men in Alameda County; YouthPOWER, a violence prevention project of the San Francisco Department of Public Health; and Building Bridges, an HIV and substance abuse prevention social marketing planning grant for African Americans in San Francisco. Mr. Roe is a member of the HIV Section and the LGBT Caucus of APHA, as well as SOPHE.

Frank V. Strona, M.P.H.

Mr. Strona has been working in gay men's health, community organizing, and substance use concerns for almost 20 years and has established himself as a nationally recognized frontline specialist in HIV/STD harm reduction techniques, sexual health, Internet interventions, and prevention education. He has served as the 2006 and 2007 community co-chair for the California HIV/AIDS Prevention Planning Group, in addition to being a member of the San Francisco HIV Prevention Planning Council. Mr. Strona has received numerous awards and recognitions for his work in gay men's sexual health promotion and the Internet.

Rosemary Thackeray, Ph.D., M.P.H.

Dr. Thackeray is an Associate Professor in the Department of Health Science at Brigham Young University. She teaches courses in social marketing, women's health, and survey and research methods. Her research interests focus on social marketing and health communication, particularly in the areas of formative research, audience analysis, and audience segmentation. Dr. Thackeray has worked with the Centers for Disease Control and Prevention, National Center for Health Marketing, and consults with the Utah Department of Health and other local health agencies on social marketing–related projects. She is the co-associate editor for the Social Marketing Department of the journal *Health Promotion Practice*.

Stephen B. Thomas, Ph.D.

Dr. Thomas is the Philip Hallen Professor of Community Health and Social Justice and Director of the Center for Minority Health in the Graduate School of Public Health at the University of Pittsburgh. He is principal investigator for EXPORT Health, an NIH-funded Center of Excellence in Minority Health and Health Disparities. Dr. Thomas has applied his expertise to address a variety of conditions from which minorities generally face far poorer outcomes, including cardiovascular disease, diabetes, obesity, and HIV/AIDS, among others. Dr. Thomas received the 2005 David Satcher Award from the Directors of Health Promotion and Education for his leadership in reducing health disparities through the improvement of health promotion and health education programs at the state and local levels and the 2004 Alyzo Smyth Yerby Award from the Harvard School of Public Health for his work with people suffering the health effects of poverty.

Heather Wagenschutz, M.A.

Ms. Wagenschutz was previously a public health educator with a tri-county health department, where she focused her presentations on sexually transmitted diseases, stress reduction, and worksite wellness. She also worked for two of the largest pharmaceutical companies in the world as an executive health care representative, specializing in Alzheimer's, mood disorders, and upper respiratory tract infections. During her time as a pharmaceutical rep, she also taught part-time at Kellogg Community College as a health and science instructor. Currently, she consults for a group of specialty physicians and is working on her doctorate in health administration.

Kathleen Young, Ph.D.

Dr. Young is an Assistant Professor in the Health Education and Master's of Public Health Program in the Department of Health Sciences at California State University, Northridge. Dr. Young also serves as the undergraduate coordinator in the Health Education Program, where she has developed and coordinated university–community partnership service learning programs with over 30 public health organizations and agencies throughout the San Fernando Valley within the greater Los Angeles area. Her research interests include tobacco control policy and women's health issues, specifically in primary prevention strategies in cancer and domestic violence. Dr. Young received the 2007 California State University-Northridge Distinguished Faculty Visionary Community Service-Learning Award.

Michael Young, Ph.D., FSSSS, FAAHB

Dr. Young is a Professor and the Associate Chair for Research and Doctoral Studies in the Department of Health Science at New Mexico State University. He is nationally known for his work in sexuality and drug education. His sexuality and abstinence education projects have been five-time recipients of the U.S. Department of Health and Human Services Award for Outstanding Work in Community Health Promotion. He is co-author of *Keep a Clear Mind*, selected by the Center for Substance Abuse Prevention for its Exemplary Program Award, and recipient of the American Association for Health Education Scholar Award and the American School Health Association Research Award. Dr. Young is a Fellow of the Society for the Scientific Study of Sexuality and a Founding Member and Fellow of the American Academy of Health Behavior.

I

Concepts and Theories Associated with Selecting and Implementing Community Health Education Methods and Strategies

1

Using Theory and Ethics to Guide Method Selection and Application

Loren B. Bensley, Jr., Ed.D.

Author Comments

This chapter is about health education theory and ethics, two essential ingredients for determining what methods to use and how to maintain integrity in the way we practice. I know you are probably thinking there are more exciting chapters—chapters that address the practicalities of how to do health education rather than the theory and philosophy of ethical practice. After all, aren't theory and ethics things you learn for a test and then forget or seldom ever use? Or, if you are a practitioner, you never have the time or the resources to apply theory to practice and, as far as ethical practice is concerned, you may think you are okay as long as you use common sense.

Realizing the above, I am challenged to write this chapter so that it is interesting, relevant, applicable, and easy to comprehend and remember. To do this, I have chosen a format that includes the daily practice of two entry level health educators and their supervisor, all of whom are employed by a county health department. Their challenges in planning and delivering theoretically based health education in an ethical manner is the chapter's focus.

As a health educator for 38 years in public schools and higher education, a consultant, a researcher, and an observer of health education in all settings—local, state, national, and international—I am convinced that the application of theory to practice ensures greater success for health education efforts. Furthermore, I am passionate about upholding the integrity of the profession by abiding by our professional code of ethics. There is nothing more professionally sacred than to behave and carry out our responsibilities in an ethical way. To do otherwise is unacceptable.

Community connections 1

Dawn has 12 years' experience as a health educator. She has served in two health departments, including the one where she is currently employed. Dawn has a master's degree in health education and is a Certified Health Education Specialist (CHES). She is also very active in the state's chapter of the Society for Public Health Education (SOPHE), serving as its president. As a supervisor, she is highly organized and considered a "pro" by her peers.

Jill is a graduate of a respected undergraduate community health education program and recently received CHES status. She has been employed by the health department for one and a half years and is currently working on her master's degree in health education at a nearby university. Her colleagues know her as a creative person with a solid understanding of professional issues. Like many health educators, she tries to balance her commitments and responsibilities to her family, employment, and graduate studies.

Mike is a recent graduate with a bachelor's degree in health education from one of the state's universities known for its excellent professional preparation program. As an undergraduate, he was active in Eta Sigma Gamma, the National Health Education Honorary, serving as chapter president. His recommendations stated he has an excellent work ethic, and he completed a successful internship as a health promotion specialist with a large corporation. Mike was hired six months ago as a health education generalist. If asked how he liked his job, he would say, "Great! I am still learning, however, what community health education is all about."

If you ask Jill, with her one and a half years' experience, she will tell you that at times she becomes frustrated and disappointed with the lack of success in motivating individuals to make changes in their health behaviors. She often feels

Introduction

This chapter has two purposes. The first is to introduce the reader to health education theory and apply it to the selection and implementation of methods. The second is to foresee ethical dilemmas in making decisions about how methods are selected and used. The role of health educators is to motivate and educate individuals, families, organizations, and communities to take action in promoting behaviors conducive to safe and healthy environments and lifestyles. Through training, health educators are empowered to change environments and behaviors to improve the quality and quantity of people's lives. The existence of this power to make a difference creates the burden of responsibility to practice theoretically sound and ethical health education. How can health educators, then, implement health education with some assurance that specific health problems are being addressed in the best possible way? By using theory and ethical principles to select and apply methods that will yield positive results without harm.

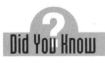

Did You Know

The health education profession did not have a unified code of ethics until 1999.

disillusioned with her chosen profession. As an undergraduate, she believed she could make a difference in people's lives by helping them live healthy lifestyles. At times there seems to be progress toward this belief, which gives her hope.

Dawn can identify with Jill's disillusionment because she went through a similar experience. It was after attending a state SOPHE conference and starting her master's degree that she realized there was more to health education than content, knowledge, and communication skills. As a nurse, Dawn had integrated her personal strengths, such as her organizational and communication skills, into her practice at the expense of applying theory to the selection of methods. She could see where Jill, like herself, would use motivational and behavioral change methods without a sound theoretical foundation. Dawn knows that Jill needs help and encouragement, as well as a working knowledge of health education theory.

Mike, on the other hand, is doing all he can to make health education work. Like many young professionals, he and Jill are hard-working, enthusiastic, and idealistic in their pursuits. Occasionally, in their quest to experience success, they may not have been aware of the importance of the process of implementing methods. For example, individuals could be misinformed, insulted, or treated unfairly by not taking into consideration basic ethical standards of practice. They did not realize this until Dawn helped them apply the Code of Ethics for the Health Education Profession to some of the dilemmas they faced. Theory and ethics were two critical components Mike and Jill had underestimated in terms of their importance in their undergraduate studies. Why? Perhaps theory and ethics did not seem that important at the time or were learned and soon forgotten.

Theory in Health Education

Health educators cannot assume, nor take for granted, that everyone is motivated and learns the same. There is no generic way to educate about health. If there were, there would be no use for this book. One of the most difficult tasks for behavioral scientists and health educators is changing individual or group behavior. It is even more difficult to help individuals or groups maintain the behavior once it is changed. The health education profession has subscribed to a number of theories that take into consideration variables that influence behavior. These theories serve as a foundation and structure from which community health education methods can be applied. Selecting methods without considering theory is like building a house without a foundation. The potential for the house to collapse will always be a threat. Likewise, methods chosen without a theoretical base will be vulnerable to failure. Can health educators afford to take these risks? Of course not—health educators are concerned about individual lifestyles that cause real or potential health problems. As a result, programs that have the greatest potential for success must be designed and implemented. The understanding and application of theory to practice is an insurance policy that this will occur.

Community connections 2

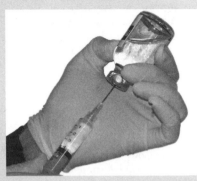

One of the health education programs Jill was concerned about was motivating low-income mothers to have their babies immunized. The methods she used were announcements in newspapers, a brochure she developed and distributed to mothers who had just delivered, and radio public service announcements. Jill remembered from her undergraduate health education planning class that the Health Belief Model addresses a belief in being susceptible to illness and that, if informed of their susceptibility, people would respond to prevention messages. The perception that their babies were at risk would surely apply to Jill's desire to motivate mothers to have their children immunized.

When the results of Jill's efforts were 40% less than the program's goal, she turned to Dawn and asked for help. In analyzing the plan, Dawn assured Jill that the choice of methods was appropriate, the group identified was at high risk, and that Jill's goals and objectives, along with her evaluation methods, were reasonable. The problem was in implementing the theoretical model. Dawn could clearly see that the Health Belief Model, as used, was incomplete. In her explanations to Jill, she pointed out that she only used one of the four principles of the model. This was

It is important to understand the meaning of *theory*. A **theory** is a general explanation of why people act or do not act to maintain and/or promote the health of themselves, their families, organizations, and communities.[1] There are over 20 theories commonly used by health educators. It is not the intent of this chapter to explain all of the theories in health education, but to discuss a limited number—those most often used. Unfortunately, theories do not work in some situations, which is why researchers and theorists are constantly trying to improve and develop new theories. In time, new theories will be developed or adapted from the behavioral sciences that will continue to help in better understanding the most effective approach for motivating people to live healthy lifestyles.

Theories can be classified in two groups, depending on their focus. Some theories focus on individuals as the units of change, whereas others focus on organizations or cultures. Theories that focus on individuals, known as cognitive-behavior models, are based on two premises: (1) Behavior is determined by cognition, or what we know, which, in turn, results in how we act, and (2) behavior is determined by perceptions, levels of motivation, self-efficacy, skills, resiliency, and environmental variables. Community models are designed to support healthy lifestyles by reducing or eliminating hazards in social and physical environments. These models center on community-level change, including community

to inform mothers that if their infants were not immunized they would be susceptible to illness. It was a fear approach used to motivate mothers. After realizing the mistake of not implementing all the components of the model, Jill asked Dawn how the model should have been applied to this situation.

Dawn explained that the program overemphasized the perceived susceptibility of harm by not protecting infants. What was missing was the perception of why and how children were susceptible. Another mistake was the failure to anticipate barriers that would discourage mothers from having their infants immunized. These might be cost, perceived threat to the infant's health if immunized, religious beliefs, or accessibility to services. The third, and probably most serious mistake, was neglecting the questions of what, where, when, and how services could be obtained. Jill did not anticipate barriers and failed

to plan services around the difficulties these barriers created. For example, she failed to make clear what the cost would be, who would qualify for free services, when infants should be immunized, the low risk of possible reactions, who could give immunizations, and where mothers could take their children to be immunized.

Dawn suggested Jill do a random sample of the targeted population to determine if they had their children immunized and, if not, why not. The results confirmed Dawn's assumptions. Jill found that 65% of mothers did not have their babies immunized because of a perceived threat to the child's health, inconvenience, lack of time, and not knowing where they could receive services. Jill realized that if the Health Belief Model had been fully applied to the methods, such as the use of media and the brochure, more information would have been conveyed that addressed these perceptions.

organization, theories of organizational change, and diffusion of innovation, and are important in planning comprehensive community-based programs.

Application of Health Education Theories and Theoretical Models

The following discussion of five commonly used theories contains a description of each theory and its practical application, using Community Connections boxes 2–6. For each scenario, imagine being in their situation.

The Health Belief Model

The Health Belief Model (HBM), as its title suggests, has to do with believing in health. This model was one of the first designed to encourage people to take action toward positive health. The model emphasizes the "role of perceptions of vulnerability to an illness and the potential effectiveness in treatment." It means health educators should take into consideration individuals' perceptions that they are vulnerable to illness that threatens their health and the actions on the part of individuals that could prevent the threat and eliminate possible illness.

The HBM is based on the belief that health-related behavior is determined by whether individuals (1) perceive themselves to be susceptible to a health problem, (2) see this problem as serious (3) are convinced they will benefit from treatment or prevention activities, and (4) recognize the need to take action and any barriers that would interfere with this action. How can this be remembered? Think of the Health Belief Model as an approach to health education that is based on the beliefs or perceptions one has regarding one's susceptibility to illness.[2]

For a person to be convinced he or she should take action to prevent illness, that person needs to answer four questions:

- Do I perceive I am susceptible?
- Is this susceptibility serious?
- Do the benefits in taking action overcome the cost in money and effort?
- Are services or help available?

The perceived need to take action is influenced by variables that affect a person's perceptions and, as a result, indirectly influence his or her health behavior. These modifying factors include level of educational attainment, cultural differences, age, personal experiences, gender, and economic status and influence the perception of susceptibility, severity of risk, benefits, and barriers.

Theory of Planned Behavior

The Theory of Planned Behavior is based on the assumption that behavior, or the intention to behave in a certain way, is determined by the person's attitude toward the behavior, subjective norms, and perceived behavioral control. In other words, if a person perceives that a given outcome will be a positive experience, that it is positively viewed by others, and that it is not difficult to perform, the person is more likely to exhibit that behavior. A person's intention to perform a behavior is also determined by social norms, such as perceptions of what others who are held in high esteem would do or expect him or her to do in similar situations.[3]

The health educator needs to identify what a person's intention is regarding performing a prescribed behavior. This could be done by identifying (1) attitudes toward the behavior—why he or she wishes to perform the behavior and what expectations, both positive and negative, are held regarding the behavior, (2) subjective norms—what significant others will think about the behavior, and (3) perceived behavioral control—how difficult it will be to perform and maintain the behavior. If an inventory of the person's intentions is positive, there will be a better chance he or she will perform the intended behavior.

Key to this theory is the concept of reasoned action. A person needs to reason, or think logically, about an intended behavior. This is a cognitive process —discovering or finding reasons or intentions to behave in a certain way.

Community connections 3

Jill had received a request from a local church to talk to a group of teenage girls about postponing sexual intercourse. Knowing that peers often influence teens, she looked for an approach that would use positive influence as a motivator. Jill knew, from her graduate classes, that there are several health education theories. Maybe there was one that would fit her needs. She asked Mike, who was not sure but suggested they search the literature to see what was available. Looking for behavioral theories, they came across the Theory of Planned Behavior. Bingo! It was what Jill was looking for. She and Mike applied the concepts of the theory to the desired behavior of postponing sexual intercourse.

The method of inquiry was used in applying the theory. Jill asked the girls questions in order to clarify the level of intent the girls had to perform the desired behavior. Questions Jill asked were what attitudes they had regarding this behavior, who they admired and respected, and what they would expect those they admired to do in the same situation. What she discovered, much to her delight, was that the girls' intentions to postpone sexual intercourse were generally positive. The questions Jill asked really worked in helping the girls define the importance of the desired behavior and in identifying who might have difficulty in performing the behavior. She felt that if these girls identified significant others and thought about what they would do under similar circumstances it would help them think twice and reconsider their actions. Jill was pleased, as the theory seemed to work. As she mentioned to Mike, "I think I really made a difference." Mike was also happy with Jill's success but reminded her that the Theory of Planned Behavior is a predictor of behavior. There are a lot of variables, such as self-efficacy, self-esteem, and communication skills, that will determine if the girls' intentions will result in the desired behavior. As a result, methods can be designed for these individuals based on theories related to the variables.

Transtheoretical Stages of Change Model

The Stages of Change Model is based on the assumption that behavior change is a process and that individuals are at varying levels of motivation or readiness to change. People at different stages in the process of change can benefit from different interventions. In other words, the methods used for a desired outcome are not generic because individuals are not always at the same stage or level of readiness. The model also assumes people may relapse or return to a previous stage. Return to the original stage can occur and often does. The model identifies five stages, or levels, of readiness that could be applied to any type of behavior change.[4]

1. *Precontemplation.* Not interested in changing behavior. (Example: Smokers who are not interested in stopping in the next six months. They may be unaware of their problem or do not consider it to be a problem.)

2. *Contemplation.* Considering changing behavior someday. (Example: Smokers who know smoking is bad for them and are considering quitting at some point but are not yet ready to do so.)

Community connections 4

Mike was given the responsibility of designing a smoking cessation program for employees of a small (80 employees) automotive parts manufacturing company. In taking on this responsibility, he was concerned that some individuals would sign up for the program with different levels of readiness to change. For example, he assumed some had stopped smoking but, within a short period of time, started again. Some would have a support system of family and friends who would encourage their efforts. Others would be lifetime smokers who would find giving up smoking very difficult. Levels of readiness would range from a sincere desire to quit to a "been there, done that" attitude. Mike needed to know in what stage the participants were. How to do this? That was the question.

Mike remembered that when he worked on a county tobacco reduction coalition, the director of the county cancer agency had mentioned his experiences in smoking cessation programs. Mike had been impressed with the materials from the cancer agency, and now he thought they might have some helpful information. All it took was one phone call. The director had material about a model called Stages of Change, which was based on the assumption that people are at different levels of readiness to change. It was just what Mike needed. In fact, questions on

smoking behavior were given as examples to determine the stages where the participants were. What a find! It just goes to show that networking pays off. Thanks to the director, Mike's job was going to be much easier.

Mike developed a questionnaire, based on examples provided by the director of the cancer agency, to determine the stages of participants' readiness. Questions focused on the following five stages of change:
1. Interest in trying to quit
2. Thinking about quitting soon
3. Ready to plan a cessation attempt
4. In the process of cessation
5. Trying to stay smoke free

Mike was able to arrange the participants into five groups according to their stage of cessation. As a result, different strategies and methods—such as personal testimonies, analysis of smoking behaviors and failed attempts, use of videos, determination and individualization of cessation approaches, use of support systems, and use of medical personnel—were designed to help the participants progress through the stages.

Mike felt good about applying the Stages of Change Model in planning the smoking cessation program. He told Dawn, "I feel like I have individualized the approach in helping people give up a very unhealthy behavior."

3. *Preparation.* Preparing for and experimenting with behavior change but lacking self-efficacy to actively engage in the process. (Example: Smokers who intend to quit within the next month.)

4. *Action.* Actively engaging in the behavior change process. (Example: Smokers who are making changes, such as reducing daily cigarette consumption, in order to stop.)

5. *Maintenance.* Sustaining the behavior change over time. (Example: Ex-smokers who have been sustaining change for six months without relapse.)

The model should be easy to remember because the key word *stage* is what the model encompasses: Individuals move through many stages in their attempt to change behaviors. Because the theory is based on stages, it is necessary to

Community Connections 5

Frustrated with the failure of individuals who signed up for their healthy eating and exercise program to change, Mike and Jill considered talking with a health psychologist who specialized in behavior change. Mike had previously met Dr. Hill, a nationally respected health education consultant who specialized in counseling clients with undesirable health behaviors. Mike suggested they call him and see if he could help them out.

"You mean, call him as a consultant?" Jill asked.

Mike responded, "Why not? The department just paid a consultant $3,500 to recommend a computer system we should have."

"You have a point, Mike," said Jill. "Let me talk to Dawn to see if she would approve it."

Mike and Jill were in Dr. Hill's office a week later, seeking advice on how to work more effectively with people who wished to lose weight. After two hours, Mike and Jill were enlightened regarding the potential of applying Social Cognitive Theory to their attempt to help participants with healthy eating and exercise behaviors.

Mike and Jill were excited about Social Cognitive Theory and its potential for individual behavior change. Dr. Hill warned them, "Changing behavior is not easy because everyone comes from different environments and experiences. If, however, you apply program objectives and methods to theory, you will have a better chance of success."

determine the stage in which an individual or group resides. Asking a few simple questions, as demonstrated in Community Connections 4, can do this.

Social Cognitive Theory

Glanz and Rimer stated that "in social learning theory, human behavior is explained in terms of a three-way, dynamic, reciprocal theory in which personal factors, environmental influences and behavior continually interact. A basic premise of Social Cognitive Theory is that people not only learn through their own experiences, but also by observing the actions of others and the results of those actions."[5]

This theory is one of the most popular among health educators. Although the definition is understandable, the theory is rather complex. A better understanding of the concept of the theory can be garnered by turning to Mike and Jill as they attempt to help a group of volunteers become more sensible regarding their choice of food and exercise lifestyles (see Community Connections 5).

Six concepts are essential to Social Cognitive Theory.[6] Each of these is defined below and then applied to methods designed for the healthy eating and exercise example.

Reciprocal determinism.   **Reciprocal determinism** means that behavior changes are determined from interactions between a person and his or her environment.

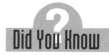

Did You Know

The first theoretical model designed for health education was the Health Belief Model, developed in the 1950s by a group of social psychologists at the U.S. Public Health Service.

The environment can influence or discourage a person in a healthy way or can be detrimental, since some environments may be healthy while others may not. Conversely, people can influence the environment so that it is more conducive to a healthy lifestyle. For example, some of the individuals in Mike and Jill's program may experience environmental factors that are supportive of healthy eating and exercise, while others may not. If there are negative forces, it may be necessary to change the environment to provide opportunities for choosing healthy foods and for engaging in exercising. Jill and Mike applied this concept by having each participant identify positive and negative forces in their work and living environments that helped or hindered their desire to lose weight.

Behavioral capability.   The concept of **behavioral capability** is based on a person's capability to change a behavior by having the knowledge and skills necessary to enact a desired behavior. Applied to Mike and Jill's program, it means that education is necessary to learn about healthy foods and their preparation, as well as about types of exercises designed for flexibility, body tone, strength, cardiovascular fitness, and endurance. Skills also need to be developed, such as analyzing labels, counting calories, preparing food, taking one's target heart rate, lifting weights safely, and planning exercises for body tone and flexibility. Methods used to accomplish this could include demonstrations, videos, print materials, self-recording sheets, and simulations.

Expectations.   **Expectations** are what a person expects as a result of modifying behavior—in other words, what he or she thinks the payoff will be. This is usually referred to as the positive value of the desired behavior.

For Jill and Mike's program, this would include expectations of improved physical appearance, becoming more physically fit, having more energy, and being more disciplined. These expected outcomes must counter the pleasures that come from poor choices such as eating foods that taste good but are unhealthy, or avoiding the pain of exercise by not exercising. This is especially true early in a program before a person experiences results or the value of his or her predetermined expectations. Personal goals that are accomplished become rewards and are considered pleasurable.

In attempting to help participants identify their expectations, Mike and Jill, in the beginning, asked them to list their expectations as a result of losing weight and becoming more fit. These could then be developed into their personal goals.

Reinforcement.   **Reinforcement** is the response to a person's behavior that will increase the continuance of the behavior. Positive reinforcement would be experienced in how individuals feel about the way they look and feel. The reinforcement of their expectations motivates them to continue with the program. External reinforcement methods used by Mike and Jill were praise, before-and-after photos, and awards.

Self-efficacy.   **Self-efficacy** means believing that one has the ability to take action and persist in one's pursuits. Accomplishing obtainable goals establishes a person's degree of efficacy. People who fail to accomplish predetermined goals become part of the history of failed attempts, causing self-defeating behavior. Mike and Jill attempted to build efficacy by identifying and sharing personal strengths of the participants. People sometimes do not realize they have strengths until they experience them through skill-building exercises, role play, or other means of gaining confidence. Strengths such as perseverance, positive attitude, and a willingness to learn can go a long way in building self-efficacy.

Observational learning.   **Observational learning** is the ability to learn by observing others. In so doing, a person can see success as well as failure and the positive or negative effects of these results. In the example in Community Connections 5, people who had been successful in both losing weight and maintaining weight loss gave personal testimonies. Mike and Jill decided they would serve as good examples of what they wanted their participants to accomplish by engaging in healthy eating and exercise. Leaders need to serve as role models so that they do not cause participants to think "I can't hear what you say because of what I see."

Diffusion of Innovation Theory

Unlike other theories that have been developed to change behavior, the Diffusion of Innovation Theory provides a process for disseminating and implementing innovations. It is the only theory discussed in this chapter that is considered solely a community-level theory; other theories addressed both individual and group change. Community-level theories are designed to help make decisions affecting large populations such as communities and institutions. These may include developing policies that affect health behavior or making decisions on purchasing products or materials. The word *diffusion* means to integrate, distribute, or spread widely. *Innovation* is something that is new or different. Applied to health education, diffusion of innovation means integrating innovative ideas, products, or programs that have proved to be successful into health education initiatives.

As new programs and materials are developed, innovative ideas and methods become available that improve the delivery of health education. Health educators need to keep abreast of new developments and apply them when appropriate.

The question is how to select the best innovations and diffuse, or integrate, them into program implementation. Diffusion of Innovation Theory establishes criteria for selecting innovations. These criteria include the following:

- *Relative advantage.* The degree to which an innovation is seen as better than the idea, practice, program, or product it replaces
- *Compatibility.* How consistent the innovation is with the values, habits, experiences, and needs of potential adopters
- *Complexity.* How difficult the innovation is to understand or use
- *Treatability.* The extent to which the innovation can be experimented with before a commitment to adopt it is required
- *Observability.* The extent to which the innovation provides tangible or visible results

Additionally, the cost of an innovation should be considered. This includes the monetary cost of purchasing the program or product as well as the time to train individuals to use the innovation.

The Diffusion of Innovation Theory also explains people's readiness to accept an innovation once they buy into it. Individuals accepting an innovation are called *adopters* and can be characterized as follows:[7]

- *Innovators.* The first to adopt
- *Early adopters.* Interested, but do not want to be the first to adopt
- *Early majority adopters.* Accept innovations once others they respect have done so
- *Late majority adopters.* Individuals who are skeptical and late to adopt
- *Late adopters (laggards).* The last to get involved, if they get involved at all

Understanding the readiness of adopters is the key to selecting the best method to motivate individuals to subscribe to a new idea, product, or program. The early adopters and early and late majority, who, combined, are the largest group, will need to be convinced that the idea, product, or program would be to their advantage.

How can this theory be remembered? The key word *diffusion*, which means to disseminate or integrate, is easy to remember, as is the word *innovation*, which could be a new idea, product, method, or program. So *diffusion of innovation* means to disseminate and integrate something new. It is important to remember that the success of an innovation being adopted is determined by specific criteria, as well as by the readiness of the adopter.

The five theories that have been discussed are commonly used by practitioners in their efforts to be more effective in helping people live healthier lifestyles. As mentioned earlier, theories serve as a foundation and structure from which community health education goals and methods can be applied.

Did You Know

Quality assurance incorporates accountability, which includes selecting community health education methods based on theoretical and ethical principles.

Community connections 6

Mike and Jill were asked by Dawn to work with local public schools on a violence prevention program. This was the result of a needs assessment compiled by a county commission on violence that indicated a 35% increase in school violence in the past five years. The most common acts identified by the assessment were bullying, fighting, and threatening violence with intent to do harm.

Mike and Jill were committed to their task and looked forward to the challenge. The problem was where to start. Should they develop a violence prevention curriculum with teacher training or should they work with schools in developing school policy? To what extent should law enforcement agencies and the county prosecutor be involved? Mike thought a curriculum with teacher training was the best approach. Jill, on the other hand, suggested they take a look at what had worked for schools that had controlled or reduced the problem of violence. Experience working with school drug education programs told her reinventing the wheel by developing new programs was not the best use of time and resources. She explained to Mike that the most cost-effective approach that had the greatest potential for success was based on a theory that provides guidance in taking different innovations and diffusing them into program needs.

Mike and Jill contacted state and national offices on violence prevention, reviewed curricula and school programs, surveyed the literature, and talked to school administrators, law enforcement personnel, parents, and students. They even went to a seminar sponsored by the state Department of Education on violence prevention. Mike and Jill gathered a great deal of information—"All good stuff," as Mike explained it. The problem was how to select a curriculum that would be most appropriate for their needs. Having identified bullying, fighting, and threatening violence as the problems to be addressed, they had to determine what approach, along with what methods and materials, to use.

They chose the Diffusion of Innovation Theory to help them with this task. In so doing, they applied the five criteria designed to select the best innovation. In particular, they identified what the schools were presently doing (relative advantage), used a focus group to determine the innovation's compatibility with schools and its degree of difficulty to use (compatibility and complexity), and conducted a pilot test to determine extent of experimentation before it was adopted and to see if there were tangible results (treatability and observability). They next looked at the characteristics of adopters to determine what to expect from administrators regarding their readiness to adopt or buy into the program. They planned their approach with methods and strategies addressing each level of adopter.

They asked Dawn for her input and approval when the program design was complete. She thought it was educationally sound and congratulated them on selecting Diffusion of Innovation as a realistic approach to developing and implementing the program.

Professional standards that respect the rights of individuals must be considered when applying theory to practice. Educators have the power to influence and thus make significant differences in people's lives. To inform and motivate people to change behavior can be a risky business unless done in an ethical way. The second part of this chapter addresses the ethical application of health education methods.

Ethics in Health Education

The study of **ethics**, or moral philosophy, enables health educators to make individual and professional decisions based on basic principles that reflect the values and morals of a society and the health education profession. These principles serve as guidelines that govern professional conduct.

The body of ethics typically centers on four principles:

- *Personal freedom, or autonomy.* One should respect people's rights. People have the right to choose and act. Sometimes freedom is overridden to prevent harm. When this occurs, it is called *paternalism.*
- *Avoiding harm, or nonmalificence.* One should not inflict harm on others.
- *Doing good, or beneficence.* One should help others or, at the least, remove harm.
- *Justice.* One should treat others equally and fairly.

In addition, *professional accountability*—being accountable to self, clients, participants, employer, profession, and society—has been generally considered as an essential ethical principle. Actions taken by health educators have the potential for good as well as harm, so health educators must be accountable.

The nature of health education is to encourage healthy behavior by employing a number of education methods and techniques. This leaves health educators in a unique position of helping, or possibly harming, others by the methods used. The responsibilities invested in them by their employers, plus their knowledge and skills, provide health educators with the power to influence people's decisions regarding their health and the health of their families, organizations, and communities. Fulfilling responsibilities and applying knowledge and skills in ethical ways are essential in the practice of health education.

What Are the Ethics of Health Education?

Unethical practice of health education leads to professional suicide. Health educators who act unethically damage their professional reputation and integrity. In their professional roles, health educators inherit the responsibility of upholding a certain code of ethics. The preamble of the Code of Ethics for the Health Education Profession states: "The health educator is to aspire to the highest possible standards of conduct and to encourage the ethical behavior of those with whom they work."[8] The preamble also states the following:

> The Code of Ethics provides a framework of shared values within which health education is practiced. The Code of Ethics is grounded in fundamental ethical principles that underlie all health care services: respect for autonomy, promotion of social justice, active

promotion of good, and avoidance of harm. . . . Regardless of job title, professional affiliation, work setting, or population served, health educators abide by these guidelines when making professional decisions.[8]

The Challenge of Making Ethical Decisions

Sometimes ethical decisions are difficult to make. Ethics are based on morals and values that often clash with each other. When this happens, a moral or ethical dilemma occurs, which often creates controversy. Most professions, such as law, medicine, psychology, and education, have established their own professional codes. These serve as standards of professional conduct that must be abided by in order to prevent bias, discrimination, wrongdoing, and harm to others.

Many professions have boards that review cases of unethical practice and reprimand individuals who are in violation of ethical practice. This situation does not exist in the health education profession, however. The enforcement of the code is left up to employers and members of the profession. It is thus the responsibility of health educators to encourage ethical behavior through example.

There is often a conflict between knowing what is ethical and demonstrating ethical behavior. It is sometimes difficult to act on what is right because of unpleasant consequences. When faced with decisions, individuals often choose a less than optimal path because doing what may be considered right might result in ridicule or in being deprived of good things. These unpleasant consequences often overpower the consequences of selecting a more ethical choice. The critical connection between knowing what is ethical and behaving ethically is *character*, or *virtue*. Character is based on personal traits such as loyalty, kindness, integrity, self-esteem, self-efficacy, and discipline. These traits provide courage and strength to make ethical beliefs become a reality. Professional character, along with the code of ethics, enables health educators to conduct themselves in an honorable and professional way. By so doing, professional standards are upheld, as well as individual integrity and respect.

Application of Article IV of the Code of Ethics for the Health Education Profession: Delivery of Health Education

Applying the code of ethics to the practice of health education is a logical way to see how it can be used in making ethical decisions. For the purpose of this chapter, examples of applying the code focus on methods, specifically as described in Article IV, Delivery of Health Education. This article has five sections that are explained here using dilemmas faced by Mike, Jill, and Dawn.

Following each dilemma, a question of ethics is raised, followed by application of the code of ethics and possible solutions.

Ethical Dilemma 1: Assuming Responsibility while Lacking Social and Cultural Sensitivity

The county in which Mike and Jill work has a substantial number of migrant workers who arrive during the harvest season and stay three or four months. During the summer, local school districts provide education programs for the children of the migrant families. One of the districts requested the county health department to assist in teaching a health education class to middle-school children, since the program was unable to hire a school health educator.

The director of the health department passed the request on to Dawn, which was the first time the department had received this type of request. Dawn was somewhat reluctant. She knew her staff had very little experience in working with migrant populations, plus she felt she could not spare staff to take on this task. At the same time, she felt an obligation to help and considered it an opportunity to establish a positive relationship with the school. Dawn decided to bring up the request at the staff meeting.

Dawn explained to her staff the nature of the request along with what she considered concerns and opportunities. Mike and Jill were excited about working with young people and saw this as an opportunity to do more with schools. They were also fortunate because each had health education interns assigned to them for the summer, which would allow them extra time to devote to the program. Besides, it was only three hours a week. They were confident they would have the time and volunteered to take on the challenge.

Jill and Mike asked the schools to send them the middle-school health education curriculum currently used during the regular academic year. After looking over the curriculum, they concluded it would meet the needs of the migrant children.

After their first meeting with the students, Mike knew he was in trouble. Jill also realized that this experience was not working as she had expected. After the second week, both she and Mike needed help. They did not connect with the students. The students were apathetic and had no interest in learning the content or participating in the methods. Something had to be done. Dawn suggested they meet with Mrs. Mendez, the director of the migrant program. Mrs. Mendez listened to Mike and Jill's dilemma. She immediately knew the problem. She confirmed her suspicion by asking Mike and Jill the following questions: Did either of them have any training in education pedagogy? Were the education materials and methods culturally appropriate? Were either of them familiar with customs and traditions of Mexican American cultures?

Were they aware of cultural differences? Had they assessed the health needs of Mexican American middle-school children? How much did they know about the students and their family's values? Did they recognize any personal bias they might have toward the culture of their students?

Mike and Jill realized they were not prepared for this assignment. For example, the methods they used—such as relying on print materials and pictures that did not depict the migrant culture and asking students to participate in discussions without considering their difficulty with the English language or taking into account their cultural values—were inappropriate.

Ethical question.   Was it ethical for Mike and Jill to assume the responsibility of teaching in the migrant program?

Application of the code of ethics.   This situation relates to the principle of justice and equality. Section 1 of Article IV of the code of ethics deals with responsibility in the delivery of health education:

> *Health educators are sensitive to social and cultural diversity and are in accord with the law, when planning and implementing programs.*

All too often, health educators fail to consider cultural differences when planning methods. This results in frustration on the part of the educator because the participants do not seem to care. Likewise, the participants feel frustration because the educator does not appear to care about them. A dilemma results because of the failure to take into consideration that people of different cultures have values, traditions, attitudes, educational backgrounds, and life experiences that make them unique. The curriculum content and teaching methods selected in the example were designed for a white, middle-class community, making them unethical to use with this population.

Solution to the dilemma.   Health educators must be aware of cultural differences of individuals and groups. To ignore this is unfair. In their excitement to work with young people, the two health educators overlooked the fact that they were of a different culture and background. This was unfortunate and should never happen. A serious attempt must always be made to determine the cultural traditions, customs, personalities, language, and other factors that make participants unique.

Ethical Dilemma 2: Incompetence in Delivering Health Education

Jill was concerned about the lack of professional preparation in health education of one of her colleagues. Mary was the senior member of the health education division, having served 22 years as a public health nurse and 5 years as a health educator. She was considered an excellent nurse and was knowledgeable about medical and public health issues under the jurisdiction of the health department. She was an excellent public speaker and related well with people. Jill's concern was that Mary did not have knowledge of health education process skills necessary to be effective. She had no background in the practice and use of strategies and methods and did not know about professional standards or theories in health education. As a result, she always used a lecture approach, supported with written materials, in her health education programs.

Jill and Mike both knew she could be a dynamic health educator if she took time to learn about the process of health education. Both were concerned that Mary's approach was not effective with many of the people she was educating. On several occasions, they tried to share ideas, programs, and professional journals with Mary, hoping she would be open to different methods. Jill decided to talk to Dawn after Mary conducted a very questionable program on HIV/AIDS that was presented to HIV-positive individuals, using her usual lecture approach. Mary also expressed her personal values, which insulted some of the participants. When Jill shared this with Mike, he said, "Forget it. Mary has more seniority and is set in her ways with no hope of change. Besides, I'm sure Dawn already realizes the problem."

Jill responded, "Health educators don't practice that way."

Mike countered, "Mary is a nurse, not a health educator."

Jill, somewhat irritated, said, "Her title is health educator, and what and how she practices reflects on the profession."

It was difficult for Jill to talk to Dawn about her colleague's incompetence. She was pleased when Dawn listened to her concerns and thanked her for bringing this to her attention. Mike, however, had been right—Dawn was aware of Mary's shortcomings but was undecided as to how to handle it.

To try to clarify the situation, Dawn asked herself the following questions: Has any harm been done as a result of Mary's approach? Is Mary aware of her lack of professional preparation? Does Mary realize she could be more effective if she understood health education theory and process?

Dawn concluded that Mary might have unknowingly done harm to individuals by not using different strategies and methods that better met individual learning needs. She was definitely out of line in the case of the HIV/AIDS program by not using more effective methods and for imparting her personal values to the participants. She also concluded that Mary was probably aware of her lack of preparation in health education, but, because of her nursing background and five years' experience as a health educator, considered herself a proficient professional. Dawn concluded that Mary was not aware, or refused to admit, that she could be more effective with a strong understanding of health education theory and methods. Dawn decided to discuss her concerns with Mary after taking into consideration the importance of maintaining the integrity of the division of health education.

Ethical question.   Is it unethical for a person to assume the role of a health educator without professional preparation in health education methods?

Application of the code of ethics.   This case of incompetence pertains to a dilemma between the principles of nonmalificence and professional accountability. The health educator meant to do well, but a lack of professional preparation may actually have resulted in more harm than good. Section 2 of Article IV of the code of ethics relates to this dilemma:

> *Health Educators are informed of the latest advances in theory, research and practice, and use strategies and methods that are grounded in and contribute to development of professional standards, theories, statistics and experience.*

Applied to the current scenario, it is clear there was an ethical violation. Mary had no professional preparation in health education; was uninformed about the latest advances in theory, research, and practice; and did not use strategies and methods grounded in professional standards. By imposing her personal values, she insulted some of the participants. Others may have been turned off by the lecture approach used.

A second answer to this dilemma is found in Article III, Section 6:

> *Health Educators maintain competence in their areas of professional practice.*

Lack of professional preparation is a serious ethical problem. Professionals not competent in the use of appropriate methods can do harm to participants and tarnish the profession.

Solution to the dilemma.   This dilemma presents a case of incompetence in the selection of proper methods due to a lack of professional preparation. It also raises the question of whether persons who are not competent should be confronted by their peers. The answer to the second question is yes. Someone needs to uphold the standards of the profession. It was important that Mary was approached before her supervisor was informed; thus, she could make a change. When that did not work, however, there were two choices. One was to forget about the problem and the other was to bring the issue to the attention of the supervisor. Professionals are expected to maintain the integrity and dignity of the profession. Article II, Section 3, addresses this issue by stating that health educators encourage and accept responsible, critical discourse. When the basic principles of accepted health education practice are not followed, the chance of intangible harm to populations and the profession exists. Unlike other professions, where ethical issues can be brought to an ethical review board, health educators have no course or recourse to follow when an unethical practice is questioned. It is up to employers and other professionals to police professional behaviors themselves.

The burden, in this case, lies on the shoulders of the supervisor. Three actions need to be taken: (1) Explain to the employee that there is a body of knowledge of the profession that governs the selection of methods and strategies; (2) provide opportunities for the employee to further her knowledge and skills; and (3) encourage the employee to work toward becoming a certified health education specialist, which would include completing additional academic training in a qualified health education professional preparation program.

The dilemma in this scenario involves an individual who lacks professional preparation and fails to keep abreast of new advances. Is this any different than other professions? No. All professions struggle with incompetent members. The test of a profession's integrity is what it does to—and for—those who are incompetent.

Ethical Dilemma 3: Absence of Accountability and Evaluation

Dawn was somewhat concerned when she read Mike and Jill's quarterly report, addressing their health education programs over the past three months. Each had planned and implemented a program and was a member of a community coalition on the prevention of child and elderly abuse. What concerned Dawn was there was no mention of an attempt to evaluate the programs. Success or failure of the methods used in the program or of new methods used in the coalition's plan should be evaluated, because the success of the methods used will directly affect the success of the program. Dawn knew that the administrator of the health department would want to have information on the results of programs. After all, he would have to answer to the county board of health and needed results of programs in order to do so. Program evaluation was also important because Dawn had recently requested an additional full-time health educator. She could use evaluation results that showed the division's health education programs were successful in accomplishing their goals and objectives. Dawn decided she needed to discuss this with Jill and Mike.

Dawn explained during their meeting the need to evaluate the methods they used, such as media and community empowerment techniques. This was important in order to determine their degree of success and discover how the methods could be improved. Evaluation also provides data that can be used to determine the effectiveness of the methods employed to help participants obtain knowledge and develop skills for use in making and carrying out decisions. Dawn explained the importance of being accountable to participants of programs, as well as to those who provide the resources for the programs.

Both Mike and Jill remembered that evaluation was important in programming but found it impractical. After all, evaluation takes time, resources, and

someone who knows evaluation design and statistics. It seemed
beyond their responsibility.

Dawn understood. After all, she had felt the same frustration as a young professional. The temptation to implement a
program, get it done, and take on the next task is a driving
force that provides excitement in being a health educator. On
the other hand, years of experience had taught her that unless
methods and programs are evaluated, the potential for repeated
failure is likely to exist. As she explained to the two young professionals, "Evaluation is not an option. It is an opportunity and
obligation—an opportunity to determine how successful our methods have
been and an obligation to determine how they can be improved."

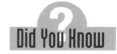

Someone who vio-
lates a professional
ethical principle and
causes harm could
be charged and prose-
cuted for malpractice.

Ethical question.   Is it unethical to design and implement programs using strategies and methods that influence individual behavior without evaluating the
effect they have on individuals and on the program's desired outcomes?

Application of the code of ethics.   The failure to evaluate programs and methods falls under the principle of accountability. Not evaluating programs and
methods reduces the educator's ability to seek the truth of their success or
failure. In a way, this leads to being dishonest to self, employers, and the
populations that health educators serve.

The code of ethics again provides direction for ethical practice in evaluating programs and methods. Article IV, Section 3, states:

> *Health Educators are committed to rigorous evaluation of both pro-*
> *gram effectiveness and the methods used to achieve results.*

It takes time and a certain amount of creativity to determine if methods
are successful in accomplishing their objectives. Health educators often assume
their methods are successful because of the positive way participants respond.
Participants may enjoy the experience, but does that mean they learned or
changed attitudes or behaviors as a result of the method?

Solution to the dilemma.   Evaluation is an essential process health educators often
fail to do. Unless a program is supported by a grant, appropriately conducted evaluation is usually rare. It is time-consuming and costly, and many health educators
do not have the knowledge or skills to conduct an appropriate evaluation.

What is the solution to the dilemma? Because the programs have already
been implemented, it may be difficult to do a more rigorous evaluation than
what had already been conducted. Possibly some type of follow-up could still
take place to determine the outcome of the program's goals and objectives,
which may serve as an indicator of whether specific methods were effective.
Can it be assumed, however, that if program goals and objectives were met, the
objectives of the methods were accomplished? To a certain extent, yes, but it

will never be known unless an attempt is made to evaluate each method. The solution is to evaluate the objectives of the methods. In other words, did the methods succeed in doing what they were designed to do?

Ethical Dilemma 4: Choice versus Coercion and Intimidation

A worksite health promotion specialist was speaking about motivational techniques at a state health education conference. Mike and Jill were attending the conference and considered this to be an opportunity to hear about how to motivate employees to develop healthy behaviors. They were serving as consultants to a worksite health promotion program in their county and were looking for new ideas to motivate participants. The session was precisely what they needed. They listened with interest to the speaker as she explained motivational techniques used in a smoking cessation program.

One of the techniques was to award a bonus at the end of the year to those who stopped smoking. This would be equal to the difference between the insurance premiums paid by the company for a smoker's health insurance and those for a nonsmoker, which amounted to $200 a year. When asked if bonuses were given for other health-enhancing behavior, such as weight reduction, physical fitness, or substance abuse counseling and treatment, the speaker replied by stating, "Insurance companies don't charge an extra premium for these health risks."

The speaker explained another motivational technique, which was to have mention of the employee's participation placed in his or her personnel file. This, of course, was with the employee's permission. Although this would not be used for promotion or bonus, it would indicate that the employee cooperated in the company's effort to control health insurance costs.

The third technique was to have managers and supervisors who were smokers voluntarily enroll in the smoking cessation program. Although this was not mandatory, the president and two vice presidents of the company were enrolled in the program and made it known that others were expected to do the same. Even the program's slogan, "From the Top Down: A Smoke Free Company," was an indication that employees were expected to participate.

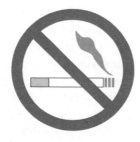

The speaker said that 80% of the smokers participated, which was attributed to leaders of the company serving as role models.

Jill and Mike began to question the techniques used by the speaker. They had a sense of uneasiness about the motivational methods used. It seemed as if the employees were being coerced to join the program. The following Monday, when talking to Dawn, they concluded that the worksite health promotion program's approach to motivation was not in compliance with ethical practice. This conclusion was drawn by putting themselves in the place of the employees and asking the following questions: Was it fair to give a bonus only to those who smoked? Why would the employer want to have information in a personnel file on an employee's willingness to participate in a smoking cessation program? Is there a subliminal message that one would be expected to participate? Does the impression that employees are expected to take part in a program become a matter of coercion rather than choice? Jill, Mike, and Dawn came to the conclusion that the methods used for motivation were suspect.

Ethical question. Is it ethical to influence health decisions based on motivational techniques designed to persuade by questionable rewards and intimidation or coercion?

Application of the code of ethics. This case is a typical example of the dilemma between the principles of justice and personal freedom. Justice, or fairness, can be applied to the first motivational method, which was to award bonuses equal to that saved by the company in insurance premiums of nonsmokers. Although an advantage for smokers, it was unfair to the nonsmoker, who deserves equal bonus opportunities for weight loss, physical fitness, substance abuse treatment, or other health-enhancing commitments.

With the other two techniques, the question of personal freedom arises. The company's approach to having employees volunteer for the smoking cessation program by recording their participation in their personnel file is questionable. Likewise, the request by the executives of the company for supervisors and managers to participate is susceptible to coercion, as is the slogan of the program, "From the Top Down: A Smoke Free Company." An employee may feel intimidated and obligated to participate. Does one really have freedom of choice? What if they choose not to participate? Might there be consequences?

How does the code of ethics address this dilemma? The code of ethics states in Article IV, Section 4:

> *Health Educators empower individuals to adopt healthy lifestyles through informed choice rather than by coercion or intimidation.*

Here lies the answer to the questions raised in the dilemma. The motivational techniques used to entice smokers were not just and fair. It was also questionable whether individuals decided to participate by informed choice rather than by intimidation and subliminal coercion. This may not have been a blatant infraction of the code, but it is enough to cause deep concern.

Solution to the dilemma.   The motivational techniques used in this case would not pass the test of ethical practice. The question is whether or not Jill and Mike's concern should be communicated to the speaker. For example, what if the speaker was not a professionally trained health educator but an exercise physiologist or some other type of professional? Should it be assumed that the code of ethics would not then apply?

An ethical solution might be to write a friendly but professional letter expressing the ethical concern. It should not be the intent to accuse the speaker of being unethical, but to emphasize the issue of freedom of choice to participate in a program. The letter should also address the issue of fairness regarding bonuses from insurance savings. Because the letter may be on stationery from the health department, it is important to have a supervisor approve the letter before it is sent.

Ethical Dilemma 5: Omitting Information to Increase Program Numbers

Each fall, the community health department offers flu shots to senior citizens and others who are considered to be at high risk. A yearly campaign is initiated to inoculate as many people as possible. A new strain of virus was expected to be of epidemic proportion, which worried Dr. Nelson, the medical director. He was further concerned about information from the Centers for Disease Control and Prevention explaining how dangerously ill elder populations could become if infected.

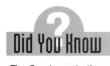

Did You Know

The Greek word *ethos*, from which the word *ethics* is derived, and the Latin word *mores*, from which the word *morals* is derived, both mean "character."

Mike was called to Dr. Nelson's office to discuss a health education campaign that would motivate senior citizens to receive this immunization. The medical director was committed to having as many people as possible inoculated, especially those most at risk. Mike was given instructions to design a media campaign plus educational programs for senior centers, local service clubs, senior residential complexes, church congregations, and other locations where older adults might be found. The medical director would take care of the medical institutions and nursing homes.

Mike felt this was a big order to accomplish in a short period of time. Luckily, Dawn had been given this responsibility in the past and had a file on previously conducted campaigns. As Mike began planning the campaign, he realized he needed to ask Dr. Nelson for more medical information to include in the media and educational programs. Dr. Nelson obliged and gave Mike the in-

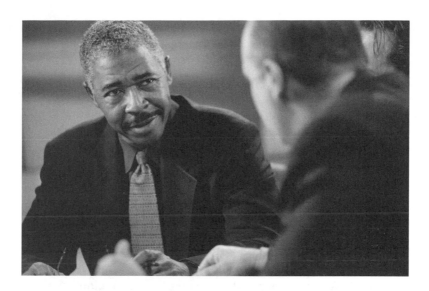

formation he requested. All the information Mike needed was included except what individuals could expect regarding possible reactions. After all, people would want to know if there was a possibility of a reaction and how serious it would be. Mike called Dr. Nelson about reactions to the immunization and what he should include in the media and educational programs. Dr. Nelson seemed evasive and did not sufficiently answer Mike's question. When Mike asked a second time, the doctor began to explain to Mike how important it was to have as many elders as possible inoculated. He said, "There were no serious reactions worth mentioning, let alone life-threatening ones." He further stated that it was his experience that if you mention possible reactions you reduce the number who would normally be inoculated by 35%.

After he hung up, Mike felt uneasy. Mike was bothered by what he believed should be included in the messages about possible reactions, so, later that day, he shared this concern with Jill, who came up with three questions: If you were encouraged to take a medication or become immunized to prevent an illness, would you want to be told about possible reactions that might endanger your health? If you became ill because of not being informed about reactions, would you lose trust in the person, agency, or institution who encouraged you to be immunized? Could the person, agency, or institution be held liable for malpractice as a result of harm that might result?

These were excellent questions, and it did not take long for Mike to answer them. On the other hand, if he pursued the issue with Dr. Nelson, his current responsibilities with the health department might be altered.

Ethical question.   Is it unethical to omit medical or other information from health education messages that could be harmful at the expense of reducing the number of participants receiving a potential life-saving service or treatment? *Application of the code of ethics.*   Turning to the basic principles of ethics, this case involves a dilemma between beneficence and nonmalifence. Failing to inform people of reactions to or complications of the immunization, even though trying to provide potential life-saving services, could possibly cause harm. Article IV, Section 5, makes the following pronouncement:

> *Health Educators communicate the potential outcomes of proposed services, strategies and pending decisions to all individuals who will be affected.*

Taking the code and applying it to the dilemma provides direction in deciding what should be done. If information were communicated about possible reactions, the campaign's success would be threatened. Which is the greater of the two risks: not explaining possible reactions to the immunization or having a substantial number of senior citizens become infected and possibly die because they chose not to be immunized?

Solution to the dilemma.   It takes character and courage to question the medical director on this issue. The strategy of explaining possible outcomes, both good as well as potentially harmful, is the ethical choice. The health educator, with the support of the supervisor, should make an appointment to again express concern about the potential harm that could be done. By so doing, he would be acting in a responsible and ethical manner.

Conclusion

This chapter has presented only an introduction to the theory and ethics applicable to community health education methods. Health education theory is still in a stage of development. In the past, health educators have relied on research from the behavioral sciences and education. Health education scholars are conducting ethical research, which focuses on making a positive impact on individual and group health behaviors. The practitioner needs to stay abreast of new theories and their application to health education methods. Doing so means being prepared to carry out our responsibilities as health educators.

Barriers to ethical practice lie in not being aware of what constitutes ethical behavior and lacking the ability to act on ethical decisions. The first is unforgiving; the second takes personal and professional courage. Health educators are faced with dilemmas that are difficult and complex. The Code of Ethics for the Health Education Profession provides guidelines for professional behavior and for doing what is right, thus upholding the standards of the profession.

KEY TERMS

action: Stage of readiness to change in which an individual is actively engaging in behavior change.

autonomy: Having the right to choose and act freely.

behavioral capability: The capability of an individual to change a behavior by having the knowledge and skills necessary to enact a desired behavior.

beneficence: Actions designed to help others.

compatibility: How consistent an innovation is with the values, habits, experiences, and needs of potential adopters.

complexity: How difficult an innovation is to understand.

contemplation: Stage of readiness to change in which an individual may consider changing a behavior.

early adopters: Individuals interested in adopting an innovation but who do not want to be the first to do so.

early majority adopters: Individuals who accept innovations once others they respect have done so.

ethics: A system of moral principles or values that governs the conduct of the members of a profession.

expectation: What is expected as a result of modifying a behavior.

innovators: The first individuals to adopt an innovation.

justice: Treating others equally and fairly.

laggards: The last individuals to get involved, if at all, in adopting an innovation.

late majority adopters: Individuals who are skeptical and late to adopt an innovation.

maintenance: Stage of readiness to change in which an individual has been sustaining the behavior change over time.

nonmalificence: Not inflicting harm on others.

observability: The extent to which an innovation provides tangible or visible results.

observational learning: The ability to learn by observing others.

precontemplation: Stage of readiness to change in which an individual is not interested in changing behavior.

preparation: Stage of readiness to change in which an individual is ready to change behavior but lacks the self-efficacy to do so.

reciprocal determinism: The theory that behavior changes are determined by interactions between a person and his or her environment.

reinforcement: The response to an individual's behavior that will increase the continuance of the behavior.

relative advantage: The degree to which an innovation is seen as better than the idea, practice, program, or product it replaces.

self-efficacy: Believing that one has the ability to take action.

theory: Knowledge, assumptions, or a set of rules or principles for the study or practice of a discipline.

treatability: The extent to which an innovation can be experimented with before a commitment to adopt it is required.

REFERENCES

1. Cottrell, R., Girvan, J., & McKenzie, J. (2002). *Principles and foundations of health promotion and education* (2nd ed.). San Francisco: Benjamin Cummings.

2. Rosenstock, I. M. (1966). Why people use health services. *Milbank Memorial Fund Quarterly, 44,* 94–124.

3. Ajzen, I. (1988). *Attitudes, personality, and behavior.* Chicago: Dorsey Press.

4. Prochaska, J. O. (1979). *Systems of psychotherapy: A transtheoretical process.* Homewood, IL: Dorsey Press.

5. Glanz, K., & Rimer, B. (1995). *Theory at a glance: A guide for health promotion practice* (NIH Publication No. 95-3896). Bethesda, MD: National Cancer Institute.

6. Bandura, A. (1977). *Social learning theory.* Englewood Cliffs, NJ: Prentice-Hall.

7. Rogers, E. M. (1983). *Diffusion of innovation* (3rd ed.). New York: Free Press.

8. Coalition of National Health Organizations. (1999). Code of Ethics for the Health Education Profession. *Journal of Heath Education, 31,* 216–217.

ADDITIONAL RESOURCES

Print

Bandura, A. (1986). *Social foundations of thought and action: A social cognitive theory.* Englewood Cliffs, NJ: Prentice-Hall.

DiClemente, R., Crosby, R., & Kegler, M. (Eds.). (2002). *Emerging theories in health promotion practice and research.* San Francisco: Jossey-Bass.

Fishbein, M., & Ajzen, I. (1975). *Belief, attitude, intention and behavior: An introduction to theory and research.* Reading, MA: Addison-Wesley.

Glanz, K., Rimer, B. K., & Lewis, F. M. (Eds.). (2002). *Health behavior and health education: Theory, research, and practice* (3rd ed.). San Francisco: Jossey-Bass.

Greenberg, J. S. (2001). *Code of ethics for health education professionals: Case study book.* Sudbury, MA: Jones and Bartlett.

Greenberg, J. S., & Gold, R. S. (1992). *The health education ethics book.* Dubuque, IA: Wm. C. Brown.

Rosenstock, I. M. (1974). Historical origins of the health belief model. *Health Education Monographs, 2,* 328–335.

Internet

American Association for Health Education. *Code of ethics for the health education profession.* Available: http://www.aahperd.org/aahe/template.cfm?template=code_of_ethics.html.

Internet Healthcare Coalition. *eHealth code of ethics.* Available: http://www.ihealth-coalition.org/ethics/ehcode.html.

2

Promoting Health Education in a Multicultural Society

Jodi Brookins-Fisher, Ph.D., CHES
Stephen B. Thomas, Ph.D.

Author Comments

We really feel that relating to people on a human level is the most important thing we can do to make a difference in people's lives. How are we to develop and implement effective programs if we do not know the people with whom we are working? It seems so basic, yet it is a point that has been overlooked for years. The focus on diversity is long overdue. We need to realize and validate the important differences in people. They should not have to be like "us" in order to receive services in this country. Unfortunately, just the opposite is often true.

This chapter addresses diversity from a practical perspective. But beyond that, we need to realize diversity in health education because it is the *human* thing to do. We should all be able to enjoy our health because we are citizens of a great country—not because of our skin color, sexual orientation, or age. Health educators can make the world a better place, and we can begin by acknowledging all of the people that make up its uniqueness.

Introduction

In the last few years, an increased emphasis on the recognition of underserved populations in the United States has played a major role in health education efforts. Community-based efforts have been initiated in response to increases in disease among particular populations (e.g., stroke among African Americans). In addition, an understanding of concepts such as *cultural awareness, cultural sensitivity, cultural competence,* and *multiculturalism* has become necessary for a health educator to be effective. It is easy to give terminology lip service, but what do these terms really mean? What must health education professionals do to effectively address the issues of diversity in the many settings in which they are expected to play their professional roles? How does an individual health educator become better prepared to work with diverse populations? This chapter addresses the need for a multicultural focus in health education and presents ideas on how to facilitate the development of a multiculturally competent health care setting, as well as lists diversity resources available to health educators.

Increasing Diversity in the United States: The Need for Multicultural Awareness in Health Education

From an ethnic and racial standpoint, the U.S. population is changing from one that is largely white to one that is more diverse. It has been projected that by the year 2030, the ethnic group with the largest percentage of increase in population will be Hispanic Americans, equating to a 187% increase. It is also projected that during the same time, Asian Americans, Pacific Islander Americans, and Native Americans will experience a 68% population growth. In contrast, only a 25% increase will occur among the white population, so that "**minority**" ethnic groups, collectively, will surpass the white population in numbers, accounting for 51% of the population.[1] This shift will result in the United States being more in line with global statistics, in which people of color comprise the majority.

Other demographic indicators also demonstrate growing diversity in America. For instance, gay and lesbian persons currently represent 2% to 10% of the U.S. population.[2] With health **disparities** being a primary focus of public health efforts, it is essential that health educators, in both the present and the future, continue to be aware of and respond to demographic changes. Growing "minority" and other hitherto **underserved** populations will need services that are appropriately delivered to them and that meet their specific needs. Regardless of the specific population to be targeted, the development of health education services will need to take into consideration the population's **culture**. This requires the focus population's input in community health assessment and improvement, program planning, implementation, and evaluation.

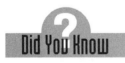

Did You Know

Suicide is the leading cause of death among gay and lesbian youth. For all others in this age group, motor vehicle accidents account for the majority of deaths.

Some U.S. populations have continued to experience problems with certain health issues. Poverty, lack of proper immunizations, heart disease, cancer, stroke, chronic obstructive pulmonary disease, pneumonia, and diabetes have continued to plague ethnic groups, while older adults continue to experience chronic diseases such as arthritis, hypertension, osteoporosis, and dementing illnesses. As the country's demographics change, it is imperative that health educators provide programming that addresses the dynamic health concerns of their diverse populations.

The Language of Diversity

Terminology pertaining to multiculturalism abounds. At times, the meaning of a particular word or how that word differs from another can be confusing. Although the following is an attempt to define the language of diversity, one should always consider the source, as words may be used interchangeably in some circumstances or settings.

- *Diversity* refers to divergence among people, rooted in age, culture, health status and condition, ethnicity, experience, gender, sexual orientation, and various combinations of these traits.

- *Cultural awareness* is the consciousness of cultural similarities and differences.[3]

- *Cultural sensitivity* has been described as "the knowledge that cultural differences exist." It is the ability to apply the understanding that stems from that knowledge in different settings and situations to ensure or facilitate a useful interaction for all parties concerned.

- *Cultural competence* is a "characteristic of those individuals who hold academic and interpersonal skills which allow an increased understanding and appreciation of another group's differences and similiarities."[1] Culturally competent individuals have made an effort to learn about other cultures and have incorporated the information to the point where assumptions about others are not made. Other definitions of cultural competence have included institutions, systems, and practitioners, with the ultimate result being the ability to respond to the unique needs of populations that differ from the majority, mainstream culture.[4]

- *Multiculturalism* has been defined as a recognition of racial and cultural diversity, respect for the beliefs and culture of others, and a recognition that all members of a society have contributions to make for its betterment.[5] It includes the concept of equality among people regardless of such factors as race, ethnicity, gender, sexual orientation, age, or ability. In addition, multiculturalism can be both a vocabulary term and a phenomenon at the individual or institutional level, inclusive of cultures outside of the majority.[6]

Multiculturalism has been an integral component in expanding the notion of education. The term *multicultural education* has been developed to refer to "the process of gaining an enhanced knowledge, understanding, and acceptance of the methods of constructive interactions among people of differing cultural backgrounds."[6] Within the health education profession, multicultural health education has been defined as learning opportunities that are carried out in relevant languages and are designed with sensitivity to culture, values, beliefs, and practices. These education activities are developed and implemented with the active participation of people reflective of the focus population and take into account their cultural diversity.[7]

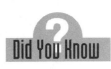

While society has become trapped in the muddied waters of "political correctness," the present and future of the health education profession require an understanding of multicultural issues beyond "correctness." For health education practitioners, the importance lies deeper than that of learning the language, it lies in equalizing the playing field for all players. In addition to knowing the terminology, health education professionals should contribute to change in societal structure for the betterment of all people in order not to miss a critical component in the development of the profession in the twenty-first century.

Being Culturally Competent in Health Education

In order to provide culturally appropriate services to diverse populations, several competency areas should be addressed. First, it is imperative that a health educator become aware of diversity and his or her role in ensuring that diversity issues are addressed in the professional setting. Next, being culturally competent results in health educators going the extra mile to ensure that their workplaces and the services they provide are inclusive of the diverse needs of the population being served. Last, building skills in creating an inclusive environment, using inclusive language, understanding culture, establishing discussion guidelines, developing facilitation skills, choosing materials that reflect diverse peoples and viewpoints, and diversifying teaching techniques and learning styles will increase the health educator's ability to meet the needs of others. Although these are not easy tasks, this section provides further ideas about how to incorporate each into one's personal and professional interactions.

Heighten Personal Awareness

Before developing and implementing programs for diverse populations, health educators must first understand their own belief systems regarding issues of diversity (e.g., race, ethnicity, religion, gender, sexual orientation, age, ability). The first step in this process involves becoming familiar with personal biases. Health educators need to be in touch with their personal biases so that they do not disrupt services and education provided in cross-cultural or transcultural (i.e., experiences with others different from oneself) settings. People have had different experiences and they naturally bring biases to interactions with others who differ from themselves. Previous social experiences and political interactions, as well as the communication and problem-solving capabilities of individuals, affect interactions with others and may lead to stereotyping or

Community connections 1

Katie, a new health educator with the local health department, was asked to give a talk to a local high school group about smoking prevention. This particular community high school had a diverse student population, with many Latino, Spanish-speaking youth. Although she felt confident in the subject matter to be presented, she realized she had very limited knowledge of, and past interaction with, those of differing ethnic backgrounds from herself. She wanted to make sure the information presented helped the young people but did not alienate them because of her lack of knowledge about them as both a population and individuals.

Over the next several weeks, Katie obtained a lot of background information for her presentation. She felt comfortable with smoking prevention messages, but still uneasy as to her ability to deliver the information within the context of the group. She decided she needed to further research smoking prevention programs and messages in the literature targeting youth in general, and would ask the high school group if she could attend a couple of its meetings. Here she would listen to the group, observe their interactions, and interview willing individuals.

misunderstanding.[5] With an understanding of personal biases, health educators have a clearer understanding of their limitations in communicating with focus populations. Health educators also must exhibit professionalism, separating their personal biases from their professional interactions, especially as they are called on more frequently to work with diverse populations. This is a difficult task, and one that should be carefully analyzed prior to programming at any level.

Along with careful evaluation of personal biases, listening, watching, reading, and participating are important in becoming a culturally competent professional. Health educators can learn the most about other cultures when they immerse themselves in those cultures. Learning about other cultures can be accomplished by attending cultural events, such as Pride Day, Cinco de Mayo, powwows, healing ceremonies, Martin Luther King, Jr., events, or other ethnic celebrations; participating in workshops or lectures about topics on different cultures; being involved in neighborhood activities in the community; and reading materials on and from people of different cultural backgrounds, especially those materials verified by the people about whom the material is written. Establishing relationships with people from different cultures is perhaps the most beneficial way to learn about other cultures. These relationships will allow free discussion and provide opportunities to listen and learn from other points of view.

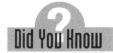

Did You Know

Hispanic as a group identifier can include individuals from all races. This fact adds to the difficulty of ascertaining which populations of people are in greatest need of health-related services.

Transfer Personal Knowledge into Professional Settings

The resulting knowledge associated with becoming aware of personal biases and learning about other cultures should be transferred into professional practice and the workplace. At a broader professional level, the following strategies can enhance a health educator's ability to understand diversity and help ensure that it is incorporated into professional practice and workplace interactions:[5]

- Determine whether current expertise addresses both regional and world-wide diversity and responsibility for human and international interactions.
- Determine whether programs enhance people's skills and knowledge about the diverse world around them so that people better understand themselves and the values of other cultures.
- Determine whether materials, curricula, services, and resources benefit all focus populations. Materials should reflect gender, racial, and other cultural differences (e.g., gender-neutral language).
- Determine whether an action plan has been developed relating to special information for underserved populations, such as migrant farm workers, immigrants, homeless persons, and people with differing sexual orientation.
- Determine whether plans incorporating Healthy People 2010 into programming have also included the needs of diverse populations.[8]
- Tailor an evaluation mechanism to suit the needs of the particular organization that measures the extent to which the health education workplace is meeting its responsibilities of responding to the diversity of its clientele, with input from the population or populations being served.

The process of becoming culturally competent is not a single-time intervention, but one that needs constant reevaluation and reappraisal both at the individual and the organizational levels. A culturally competent health educator is in a position to determine the extent of the cultural competence of the professional setting, assess and document the strengths and weaknesses of the organization, and focus on areas for improvement in both the workplace and programming.

Create an Inclusive Environment

Creating an educational environment inclusive of the diversity among participants can be one of the greatest challenges in health education programming. In doing so, several areas of concern should be addressed, including (1) the use of language and verbiage, (2) understanding the focus population culture, (3) discussion guidelines, (4) facilitation skills, (5) use of materials, and (6) teaching techniques and learning styles. These ideas will help to infuse

Community connections 2

Upon completing her research regarding Latino youth, Katie discovered that youths often thrive in educational environments that facilitate cooperation rather than competition and that allow for group work. As far as smoking prevention messages, there were a few ideas, but not many targeted at Hispanic youth. She decided that she would incorporate group activity into the presentation after consulting with the youth group.

Upon interviewing Latino youths from the high school group, she discovered that very few could identify services or resources available to them for smoking prevention. She decided to explore her own agency's ability to meet Latino youth needs and its response to youth as they utilized health department services. She found that although the health department was often empathetic to people with diverse cultures and backgrounds, they did not have specific resources available to youth about smoking, and that the pamphlets that were available were really directed to white populations. She decided to further explore the resources in the community in order to develop a resource list. That way, when young people utilized health department services, the providers could have a referral sheet for existing resources upon request. She also decided to revise the smoking prevention information available to Latino youth to make it more appropriate, attractive, and applicable to them.

culture into the educational environment and will help ensure that method selection has taken culture into account.

Use Inclusive Language

Health educators need to consider the importance of **inclusive language** when presenting information to individuals and community groups. Language is one of the most important methods for communicating, yet can be the hardest to change for inclusiveness. Both oral and written communication must be clearly understood by diverse populations. Strategies for ensuring inclusiveness include oral and written communication that is gender neutral (e.g., using words such as *partner* and *spokesperson*), in the appropriate language, and at the appropriate literacy level. Reading-level-analysis programs and learner verification procedures should be used with written materials. Members of the focus community should be involved in developing materials in different languages. Translation and retranslation should be carried out to ensure that the appropriate message is conveyed. Pictures and words conveying health messages should be used as much as possible and where appropriate. If language issues are not considered, health educators risk not connecting with the focus population at the most basic level.

Understand the Focus Population Culture

Another area of challenge is becoming aware of the culture, beliefs (especially health beliefs), and values of the focus population. It is very difficult for someone living outside the cultural parameters of a community to understand that population's culture if it has not been personally experienced. Culture in itself is diverse, and generalizations from past experiences will not necessarily hold true for any particular focus population or help a health educator with a current program or event. Even when the health educator is properly prepared, cross-cultural interaction may include participants' previous experiences that may impede the educational process. Although this may be frustrating, the health educator should remain motivated and interested in the participants' points of view. If needed, community resources and organizations that are culture-specific can be utilized for troubleshooting problematic areas.

Establish Discussion Guidelines

Group discussion guidelines (e.g., for use with focus groups or classes) should be determined and stated at the beginning of any program or event, and should be maintained by the facilitator and group members. Discussions among groups should be sensitive to diversity. Guidelines for inclusiveness may include any or all of the following: (1) respecting the confidentiality of all participants' comments and actions, (2) being sensitive to different personal experiences of group members, (3) being sensitive to different levels of expertise among the group, (4) avoiding assumptions about the cultural or ethnic backgrounds of other group members, (5) allowing privacy (i.e., the right to pass in any discussion or activity), and (6) other guidelines that the group deems important in order to facilitate tolerance and respect for each person's point of view.

Develop Facilitation Skills

Health educators should be facilitators of acceptance and respect in any setting. Good facilitation skills require negotiation, the ability to deal with controversy, being approachable and open, and being objective and impartial. If proper facilitation occurs, a health educator can be a role model for inclusiveness.

Choose Materials Wisely

Efforts should be made to select pieces from many perspectives when determining which materials to include in programming. For instance, articles by women and people of color can culturalize a curriculum. By remembering there is diversity among participants, health educators will utilize materials from more than one viewpoint. It may also be necessary while preparing curricula to use focus group discussions to determine what teaching materials and methods are appropriate and acceptable for the population at hand.

Diversify Teaching Techniques and Learning Styles

It is always easiest to teach how one prefers to be taught, but this may not reach all participants. Education should include various methods (e.g., lectures, small groups, role plays, computer exercises) to be inclusive of the

Community
connections 3

Feeling more prepared for her presentation because she had learned more about her focus population and its culture, Katie began to gather materials for the presentation. Although she prided herself in her ability to adapt to different presentations, she knew if she was to be truly effective with her group she would need to ensure she was attentive to cultural considerations. She thought a learning environment with group activity and culturally appropriate materials were crucial (i.e., materials correctly translated into Spanish that were appealing to the group). These ideas, although somewhat easy to infuse into the presentation, might make all the difference in helping her population relate to her and connect with her smoking prevention messages.

various learning styles among participants. Because learners may be visual, tactile, or audio-oriented, a variety of teaching methods should be incorporated to accommodate different preferences. Values clarification exercises are also beneficial in heightening cultural sensitivity because they help further participant awareness of personal values, while allowing others to state their values. As stated by Noreen Clark, dean of the School of Public Health at the University of Michigan:

> As a society we have to get agreements on what is important, what we value. . . . It's not a matter of your values being better than mine . . . it's a matter of creating a society where both our values coexist.[9]

Tips and Techniques for Incorporating Cultural Competence into Professional Practice

As health educators attempt to positively change themselves and the environments in which they work, they should be aware of a few issues that will aid in the process of establishing multicultural competence in the heart of professional practice.

Take Small Steps toward Change

Becoming a culturally competent health educator will take time. Old habits are hard to break, so effort must be made to institute change over time. It is important to remain oneself throughout the process, as humanness in the effort of trying to be culturally sensitive is an admirable quality. People will be aware of a fake persona anyway, so truthfulness is the best policy. Additionally, as small steps are taken toward inclusiveness, a trust in others must be established. Each client or participant is a unique individual, so care should be taken to not judge

Table 2-1	Characteristics of a Multiculturally Competent Health Educator

- Acquires knowledge about individuals and groups of people different than oneself
- Participates in cultural events
- Empathizes with humankind
- Competent in process and content areas of health education
- Facilitates discussion about the importance of culture among varying individuals and groups
- Provides a safe environment for exploring the meaning of culture
- Provides an inclusive environment
- Speaks in gender-neutral language
- Promotes not only tolerance, but acceptance
- Strives to reduce health disparities
- Empowers diverse populations to help themselves
- Models the importance of diversity in personal and professional settings
- Includes cultural considerations in all programming and activities

based on past experiences. With each successful venture at attaining cultural sensitivity, the health educator will become more culturally competent (see Table 2-1 for traits of a culturally competent health educator).

Infuse Cultural Issues into Facilitation

Although the information presented in Table 2-1 will help equip the health educator with facilitation skills, other tips are also important.[5] Cultural differences can be brought into the discussion through a planned activity regarding a health topic. For example, special remedies for dealing with common illnesses might be discussed, or ethnic or more readily available or obtainable foods might be evaluated for nutritional content. By providing these types of opportunities, health educators are encouraging expression of, and acceptance for, differences in culture, food or other preferences, and socioeconomic class, while allowing for exchange of ideas and even the fostering of relationships between people in a nonthreatening environment. Participants may disagree on a concept being presented. As the facilitator, the health educator should be careful to not support or oppose one view. By being open in discussions, the health educator establishes a climate of caring and acceptance. Inclusive language and use of variety in examples will also improve facilitation skills.

Know Limits

Health educators may find at times that their personal values intrude in professional settings. If this is a continual problem, then refer clients to another competent professional who is better able to deal with the issue. This is not to say the health educator should avoid all potential clients that cause internal struggle, because continued effort at working with others may help the health educator sort through conflicting personal values and professional obligations.

Overcoming Challenges to Becoming Multiculturally Competent

There are many challenges to becoming a multiculturally competent professional and ensuring a multiculturally competent workplace. Both personal and professional barriers, as well as outside opposition, may impede a well-intended effort. This section includes ideas for reducing barriers and lessening community resistance.

Reduce Personal Barriers

Perhaps the biggest barrier to attaining cultural competence at the personal level is a lack of awareness. Getting beyond one's paradigm and life focus is difficult, and occurs best when awareness is first heightened. Awareness at a global level encourages sharing of wealth, prosperity, and economic development among all U.S. citizens. It is a difficult process, as expressed in the following sentiments:

> Simply put, at a time when the economy is weak and many politicians are employing old strategies of blaming minorities for getting more than their fair share, it is not difficult to understand the resistance that many people express towards texts and programs, that, in their minds, merely "rewrite" history. For these people, all this talk about multiculturalism is little more than an attempt to create a narrative that makes them less than heroic by virtue of acknowledging the significance of others, others who have been oppressed and who have been hitherto viewed not as important but rather as problematic. Because of this, educators cannot underestimate the importance of the reevaluation of the status of individuals and groups of people; many will be compelled to see their own significance challenged, if not threatened with erasure, as others gain a new place in both texts and the nation.[10]

Health educators should adhere to the Code of Ethics for the Health Education Profession when dealing with personal barriers.[11] Article IV, Section 1, specifically addresses the need to be sensitive to social and cultural diversity. By following the code of ethics, health educators will ensure they are abiding by professional expectations rather than personal beliefs when conflict arises. Reviewing literature in related disciplines may also help a health educator increase cultural awareness. Health educators should avail themselves of the various opportunities that present themselves to become more educated on cultural awareness and the provision of culturally appropriate care, such as attending conferences and symposia and reading the growing body of literature available. The reader is referred to Marin and colleagues[1] and Buckner[5] for more information on the importance of cultural diversity in health education programming. Finally, the health educator can combat personal resistance by referring to several organizations and resources that can help professionals become more culturally aware and competent (see Table 2-2 and the Additional Resources list).

Lessen Professional Barriers

In the health education field, the greatest barriers to multiculturalism confronting health educators are a lack of the following: research, available health education programming specifically targeting diverse populations,

Table 2-2	Organizations Promoting Multicultural Health Education

American Association for Health Education
1900 Association Drive, Reston, VA 20191-1599
1-800-321-0789
(Specifically, two publications exist: *Cultural awareness and sensitivity: Guidelines for health educators*, and *Cultural awareness and sensitivity: Resources for health educators*.)

American Public Health Association
1015 15th Street NW, Washington, DC 20005
202-789-5600
(APHA has specific caucuses to address diversity issues.)

American School Health Association
7263 State Route 43 or PO Box 708, Kent, OH 44240
330-678-1601

Society for Public Health Education
1015 15th Street NW, Suite 410, Washington, DC 20005
202-408-9804

and preprofessional training. Much of the research in health-related fields has predominantly used white males as the point of reference. Additionally, research has shown that traditional health education approaches are not as effective with underserved groups of people as with the rest of the population.[1] Few professionally trained health educators have received education regarding multicultural issues because few programs nationwide have incorporated a multicultural emphasis into their course content, although this is changing. These barriers may affect a health educator's ability to effectively work with the many diverse focus populations for which programs are designed.

Even in a profession in which most individuals consider themselves open-minded, the road to cultural competence has been slow. Many organizations and agencies still face barriers that impede their ability to effectively incorporate culture into programming, method selection, and material development. At the institutional level, health education agencies can avoid barriers by (1) being aware and accepting of cultural differences and similarities; (2) having the ability for cultural self-assessment (i.e., for assessing how culturally competent the organization is); (3) having the required awareness, understanding, and knowledge of focus populations; (4) developing skills that facilitate diversity; and (5) being sensitive to dynamics inherent with cultural interaction.[1]

To improve the status of research regarding multicultural issues in health education, more researchers need to see cultural diversity as important. For instance, one study found that only 78 titles of 774 articles that appeared in prominent health education journals over a four-year period alluded to a multicultural emphasis.[12] More research projects will need to be specific to focus populations and must be run by adequately trained health educators. To avoid barriers to multiculturalism, professional research should adhere to a number of guidelines, including the following:[1]

- Demographic information must be collected on all focus populations.
- Better means of reaching underserved populations through interventions must be developed and implemented.
- Peer education must be utilized.
- Studies need to include not only health problems but also social and contextual indicators of their incidence and prevalence.
- Evaluation components should address both process as well as impact indicators.

Approaches that are more useful than traditional health education programs in helping underserved populations include peer education, lay health workers (e.g., family members, significant others in the communities), interaction with health care providers, self-help groups, and school-based interventions. When implementing any of these approaches, cultural issues should be addressed by taking into account the values, expectancies, norms, beliefs, and behavioral preferences of the focus group.[1]

Along with a multicultural focus, a mindset of advocacy must be instilled in professionally prepared health educators, since they will be in positions to work with people (e.g., administrators, legislators) who have a profound impact on other groups' causes. Colleges and universities training future health educators should incorporate skill building and training in areas of community organization and empowerment, advocacy, volunteerism, and diversity in order to prepare students for the realities of changing demographics. Developing culturally sensitive programs will increase the level of culturally competent health educators.

Plan for and Dissipate Community Resistance

Community resistance may also be a barrier to incorporating cultural diversity at the agency level, especially when dealing with multicultural issues that ignite debates among those with different value systems. For example, inclusion of a gay and lesbian youth support program in a school district may initiate controversy because of differing belief systems among educators, administrators, parents, and students. Religious values and lack of information about an issue may also contribute to the resistance.

It is important to be able to handle community opposition to multicultural programming. Opposition to multicultural programming may even include the focus population itself. For example, Native American populations who have had negative past experiences with health education programs may not be supportive of additional programming. Finding out why the focus population or populations feel as they do, and making sure that the program is developed incorporating their perspectives, will increase the likelihood of program success.

Overcoming community opposition can be accomplished by developing relationships with key individuals associated with the focus population. These key individuals and groups will provide insight into community norms, values, and belief systems. By believing in what the agency is trying to accomplish, they will help the health educator create a successful plan to reduce or eliminate opposition.

Whenever possible and appropriate, broad-based coalitions or partnerships concerning a particular health issue should be developed. By beginning with a common point of interest (i.e., the health issue), individuals will focus on the issue at hand rather than individual biases about the focus population. For example, if a coalition is organized to promote sexual abstinence, including abstinence among gay youth, the group should focus on the issue at hand instead of personal views about homosexuality.

It is always better for a program to work with the opposition than to exclude them. By finding a common concept for agreement (e.g., reducing risks for a specific disease), barriers such as conflicting values and personal stereotypes will begin to break down. An attempt at working together shows empathy and concern on the health educator's part. Once the opposition is heard, they may be satisfied and no longer be a threat to the program. Some groups, however, will refuse to agree with other positions and will not be willing to compromise. When this occurs, partnerships will not likely work for either party involved.

Expected Outcomes

By following the suggestions described previously, health educators can expect to enhance their cultural competency. This, in turn, will lead to more culturally competent institutions, organizations, programs, and research. By including the focus populations throughout program development, materials and resources will be inclusive of their point of view and more likely to be utilized in the future.

Community Connections 4

After the presentation about smoking prevention, many of the young people stayed to ask Katie further questions. Her preparation had paid off. By carefully selecting methods for the presentation that incorporated the unique cultural considerations of the youth group, her messages were well received. Besides imparting information on an important risk factor for disease prevention to a group of young people, she also had increased her comfort level regarding different populations. The youth knew she was open and respectful, and in turn, they encouraged her continued involvement in the health lecture series at their group meetings. Indirectly, she had also established a trusting bond between the health department and a group of traditionally disenfranchised youth.

Another outcome is mutual trust and respect between groups that traditionally have had turbulent relationships. Many minority groups distrust the more dominant, or **majority**, populations (i.e., those populations with power in the social structure) and their services. Ensuring cultural diversity in programming can build relationships with mutual understanding. The power of reestablishing trust relationships is not to be underestimated in the context of relationships between individuals and the institutions represented by other individuals.

A very important outcome of obtaining cultural competence at the individual and professional levels is the development of health education programs, including method selection, that are embraced by the community to the extent that they are institutionalized by the focus population. The focus population is more likely to take ownership because it has been empowered and involved in the process.

The goal of all the aforementioned is to pave the way for the elimination of disparities in health outcomes across populations within the United States. Clearly, barriers to continuous, quality care are very important reasons for the continued disparities in health status and outcomes of members of underserved populations. Thus, at the personal, professional, and community levels, greater awareness of diversity issues must be achieved, paving the way for new directions in programming for diverse populations. The goal of multicultural diversity can best be summarized by the following:

> We [health educators] have to begin with developing an awareness
> and knowledge of culture which implies a non-judgmental acceptance
> of the worth of all ethnic groups—a willingness to see people as much
> as human beings as members of a particular group. . . . The final
> stage is to be able to perform a specific task while taking culture into
> account such that the outcome is better than it would have been had
> the role of the client's culture not been considered.[9]

Conclusion

Society demographics are changing, which directly affects the practice of health educators. New strategies need to be inclusive of cultural diversity and should be implemented by culturally competent health educators. The health education profession must continue to examine its professional preparation programs, research, literature, programming and curricula, methods, and evaluation strategies to ensure the inclusion of cultural diversity.

The goal of attaining a multiculturally competent profession begins with each individual health educator. By each individual examining his or her own biases, beliefs, and values and determining how these transfer into the professional setting, he or she can devise more inclusive ideas and activities if needed. Once every health educator is responsive to the diverse needs of his or her focus populations, workplaces can then be transformed into respectful and inclusive settings. Above all, the health education profession can be responsive to Buckner's challenges[5] to be at the forefront of meeting the needs of our ever-changing American population.

KEY TERMS

culture: Similar ideas, beliefs, values, and perceptions among people of a particular group.

disparity: The vast differences that exist between populations in terms of access to services, morbidity and mortality statistics, availability of resources, and the like.

inclusive language: Using language that does not leave out a particular group or population. For example, referring to the top position in a local agency as the *chairperson* rather than *chairman*.

majority: The group that holds the power in a population. This may or may not mean they have the greatest number of individuals in the community (e.g., white men hold the power in American political arenas, although they may not account for the most people in the community).

minority: A government-invented word used to categorize people. This term is often seen as inferring "lesser than" or somehow inferior; therefore, its use is on the decline.

underserved: Populations that do not have the same amount of services, resources, and so forth needed to deal with individual and community health issues compared with other populations.

REFERENCES

1. Marin, G., Burhannsstipanov, L., Connell, C. M., Gielen, A. C., Helitzer-Allen, D., Lorig, K., Morisky, D. E., Tenney, M., & Thomas, S. (1995). A research agenda for health education among underserved populations. *Health Education Quarterly, 22,* 346–363.

2. Greenberg, J. S., Bruess, C. E., & Conklin, S. C. (2007). *Exploring the dimensions of human sexuality* (3rd ed.). Sudbury, MA: Jones and Bartlett.

3. Redican, K., Stewart, S. H., Johnson, L. E., & Frazee, A. M. (1994). Professional preparation in cultural awareness and sensitivity in health education: A national survey. *Journal of Health Education, 25,* 215–217.

4. National Alliance of Black School Educators. (1984). *Saving the African-American child.*

5. Buckner, W. P., Jr. (1994). Promoting multicultural sensitivity among educators. In P. Cortese & K. Middleton (Eds.), *The comprehensive school health challenge: Vol. 2* (pp. 661–686). Santa Cruz, CA: ETR Associates.

6. Staddon, D. T. (1992). *Multicultural resource manual.* Mt. Pleasant, MI: Central Michigan University Printing Services.

7. MacDonald, J. L., Thompson, P. R., & DeSouza, H. (1998). Multicultural health education: An emerging reality in Canada. *Hygiene, 7,* 12–16.

8. U.S. Department of Health and Human Services. (2000). *Healthy People 2010.* Washington, DC: Author.

9. Clark, N. M. (1994). Health educators and the future: Lead, follow, or get out of the way. *Journal of Health Education, 25,* 136–141.

10. Scapp, R. (1993). Feeling the weight of the world (studies) on my shoulders. *The Social Studies, 84,* 67–70.

11. Coalition of National Health Organization. (2000). The Code of Ethics for the Health Education Profession. *Journal of Health Education, 31,* 216–218.

12. Brookins-Fisher, J., & Rieckmann, T. (1996). The presence of multiculturalism in titles of selected health education journal articles. *The Health Educator, 28,* 3–7.

ADDITIONAL RESOURCES

Print

Banks, J. A. (1997). *Teaching strategies for ethnic studies* (6th ed.). Needham Heights, MA: Allyn & Bacon.

Banks, J. A., & McGee, C. A. (1997). *Multicultural education: Issues and perspectives* (3rd ed.). Needham Heights, MA: Allyn & Bacon.

Brainard, J. M. (1996). *Cultural diversity in the health classroom.* New York: Glencoe.

Campinha-Bacote, J. (2002). The process of cultural competence in the delivery of health care services: A model of care. *Journal of Transcultural Nursing, 13,* 181–184.

Downes, N. J. (1997). *Ethnic Americans for the health care professional* (2nd ed.). Dubuque, IA: Kendall/Hunt.

Doyle, E. I. (1995). *In the rough: A teaching strategies directory for cultural diversity in health education.* Denton, TX: Texas Woman's University.

Gordon, A., & Williams-Brown, K. (1996). *Guiding young children in a diverse society.* Needham Heights, MA: Allyn & Bacon.

Heilman, E. E. (2004). Hoosiers, hicks, and hayseeds: The controversial place of marginalized ethnic whites in multicultural education. *Equity and Excellence in Education, 37,* 67–79.

McIntosh, P. (1995). White privilege and male privilege: A personal account of coming to see correspondence through work in women's studies. In M. L. Anderson & P. H. Collins (Eds.), *Race, class, and gender.* Belmont, CA: Thomson/Wadsworth.

Rickard, M. L. (2005). Hispanic growth in America: How can health educators respond? *The Health Education Monograph Series, 22,* 2–5.

Sebastian, J. G., & Bushy, A. (1999). *Special populations in the community.* Gaithersburg, MA: Aspen Publishers.

Simmons, R., Bennett, E., Ling Schwartz, M., Tung Sharify, D., & Short, E. (2002). Health education and cultural diversity in the health care setting: Tips for the practitioner. *Health Promotion Practice, 3,* 8–11.

Spector, R. E. (2004). *Cultural diversity in health and illness* (6th ed.). Upper Saddle River, NJ: Pearson Prentice Hall.

Trevino, R. P. (2005). Social capital and health: Implications for working with minority and underserved populations. *The Health Education Monograph Series, 22,* 12–18.

U.S. Department of Health and Human Services, Substance Abuse and Mental Health Services Administration, Center for Mental Health Services. (2001). *Cultural competence standards in managed mental health care services: Four underserved/underrepresented racial/ethnic groups.* Washington, DC: Author.

Internet

CDC on the Move against Health Disparities. Available: http://www.kaisernetwork.org/health_cast/hcast_index.cfm?display=details&hc=52.

The Center for Research on Ethnicity, Culture and Health. Available: http://www.sph.umich.edu/crech/.

Cross Cultural Health Care Program. Available: http://www.xculture.org/index.cfm.

House, J. S., & Williams, D. R. Understanding and reducing socioeconomic and racial/ethnic disparities in health. Available: http://books.nap.edu/books/0309071755/html/82.html#pagetop.

Midwest Latino Health. Available: http://www.uic.edu/jaddams/mlhrc/mlhrc.html.

Minority Health. Available: http://www.iom.edu/CMS/.

National Heart, Lung, and Blood Institute Strategic Plan to Address Health Disparities. Available: http://www.nhlbi.nih.gov/resources/docs/plandisp.htm.

Native American Cancer Research. Available: http://natamcancer.org.

3

Developing Professionalism as a Health Educator

Kathleen J. Young, Ph.D.
Mike Perko, Ph.D., CHES, FAAHE

Author Comments

This chapter is about professionalism in health education. What does it mean to be a professional entering the workforce? When does it begin? Does the art and practice of professionalism ever end? This chapter provides the new and seasoned community health education professional with concepts and building blocks of professionalism. Both of us are community health education academics and practitioners who have (collectively) spent over 40 years honing the craft of professionalism not only within our personal careers but also as mentors for our students. We hope this chapter will help those entering the field of health education, as well as those who already have an established community health education career.

Introduction

This chapter both defines and introduces professionalism as a fundamental and important concept for the community health education practitioner. It also addresses important questions about professionalism, such as: Does one simply become a professional on the day she or he walks across the stage, diploma in hand? Can professionalism be taught, or is it something that just happens? and Does the health education profession help guide its members regarding professionalism through established standards and benchmarks? Information concerning key areas in which professional development changes during the span of one's career is provided. Various elements of professionalism and strategies to develop and utilize to enhance one's professionalism are presented and discussed.

Defining Professionalism

The notion of professionalism seems at first easy to define. Being a professional means upholding the standards and conduct expected of one who has been trained in a profession. Professionalism, however, is much more intricate and complex. If one types, "What is professionalism?" into an Internet search engine, roughly 1.9 million hits turn up to help define, explain, argue for, and apply this term. The *Random House Unabridged Dictionary* defines **professionalism** as "professional character, spirit, or methods."[1] Brandeis believed a profession had three features: (1) training that was intellectual and involved knowledge, as distinguished from skill; (2) work that was pursued primarily for others and not for oneself; and (3) success that was measured by more than the amount of financial return.[2] More recently, Ball noted that professionalism contains five key factors: character, excellence, attitude, competency, and conduct.[3]

Throughout the literature on professionalism, certain traits are consistent across many disciplines in regard to its practice; among these are excellence, duty, advocacy, and service. Professionalism is defined in many ways, yet a central theme in all of these definitions suggests that professionalism is fluid, meaning that it rests on a continuum of practice through one's career and requires an individual—regardless of the individual's discipline—to maintain high standards of excellence.

A Historical Look at Professionalism

The emergence of "professions" and the beginning of professionalism occurred roughly in the sixteenth century, when society saw value in the practice of theology, law, medicine, and university teaching. According to the ideal, a profession was a dignified occupation espousing three fundamental attributes: knowledge, organization, and the ethic of professional service.[4] Professionalism as a field of study has been systematically researched and incorporated into such diverse fields of study as architecture, engineering, computer science, and the medical and allied health professions.

Probably the occupation most studied in terms of defining and operationalizing professionalism is the medical profession. The Hippocratic Oath has guided physicians' professional conduct for 2,500 years; in 2002 the Medical Professionalism Project and its publication entitled *The Charter on Medical Professionalism* ushered in professionalism standards for the twenty-first century.[5] Focusing on new medical and health care challenges in virtually all cultures and societies, this project highlights the continuing evolution of professionalism and its importance to those who are served.

Throughout the years, literally thousands of research articles have been written to define the complex characteristics of various professions, but no singular definition has captured the true essence of professionalism.[4] From this vast body of work, however, have emerged terms that best represent the culture of professionalism. These are stated here to define what it means to be a professional: altruism, accountability, advocacy, duty, ethical and moral standards, excellence, honor, integrity, respect, and service.

The Community Health Education Profession

As a term directly related to community health education practice, professionalism has not been operationally defined. A good starting point may be Fromer's descriptive criteria defining the qualities of those who choose health (including health education) as a *profession:*[6]

- The health profession is worked at full time and is the principal source of income.

- Health professionals see their work as a commitment to a calling.

- Health professionals are set apart from others by signs and symbols that are readily identifiable.

- Health professionals are organized with their peers for reasons other than money and other tangible benefits.

- Health professionals possess useful knowledge and skills based on an education of exceptional duration and difficulty.

- Health professionals exhibit a service orientation that goes beyond financial motivation.

- Health professionals proceed in their work by their own judgment. They are autonomous.

Even though professionalism is not defined for health educators, there are clearly defined ethical codes of conduct that govern practice that directly affect health education professional actions. Both the health education profession's Unified Code of Ethics and Certified Health Education Specialist Competency Areas provide guidelines for professional behavior.[7,8] These are further discussed later in this chapter.

Overarching this is the notion that the entire field of community health education has a professional edict to promote and safeguard the health of the citizens in its care. Health is a primary public good because many aspects of human potential, such as employment, social relationships, and political participation, are contingent on it. In view of the value of health to employers, business, communities, and society in general, creating the conditions for people to be healthy should be a shared goal of professionalism among those in the health discipline. As Dr. David Birch, past president of the American Association for Health Education, and chair of the Department of Health Education at Southern Illinois University-Carbondale, points out in Table 3-1 (personal communication, May 2, 2007), certain qualities in those that practice health education help to ensure an ethical and professional career.

Table 3-1	Qualities That Bring Professionalism to Health Education

- *Be passionate about what you do.* Love what you do and believe in the importance and impact of your work if it is done with passion (it should be much more than a job).
- *Caring.* Genuinely care for the well-being of the individuals you work with—your colleagues, students, program participants, and so on.
- *Respect.* Treat others with respect—you might be older, more experienced, or more informed, but all should be equal in terms of respect.
- *Lifelong learning.* Realize that to be the "best you can be," you need to continue to learn about life and all those things that are important to your profession.
- *Honesty and transparency.* Little should be done in private (though at times there is a need for privacy).
- *Dependability.* If you make a commitment, follow through to the best of your ability. If you can't, be honest and transparent about your inability to follow through.

Professionalism: Beginning Steps to Career's End

If professionalism is indeed defined as "professional character, spirit, or methods," professionalism begins with one's involvement as a student and the ability to envision oneself as a practicing community health educator. This might occur in the first core course in a professional preparation program or when declaring a major. According to Dr. James Eddy, 2006 AAHE Scholar (personal communication, April 18, 2007), "Being a professional in community health begins the first time a student calls himself or herself a health educator. The thinking, actions, and words used from then on should reflect the history and competency-based practice that health education is recognized for. Once those first steps are taken, the process has begun." Throughout one's career, professionalism evolves; there is never any single event or time at which one can no longer learn. There are many facets to professional growth, several integral to the development of the community health educator. By participating in the mentoring process, joining a health education professional organization, volunteering, developing a portfolio, practicing health education competencies and ethics, developing a health education philosophy statement, establishing both cultural and technological competence, and participating in the community, one will grow as a professional.

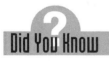

Everything you do is a reflection of your professionalism. Your attire, your emails, your language, and your blog all reflect on you and your image in the profession. Make these as professional as possible.

Participate in the Mentoring Process

One of the most satisfying and traditional ways in which young professionals begin learning about professionalism is to seek out those whom they identify as mentors. This process should be encouraged to start during undergraduate studies and continue throughout professional life. Whether the mentor relationship is formal or informal, the best mentors all share the same qualities: respect for each other, a shared vision to reach a common goal, trust, acting as a pipeline to new experiences and growth, creating a safe place where mistakes can be made, providing challenges, listening, giving advice, imparting wisdom, and providing inspiration. The mentor will become a lifelong friend and colleague.

The opportunities of **mentorship** for the mentee are numerous. Meeting with a seasoned professional allows the mentee to ask for advice, learn about the job, and participate in networking opportunities. Involvement with a professional mentor does not connote incompetence, but rather the conscientious commitment of excellence to one's career.

Professional mentorship programs have evolved to help newer professionals seek out a compatible mentor. For example, the Cleveland MetroHealth System instituted a successful Mentor/Protégé Program for health professionals in training, and defines *mentor* as "a wise, loyal advisor or coach."[9] Mentors, therefore, are critical to newer professionals as they establish their careers. The importance of mentorship also is recognized at the university level, where mentor programs are frequently offered. Many universities and colleges across the United States offer formal mentoring programs for students either entering a new major or exiting as a new professional into the workforce. Professional organizations also cultivate new professionals with mentoring opportunities. One example of this is a program within the Health Education Association of Utah. Central to this mentorship program is the commitment to develop professional relationships in Utah's public health fields.[10] Goals of this program are to

- Create an opportunity to align students and professionals with common interest
- Expose students to different areas in the health field
- Increase professional membership in the Health Education Association of Utah

Mentorship opportunities also are available for the seasoned professional. As in the previous examples, experienced and well-established health education professionals in various community health settings (e.g., community-based organizations and agencies, hospitals, local and state health departments) serve as mentors to the prospective or new professional.

Mentors have as much to gain from these relationships as their protégés. The one-on-one exchange creates an opportunity for the "senior" professional to assess and reevaluate his or her progression and to reflect on his or her current work methods.[11] Mentorship should always be embraced as a verb (for both the mentee and mentor), meaning mentorship is an "action" taken on the continuum of the professional spectrum.

Join a Health Education Member Organization

Becoming a member of a health education organization introduces both the new and the seasoned professional to the values of being invested in one's profession. Benefits of membership and involvement in health education professional organizations are evidenced in the literature.[12–15] Benefits include receiving professional journals about the research, methods, and processes of health education; attending and possibly presenting research at state, regional, and national conferences; and networking with others who can help shape and support professional growth. Table 3-2 lists select organizations that a health educator might consider joining.

Professional and member organizations provide the health professional with many opportunities. Health education and promotion associations cover a wide range of disciplines, including health education, health promotion, public health, nursing, and the behavior sciences.[12] The purpose of membership and involvement in a health education professional organization is to expand one's professional vision, network with a variety of health professionals (established and new), and advance oneself in the profession.[12] Opportunities for involvement exist at all levels, because many of the national organizations have regional and state affiliations.

Volunteer

At any level, volunteer opportunities are a part of community health education practice that can provide excellent formal and informal professionalism experience for new and seasoned health educators. By volunteering one's time and skills, the notion of professionalism is reinforced; that is, being a professional is not about looking the part but about actually doing the job. An expected role of any professional is that one has a social responsibility to the community in which he or she lives. The playwright George Bernard Shaw (1865–1950) remarked, "I am of the opinion that my life belongs to the community, and as long as I live it is my privilege to do for it whatever I can." Local organizations that benefit from volunteer assistance, such as the American Heart Association, American Cancer Society, and American Red Cross, are examples of good places to begin volunteering.

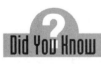

Did You Know

In every state, women volunteer at a higher rate than men. Nationally, women who work volunteer at higher rates than women who are not working in the labor force.

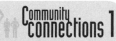

Community connections 1

Sureka is a recent community health education graduate of Springville University who was hired by the Springville Department of Public Health to develop a health literacy campaign aimed at mostly rural residents of Springville County. Sureka received straight A's in her community health education major, and in her two-piece gray suit and very smart shoes, she interviewed very well. Given that she had worked so hard on her grades at Springville University, however, she had not joined the Eta Sigma Gamma chapter and had not really sought out a mentor (she always made good grades and did not think she really needed one), nor spent any time outside of her studies to participate in community health education activities. In her first week on the job, Sureka was given three tasks regarding the health literacy campaign: (1) gather information that would best help county residents benefit from the health literacy campaign, (2) attend meetings with a group of rural physicians invested in preventive care in the area, and (3) present the information to a local foundation known for funding Springville causes.

Table 3-2	Select Health Education Professional Organizations
Association	Description
Eta Sigma Gamma (ESG) www.bsu.edu/esg	Founded in 1967, Eta Sigma Gamma is the national professional health education honorary. Being inducted as a member of ESG represents professional opportunities to hold elective office at ESG collegiate chapters, obtain scholarships based on academic achievement, advocate on behalf of the profession, and serve the needs of local communities where chapters reside. Leaders at all levels of community health began their careers in ESG.
American Association for Health Education (AAHE) www.aahperd.org/aahe	The American Association for Health Education is a membership organization representing 7,500 health educators and health promotion specialists and is the oldest and largest health education association. AAHE advances the profession by serving health educators and other professionals who strive to promote the health of all people, and serves professionals in all settings, such as health care, community/public agencies, businesses, schools (pre-K–12), and institutions of higher education.
American School Health Association (ASHA) www.ashaweb.org	The American School Health Association is an organization for professionals working in schools who are committed to safeguarding the health of

(Continued)

Table 3-2	Select Health Education Professional Organizations (Continued)
Association	Description
	school-aged children and youth. It represents a multidisciplinary organization of administrators, counselors, health educators, physical educators, school food service personnel, school psychologists and social workers, school nurses, and school physicians who advocate for high-quality school health programs.
American Public Health Association (APHA) www.apha.org	The American Public Health Association's mission is to be a strong advocate for health education, disease prevention, and health promotion directed to individuals, groups, and communities in all activities of the association. Its primary mission is to set, maintain, and exemplify the highest ethical principles and standards of practice on the part of all professionals and disciplines whose primary purpose is health education, disease prevention, and/or health promotion. To meet this mission it seeks to be a strong advocate for health education, disease prevention, and health promotion directed to individuals, groups, and communities in all activities of the association.
Society for Public Health Education (SOPHE) www.sophe.org	The Society for Public Health Education (SOPHE) is an independent, international, professional association made up of more than 4,000 professionals and students with formal training and/or interest in health education and health promotion throughout the United States and some 25 foreign countries. Members work in schools, universities, medical/managed care settings, corporations, voluntary health agencies, international organizations, and federal, state, and local government. SOPHE is the only professional organization devoted exclusively to public health education and health promotion. Its primary mission is to provide leadership to the profession of health education and to contribute to the health of all people through advances in health education theory and research, excellence in health education practice, and the promotion of public policies conducive to health.

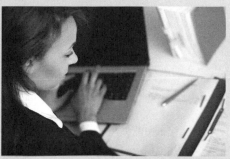

Community connections 2

In an effort to develop her health literacy knowledge, Sureka spent most of her time at work on her computer searching for information about health literacy (something she knew little about) and reading her college health textbooks. She had thought about joining a health education member organization that had a Special Interest Group (SIG) devoted to health literacy but decided against it, figuring that most organizations are the same, and besides, who had time to chat with these SIG people on something called a listserv? She had work to do. People in her office assumed she was doing a good job because she was always at her desk, well dressed, and pleasant at work; they didn't know for sure because she never went to lunch with her co-workers, preferring to eat at her desk while working. Ultimately, she had to cancel a few meetings with the rural physicians group because she had found some really good Web sites on health literacy and did not want to lose her "momentum and focus" in trying to learn as much as she could. In fact, she ended up failing to attend any meetings at all.

Volunteerism is not driven by financial rewards, but from one's own sense of purpose and motivation. Work of this nature often solidifies for the practitioner the importance of making a difference in the community or professional field and the role he or she plays in it.

Develop a Career Portfolio

A **career portfolio** is a compilation of various pieces of one's work in both academic and nonacademic settings. The portfolio should represent a selection of items that present and demonstrate both competencies in particular subject areas and examples of work created in the health education setting. A portfolio should be updated and reflect current items of work that one has created or participated in, and that represent performance measures (evaluations). A portfolio may be in a hard copy (such as a folder or briefcase) or electronic (such as a CD-ROM) version. The main purpose of a professional portfolio is to be able to display a selection of work that demonstrates competency in different areas of health education. Table 3-3 lists possible portfolio content item examples. Additional information and portfolio tutorials can be found in the "Additional Resources" at the end of the chapter.

Practice through Health Education Competency Areas

Basic competencies in the discipline of health education are needed to compete in the professional world. Health education is a profession requiring the ap-

Table 3-3	Examples of Portfolio Items

Table of contents

Letter of application

Résumé

Unofficial transcripts

Philosophy statements

Work and school example items, such as a health brochure you designed, three- to five-minute teaching or training video, training manuals you have developed, teaching lectures, pieces of research you conducted (data loading and analysis), etc.

Student teaching evaluations, work evaluations, and/or recommendations

Photographs of work projects or "works in progress"

Honors and awards

Types of certifications (e.g., CPR, CHES)

Second-language competencies

plication of moment-to-moment multitasking in various content areas. Health educators must be proficient in health content areas as well as in program development, implementation, and evaluation.[8]

Specific skills through defined responsibilities and corresponding competencies represent the scope and practice of entry-level health educators. These responsibilities are the culmination of the work of the National Task Force on the Preparation and Practice of Health Educators. The task force first published these roles in the Framework for the Development of Competency-Based Curricula for Entry Level Health Educators in 1985.[16,17] Today the National Commission for Health Education Credentialing (NCHEC) identifies seven overarching responsibilities, as highlighted in Table 3-4.

Certified Health Education Specialist (CHES) certification is available through the NCHEC for those health educators who wish to show they have proficiency in these seven competency areas. To become CHES certified, a new or seasoned health education professional must possess "a bachelor's degree,

Table 3-4	CHES Responsibility Areas

I. Assess individual and community needs for health education

II. Plan health education strategies, interventions, and programs

III. Implement health education strategies, interventions, and programs

IV. Conduct evaluation and research related to health education

V. Administer health education strategies, interventions, and programs

VI. Serve as a health education resource person

VII. Communicate and advocate for health and health education

master's or doctoral degree from an accredited institution of higher education and one of the following: An official transcript (including course titles) that clearly shows a major in health education (e.g., Health Education, Community Health Education, Public Health Education, School Health Education)" or "an official transcript that reflects at least 25 semester hours or 37 quarter hours of course work with specific preparation addressing the area of responsibility."[8] The NCHEC has provided further clarification of the scope and practice of health educators, identifying a complete list of the responsibilities, competencies, and subcompetencies for each responsibility. Information concerning the cost and examination dates for the CHES can be found on the NCHEC Web site (www. nchec.org/aboutnchec.re.html). Further competencies for the seasoned health educator are currently under consideration.

Develop a Philosophical Foundation for Practice

Throughout one's career, people, events, and history will serve as guides on the professional path. Planning and goal setting will also play a significant part. Perhaps, however, the single aspect of the professional's portfolio that should not be left to chance is the development of a philosophy of health education. The word *philosophy* roughly translates to "love of wisdom." Gambescia posed some meaningful philosophical questions aimed at helping those invested in their own professionalism.[18] These questions perhaps best help the community health education professional determine his or her philosophy (or "mission," as some professionals prefer to call it) statement:

- Who are we?
- What areas of the human condition do we choose to affect?
- Why do we do the things we do, and the way we do them?
- What difference is it making?

Gambescia also posed three themes for consistent reflection that encourage professionalism:[18]

- How do I know what I know?
- What should I do; how should I behave?
- How do I interact with others?

Clearly, these questions take health educators outside of the "training" areas and can take some deep reflection time to answer. Nonetheless, they help the new and seasoned professional alike stay true to the core of the health education field. All community health education professionals should possess a philosophy statement. Professional health education organizations also have philosophi-

Table 3-5	Health Education Organization Mission Statements
Health Education Organization	Mission/Philosophy
AAHE	"The American Association for Health Education (AAHE) envisions health education as a dynamic collaborative process directed at protecting, improving and promoting the health of all people."
The Public Health Education and Health Promotion (PHEPH) Section of APHA	"To set, maintain, and exemplify the highest ethical principles and standards of practice on the part of all professionals and disciplines whose primary purpose is health education, disease prevention, and/or health promotion."
SOPHE	"The mission of the Society for Public Health Education is to provide leadership to the profession of public health education and to contribute to the health of all people and the elimination of disparities through advances in health education theory and research, excellence in professional preparation and practice, and advocacy for public policies conducive to health."

cal statements that guide them in their mission to members and the public. Table 3-5 provides examples of organizational philosophy statements.

Practice Ethical Behavior

Ethics are a core aspect of professionalism. In health education, ethical dilemmas are a part of the job; controversial and often intensely debated topics are part of the professional landscape. Potentially controversial areas in health education include school-based (K–12) sexuality education, college and university tobacco-free policies, the role of genetic education in the health education curriculum, and access to universal health care. For a field of study, ethics provides a more objective view that there is a professional action to take based on a profession's views.

Ethics are based on reason and philosophical principles, not popular opinion. In 1953, Kleinschmidt and Zimand wrote, "it is very important that the health professional consider seriously what he/she is doing to the minds of people when they undertake to influence them."[19] This statement is particularly relevant to the role that a health educator possesses as a potential "change agent" of health behaviors while working with the public. The community health educator must be cognizant of his or her role and what ethical standards must be adhered to during community health education interactions.

In order for community health educators to keep ethics at the forefront of their practice, codes of ethics have evolved and been adopted within the profession. Currently a Unified Code of Ethics, under the auspices of the National Coalition of Health Education Organizations (NCHEO), guides the health education profession. After many years of work involving multiple health education organizations, including the American College Health Association, Health Education Section; American Public Health Association, Public Health Education and Health Promotion Section; American Public Health Association, School Health Education and Services Section; American School Health Association; American Association for Health Education; Association of State and Territorial Directors of Health Promotion and Public Health Education; Society for Public Health Education; Society of State Directors of Health, Physical Education, and Recreation; and Eta Sigma Gamma, the Unified Code of Ethics was approved and ratified in 1999.[20]

The NCHEO Unified Code of Ethics begins by stating, "The Health Education profession is dedicated to excellence in the practice of promoting individual, family, organizational, and community health. This Code of Ethics provides a framework of shared values within which Health Education is practiced. The responsibility of each health educator is to aspire to the highest possible standards of conduct and to encourage the ethical behavior of all those with whom they work."[20] Subscribing to and following the code of ethics is the foundation of professionalism. The code of ethics has been developed as the standard for professionalism to help the community health educator separate personal values and beliefs from professional behavior when needed. It is best for both the practicing community health educator and the profession if personal values and professional behaviors are congruent. For further information concerning the role of ethics in health education, refer to Chapter 1, "Using Theory and Ethics to Guide Method Selection and Application."

Develop Multicultural Competence

Given the important role of culture in the health status of individuals, it has been argued that understanding cultural concepts is vital to the delivery of health-related programs, including health education.[21] **Cultural competency** is defined as the "ability of an individual to understand and respect values, attitudes, beliefs, and mores that differ across cultures, and to consider and respond

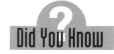

Did You Know

You are who your résumé says you are. Be sure you have a complete, attractive résumé that is tailored for its intended purpose. A sloppy résumé reflects poorly on your professionalism—it only takes one typo on a résumé to send it to the trash.

Community connections 3

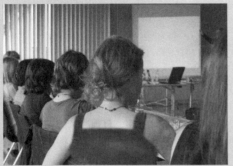

Sureka worked long hours and eventually pulled together all that she could on health literacy and rural populations. She felt really good about it—if she were still in school, she knew she would have aced this project. When it came time to present her findings to the local foundation, she was a few minutes late, but had a good excuse, since her printer had jammed as she was putting the finishing touches on the presentation an hour before the foundation meeting was to begin. She did, however, look very seasoned, with her leather briefcase and her laser pointer. She began to present to the foundation board a broad overview of health literacy in rural settings—her PowerPoint slides full of colorful graphs and fancy icons (she had put hours into the animation). Halfway through, one of the board members asked her if she would mind presenting on the specific needs of the rural residents of Springville. Sureka quickly said that the programs she was presenting were very successful and would work in any rural population. When Sureka was asked if she had actually been out in the rural community to know for sure, she replied that she hadn't had time because she was too busy getting this presentation ready. When asked if she had met with any key stakeholders, such as the rural physicians group, she again pleaded her case that she had been too busy. At this point the board member thanked her for her time and said that would be all. No funding was provided for her program.

appropriately to these differences in planning, implementing, and evaluating health education and promotion programs and interventions."[22] To be effective, health educators must attain a high level of multicultural competence.

In the latest release by the American Association of Health Education (AAHE) on Cultural Awareness and Sensitivity: Guidelines for Health Educators, particular attention was given to the challenges faced by health care organizations and health care educators in trying to reach diverse populations.[21,23] In this document, the AAHE has indicated that health educators must become far more culturally aware and sensitive.[21] Futhermore, *Healthy People 2010* has noted the need for culturally competent interventions to assist in reducing the health disparities in the nation.[21,24]

The community health educator who demonstrates cultural awareness and sensitivity to a focus population will significantly determine the level of participatory success.[25] In order for the new and seasoned community health education professional to better craft these skills, the professional must develop a philosophy about what it means to be culturally competent. It is when the community health educator has established a personal philosophy and commitment of incorporating diversity awareness into practice that the initial steps of "competency" have taken root. Becoming culturally competent is a lifelong endeavor and rests forever on the continuum of professional behavior. Being culturally competent is essential not only to the profession but also to potential clients, institutions, and public health communities in which the health educator serves.[21] Refer to Chapter 2, "Promoting Health Education in a Multicultural Society," for specifics and additional information regarding multicultural competence for the community health education professional.

Establish Technological Skills and Competency

The use of computer technology has become an essential aspect of the health education profession. A significant role of the community health educator is to adequately disseminate health information. Within the responsibility of disseminating health information, the community health educator must be able to use electronic media, primarily via computers and the Internet, to be effective.[26] Additionally, information technology has affected health education in the areas of medicine, classroom instruction, teaching, and distance education. Community health educators use information technology in various ways, from the dissemination of health information and health-related services to distance education course offerings for students residing in rural areas. Additionally, community health educators understand the importance of assistive technology for a client with a disability.

Electronic networking has also become a primary communication medium for targeted audiences in health education.[27] An example of this is electronic mailing lists (email), which many health educators use to enhance the environment of different settings.[28] Another communications technology for the new and seasoned professional is the use of listservs. For example, the Health Education Directory listserv (HEDIR) is a popular and helpful professional listserv for the new health education professional. Table 3-6 lists some of the basic competencies for the new and seasoned community health education professional regarding technology.[29]

Netiquette (network etiquette), or Internet etiquette, is a central practice of professionals when using computers. It is important for the health education professional to become aware of the basic rules and procedures as well as new updates when they are announced. A few basic guidelines should be followed when using online communication media such as email. First, a professional email address should be created. Second, understand and practice the rules of email, such as using uppercase letters in a posting with caution (this is considered shouting and potentially rude to the recipient). Next, professional emails should be responded to within two to five business days. Finally, remember

Table 3-6	Basic Technology Competencies for the Health Education Professional

- How to create, maintain, and edit a Web page
- Ability to use PowerPoint in an interactive mode (e.g., Producer)
- Ability to access databases to obtain pertinent data, such as CDC WONDER, Census, and PubMed, as well as several of the public health–specific databases
- Ability to analyze data without a high-powered statistical program such as SPSS
- How to convert files into PDF format
- How to link and input audio, video, and graphics
- Theories on using technology to deliver educational programs
- Ability not to dismiss anything novel because one does not like it

to write an email that you can live with, because it is a piece of documentation saved in cyberspace forever.

Participate in Service Learning

As the practice of health education has become more community focused and participatory, the integration of service learning activities into educational programs has increased.[30] Service learning activities provide health education professionals with opportunities to participate in community organizing and building, as well as to practice many of the NCHEC-identified responsibilities for professional development.

Service learning is a collaborative partnership between an institution and the communities it serves. It is one of the most applicable forms of experiential learning for the health education professional. Many of the core concepts of service learning are at the heart of the discipline of health education. Service learning provides both the new and seasoned health education professional with the immediate opportunity to participate in formalized community health activities while actively engaging in a needed service for a community. Most important, service learning provides both the prospective (e.g., student) and seasoned (e.g., supervising faculty) community health educator with the means to connect with various levels of "community." This develops a bridge of potentially authentic partnerships between prospective and seasoned health education professionals and their community members. Authentic partnerships between the academic setting and its community base are critical in building the bridges of collaboration and community organizing and building.[31]

Furthermore, many service learning elements are aimed at assisting the health educator in overall professional development, such as leadership,

Community connections 4

In looking back at her behavior at work, Sureka could see that her efforts, although well intentioned, were more about acting professional than *being* a professional. She showed up to work on time, worked hard, dressed appropriately, and was pleasant. These are all very important attributes of being professional, but she missed any number of opportunities for true professionalism. By not getting out into the community, failing to meet with the rural physicians or join an organization for resources and networking, and not socializing with coworkers, she had failed to demonstrate professional qualities that would have paid off. She decided to join her state's health education professional organization and consult with another staff member on her team about how to better prepare for next time.

interdisciplinary teamwork and collaboration, public speaking, coalition exposure and development, media advocacy, and public policy strategy development.[32] Central to service learning is the potential not only to address and meet many of the seven NCHEC responsibilities but also to build on critical elements of learning that are based on civic engagement, social activism, and community advocacy.[31] According to Clark, service learning also provides the new careerist with opportunities to identify and build a professional identity.[33]

The authors of this chapter would suggest a broader impact, in that while the student (prospective health educator) develops a sense of professional identity, service learning involvement also provides all participating parties (student, supervising faculty, and community member) with the opportunity to independently reflect, assess, and reshape the future direction of his or her professional practice. In doing so, character development (integrity, professionalism, and ethics) becomes central to each member involved in the service learning experience.[31]

Partake in Civic Involvement

In President John F. Kennedy's inaugural address, he stated, "My fellow Americans, ask not what your country can do for you—ask what you can do for your country." As a nation, we have read, heard, and reviewed this quote for over 40 years in an attempt to understand and practice what this president believed in: active citizenship and civic involvement. As a community health education professional, there are various ways to serve one's community or the larger state and global communities. Activities can range from political causes to nonpolitical causes.

Civic involvement is an excellent way to develop or expand a professional résumé. Civic involvement also provides the community health education professional with many opportunities for external visibility. Benefits of civic involvement include the following:[34]

- Building political and social engagement
- Building citizenship
- Increasing civic development
- Enhancing leadership qualities
- Networking

These are just a few of the benefits of civic involvement. It is important to remember that giving to others and creating social change for the betterment of society and humanity at large are the most important ways to grow both personally and professionally.

Receive Continuing Education for Lifelong Learning

Continuing education units (CEUs) are designed for the working professional to advance knowledge in a particular discipline, maintain credentials, advance in salary, and possibly advance to the next level of an academic degree (e.g., M.S, M.P.H., Ph.D.). For example, one may enroll in a three-unit technology CEU class in order to better prepare for various technology competencies at work. An employer may require the prospective community health education professional to be CPR and First Aid certified. The requirements and reasons are endless. Regardless of the individual goal or work-related requirement for enrolling in continuing education units, the benefits of CEU engagement are plentiful for both one's personal and professional growth. CEUs can be obtained in a variety of ways, including online courses, journal articles, and conference sessions.

Conclusion

One of the most significant benefits of taking an active role in one's professional growth is the opportunity to establish oneself as a community health education professional. Although professionalism is on a constant participatory continuum, it can be a positive endeavor with the assistance of other professionals who are committed to the excellence of the health education profession. Regardless of one's level of experience as a community health educator, there are a host of different professional building blocks for growth in professionalism, whether one is beginning the process (as a newcomer) or is continuing to refine one's practice as a seasoned careerist in the field of community health education.

KEY TERMS

career portfolio: A compilation of various pieces of one's best work in both academic and nonacademic settings.

Certified Health Education Specialist (CHES): Those who have met the standards of competence established by the National Commission for Health Education Credentialing (NCHEC) and have successfully passed the CHES examination.

cultural competency: The ability of an individual to understand and respect values, attitudes, beliefs, and mores that differ across cultures, and to consider and respond appropriately to these differences in planning, implementing, and evaluating health education and promotion programs and interventions.

ethics: A system of moral principles or values that governs the conduct of the members of a profession.

mentorship: A developmental relationship between a more experienced mentor and a less experienced partner (referred to as a mentee or protégé).

professionalism: To possess professional character, spirit, or methods.

service learning: A teaching and learning strategy that integrates meaningful community service with instruction and reflection to enrich the learning experience, teach civic responsibility, and strengthen communities.

volunteerism: The willingness of people to work on behalf of others without the expectation of pay or other tangible gain.

REFERENCES

1. *Random House Webster's Unabridged Dictionary*. (1997). New York: Random House Information Group.
2. Brandeis, L. D. (1933). *Business: A profession*. Boston: Hole, Cushman, and Flint.
3. Ball, J. (2001). *Professionalism is for everyone*. Available: http://www.goalpower. com/Keynotes-Seminars/Professionalism-Is-for-Everyone-program.html. Accessed 5/12/07.
4. Lawson, W. D. (2004). Professionalism: The golden years. *Journal of Professional Issues in Engineering Education and Practice, 130*(1), 26–36.
5. Brennen, T. (2002). Medical professionalism in the new millennium: A physician charter. *Annals of Internal Medicine, 136*, 243–246.
6. Fromer, M. J. (1981). *Ethical issues in health care*. St. Louis, MO: C.V. Mosby.
7. Coalition of National Health Education Organizations. (1999). *A unified code of ethics*. Available: http://www.cnheo.org/. Accessed 7/2/07.
8. National Commission for Health Education Credentialing. (2007). *About NCHEC*. Available: http://www.nchec.org/aboutnchec/rc.html#1. Accessed 6/24/07.

9. Cleveland MetroHealth System. (2007). *Case Western Reserve University Department of Anesthesiology's mentor/protégé program.* Available: http://www.metrohealth.org/body.cfm?id=308. Accessed 7/4/07.

10. Health Education Association of Utah. (2007). *HEAU mentorship program.* Available: http://www.heau.org/mentorship.php. Accessed 6/2/07.

11. Wagner, R. (2001, December 7). Why you'll want a mentor outside the ivory tower, too. *Chronicle of Higher Education.* Available: http://chronicle.com/jobs/2001/12/2001120702c.htm. Accessed 6/30/05.

12. Young, K., & Boling, W. (2004). Improving the quality of professional life: Benefits of health education and promotion association membership. *California Journal of Health Promotion, 2*(1), 39–44.

13. Logemann, J. (1994). Why should I belong to a professional organization like ASHA? *Journal of School Health, 36*(11), 113–122.

14. Desmond, S. A., & Symens, A. M. (1997). Promoting graduate students' membership in professional organizations. *Teaching Sociology, 25,* 176–182.

15. Hall, E. R. (1993). Increasing student involvement in professional organizations, and the pursuit of excellence in nursing. *Journal of the Society of Pediatric Nurses, 6*(3), 147.

16. Cottrell, R., Girvan, J., & McKenzie, J. (2005). *Principles and foundations of health promotion and education* (3rd ed.). San Francisco: Pearson Benjamin Cummings.

17. Frauenknecht, M. (2003). *The need for effective professional preparation of school-based health educators* (ERIC Document Reproduction Service No. ED482701).

18. Gambescia, S. (2006). Message from outgoing president. *SOPHE News/Views, 33*(6), 3.

19. Kleinschmidt, H. E., & Zimand, S. (1953). *Public health education: Its tools and procedures.* New York: Macmillan.

20. National Coalition of Health Education Organizations. (1999). *Code of ethics: Introduction.* Available: http://www.cnheo.org/code1.pdf. Accessed 7/7/07.

21. Luquis, R., Perez, M., & Young, K. (2006). Cultural competence development in health education professional preparation programs. *American Journal of Health Education, 37,* 233–241.

22. Joint Terminology Committee. (2002). Report of the 2000 Joint Committee on Health Education and Promotion Terminology. *Journal of School Health, 72*(1), 3–7.

23. Association for the Advancement of Health Education. (1994). *Cultural awareness and sensitivity: Guidelines for health educators.* Reston, VA: Author.

24. Luquis, R., & Perez, M. (2003). Achieving cultural competence: The challenge for health educators. *American Journal of Health Education, 34,* 131–138.

25. Huff, R., & Klein, M. (1999). *Promoting health in multicultural populations: A handbook for the practitioners.* Thousand Oaks, CA: Sage Publications.

26. Kotecki, J., Siegel, D., & Javed, N. (1998). Outsourcing your web presence: Questions and considerations for the health professional. *Journal of Health Education, 29,* 195–197.

27. Dorman, S. (1998). Assistive technology benefits for students with disabilities. *Journal of School Health, 68,* 120–122.

28. Dorman, S. (1999). Electronic mailing lists. *Journal of School Health, 69*(1), 39–41.

29. Kittleson, M. J. (2003). The future of technology in health education: One person's vision. *California Journal of Health Promotion, 1*(1), 113–122.

30. Campus Compact. (2003). *Campus Compact annual membership survey.* Available: http://www.compact.org/newscc/states2003/. Accessed 6/27/05.

31. Young, K., & Spear, C. (2005). Addressing health education responsibilities and competencies through service learning. *California Journal of Health Promotion, 3*(3), 17–23.

32. Minkler, M. (2005). *Community organizing and community building for health* (2nd ed.). New Brunswick, NJ: Rutgers University Press.

33. Clark, P. (1999). Service-learning education in community-academic partnerships: Implications for interdisciplinary geriatric training in the health professions. *Educational Gerontology, 25,* 641–660.

34. Eyler, J., & Giles, D. (1999). *Where's the learning in service-learning?* San Francisco: Jossey-Bass.

ADDITIONAL RESOURCES

Internet

American Association of Public Health Student Association. Available: http://aphastudents.org/nmp.php.

Barrett, H. C. (2000). *How to create your own electronic portfolio based on the "5-by-5 model" of electronic portfolio development.* Available: http://electronicportfolios.com/portfolios/howto/index.html.

Boston College, Career Center. Available: http://www.bc.edu/offices/careers/skills/resumes/portfolios/.

The Goals Institute. Available: http://www.goalpower.com/.

4

Health Communication

Gary L. Kreps, Ph.D.
Michael D. Barnes, Ph.D.
Brad L. Neiger, Ph.D., CHES
Rosemary Thackeray, Ph.D., M.P.H.

Author Comments

Having worked on health communication campaigns in community health education settings for a collective 60 years, we have found the work to be both exciting and challenging. We know that when health communication interventions are developed and implemented properly, they can influence health knowledge, attitudes, awareness, norms, and values, which are instrumental to changing health behaviors to improve health and reduce both chronic and infectious diseases. But developing and implementing health communication interventions properly is surprisingly complex. Effective health communication is so much more than writing a press release or a pamphlet. It involves careful planning; strategic analysis; thoughtful selection of strategies, settings, channels, and communication methods; and continual return to the consumers to ensure they receive the intended messages, understand them, respond to them positively, and adopt the intended health behaviors.

Accordingly, this chapter presents health communication interventions as a consumer-based health promotion process composed of several interrelated stages. We believe that if you understand the health communication process presented in this chapter, you will soon realize how powerful health communication is for any health education method you select for implementation. You will soon begin to think about health interventions more strategically and apply sound communication principles to all of your health education methods. This chapter has been written to reflect the best thinking that health communication has produced in the past 20 years. It will help you gain an appreciation for how intricate a process it really is.

Remember, success in health communication intervention begins with the consumer. The more you invest in your target audience before, during, and after your interventions, the more effective you become in influencing change. Combine this investment in your audience with a willingness to think strategically about health communication and a daringness to be creative, and you will soon realize how influential your work can become. Good luck in your efforts!

Introduction

Health communication has become increasingly central to health promotion efforts during the last 20 years. For example, health communication played a primary or contributing role in the completion of 219 of 300 objectives within Healthy People 2010, which for the first time introduced a chapter dedicated to the role of health communication in promoting public health.[1] Yet, health communication is a very broad field of study that includes analysis of the interactions between health care providers and consumers in the delivery of care, the ways consumers seek relevant health information, the provision of social support, the preserving and sharing of health information using different media and information technologies, the sharing of health information for informed health care decision making, the use of communication to coordinate interdependent activities between health care providers, the administration of personnel and resources within complex health care systems, and the development of health communication campaign interventions for health education and health promotion. This chapter examines the role of health communication campaign interventions for promoting public health. When used appropriately, **health communication interventions** can influence attitudes, perceptions, awareness, knowledge, and social norms, which all act as precursors to behavior change.[2] Strategic health communication efforts are effective at influencing behavior because they draw on social psychology, health education, mass communication, and marketing to develop and deliver influential health promotion and prevention messages that appeal to unique audience capabilities and orientations.[3]

An early work that influenced the development of health communication interventions was produced by the Office of Communications at the National Cancer Institute (NCI) and titled *Making Health Communication Programs Work: A Planner's Guide*.[4] This guide stated that disciplines such as health education, social marketing, and mass communication were all important parts of health communication. It is not uncommon to hear it proposed that health communication may even be a better name for the profession than health promotion or health education—that everything done in health promotion involves communicating for health.[5] In fact, health communication has been broadly defined by Everett Rogers, a pioneer in the communication field, as any type of human communication concerned with health.[6] Kreps, Bonaguro, and Query describe health communication as an interdisciplinary area of study concerned with the powerful roles performed by human and mediated communication in health care delivery and health promotion.[7]

Health communication intervention specialists carefully examine the ways health issues are perceived by select audiences, how different audiences access health information, and what message strategies (campaigns) are likely to be most salient for these audiences.[8,9] For example, *Healthy People 2010* defines health communication as "the art and technique of informing, influencing, and motivating individual, institutional, and public audiences about important health issues."[10] The National Cancer Institute and the Centers for Disease Control and Prevention (CDC) define health communication as "the study and use of communication strategies to inform and influence individual and community decisions that enhance health."[11] Still others speak of the concept by emphasizing the various forms of its applications, including media advocacy, risk communication, entertainment education, print material, and interactive communication.[12]

It is a mistake to think about a health communication intervention as only a narrow strategy or activity such as a press release or the type of interpersonal communication that might occur between a health educator and a client.[13] These are just a couple of the communication methods or tools that are used in health communication interventions. In effective health promotion efforts, a great deal of communication strategy and research lies behind the use of these communication tools. Health communication campaign interventions must be guided by evidence-based strategies if they are going to be effective.[3] It is best to view health communication campaigns as a comprehensive process that strategically frames the implementation of health promotion interventions. The way health communication interventions are viewed has a major influence on the ways they are used and the impact they will have. Because of the complexities of health promotion, it is best to develop strategic health communication intervention processes that actively adapt to the unique features of the different audiences targeted in health promotion campaigns.[9] This chapter presents health communication interventions as a consumer-based process with several sequential and interrelated phases. In this sense, health communication intervention is a process that can help guide the development of a wide variety of methods used in community health education.

Health Communication as a Process

Experts in health communication confirm the need to define health communication as a systematic and strategic process.[3] This means that the mere transmission of information or data does not equal effective communication.

To the contrary, those who plan and implement health communication campaigns must use strategic approaches based on established communication and behavioral theories, as well as incorporate consumer feedback to create targeted interventions and messages.[13]

Three well-respected and influential institutions that have assumed leadership roles in health communication have very similar outlooks regarding what health communication interventions are and how they should be applied. The Office of Communication at the CDC released a CD-ROM tool in 1999 called *CDCynergy*, which was updated and re-released in 2001.[14] *CDCynergy* is a six-phase multimedia tool that can be used to systematically plan health communication interventions within a public health framework.[15] Before *CDCynergy*, the CDC used a ten-step framework for developing and implementing health communication campaigns.[16] A health communication campaign model presented in the NCI planner's guide involves six steps.[4] Finally, a health communication campaign model developed by the Center for Communication Programs in the School of Hygiene and Public Health at Johns Hopkins University also promotes a six-step process.[17] These models or approaches present health communication as a comprehensive and strategic process.

Although these health communication campaign models vary in terminology and sequence, they share several common features. All three models involve analysis of the health problem as well as consumer characteristics that contribute to the problem. They include strategic design of communication based on analyses of consumers themselves, market factors, and communication settings, channels, and methods that are most consistent with the needs of the target audience and most likely to result in accomplishing predetermined goals and objectives. They also involve pretesting communication components with intended target audiences before full-scale implementation occurs. These models involve effectively managing the implementation process and performing adequate evaluation to ensure that the quality of communication methods is acceptable and to measure the impact of communication methods with respect to behavior change and disease outcomes. In essence, this means that health communicators must carefully analyze an audience and strategically develop appropriate methods to bring about desired outcomes.[3]

Rarely is a community health problem solved by using only one method or solution. Rather, a multicomponent approach is most useful in finding answers to public health issues. Therefore, health educators can use health communication interventions to support a variety of other methods presented in this text, such as legislative advocacy, media advocacy, community empowerment, media tools, and building and sustaining coalitions. For example, health educators can use health communication methods such as press conferences or one-on-one interactions with legislators to gain support for enacting policies (e.g., a mandatory motorcycle helmet law).

Health Communication Campaigns

Promoting public health and preventing the spread of dangerous health risks are integral functions of communication in modern society. Whether focusing on the prevention and control of acquired immunodeficiency syndrome (AIDS), cancer, heart disease, or violence in neighborhoods, a fusion of theory and practice in communication is urgently needed to guide effective health communication promotion efforts. Health communication campaigns involve a broad set of communication strategies and activities that health promotion specialists engage in to disseminate relevant and persuasive health information to groups of people who need such information to help them lead healthy lives.

Health communication campaigns are carefully organized and conducted strategic public information dissemination efforts designed to help groups of people resist impending health threats and adopt health-promoting behaviors. Typically, health communication campaigns are designed to educate specific groups (target audiences) about imminent health threats and risky behaviors that are potential hazards that might harm them, raising public consciousness about important health issues. Health campaigns are designed to both increase awareness of health threats and to move target audiences to action in support of public health. For example, health communication campaigns often encourage target audience members to engage in healthy behaviors to resist serious health threats, such as adopting healthy lifestyles (influencing exercise, nutrition, stress reduction, and other behaviors), avoiding dangerous substances (such as poisons, carcinogens, tobacco, or other toxic substances), seeking opportunities for early screening and diagnosis for serious health problems, and availing themselves of the best available health care services, when appropriate, to minimize harm.

Campaigns are designed to influence public knowledge, attitudes, and behaviors. Yet achieving these goals and influencing the public is no simple matter. There is not a direct relationship between the messages sent to people and the reactions these people have to campaign messages. Not only do people interpret messages in unique ways, but also they respond idiosyncratically to the messages sent to them. For example, it might seem like a very straightforward health promotion goal to ask drivers to use their seat belts when they drive. A very simple communication campaign might develop the message "Wear your seat belt when you drive!" For this message to influence drivers' beliefs, attitudes, and values, the campaign planner must take many different communication variables into account. Is this message clear and compelling for its intended audience? How are audience members likely to respond to this message? Will they pay attention to it? Will they adjust their behaviors in response to it? Campaign planners must do quite a bit of background research and planning to answer these questions. Effective communication campaigns must be strategically designed and implemented. They use carefully designed messages that match the interests and abilities of the audience for which they are designed, and convey these messages via the communication channels that target audience members trust and can easily access.

The Strategic Health Communication Campaign Model

Health communication is a process with several sequential and interrelated stages. Each stage aids in properly selecting and implementing health communication methods. The Strategic Health Communication Campaign Model developed by Maibach, Kreps, and Bonaguro (Figure 4-1) is a synthesis of models, principles, and theories that have been presented over the last 20 years and represents the best of health communication's collective thought.[3] The Strategic Health Communication Campaign Model identifies communication strategies that incorporate multiple levels and channels of human communication. The model suggests that a wide range of different prevention messages and campaign strategies targeted at several audiences will have to be employed to influence health knowledge, beliefs, values, and behaviors.

Effective health communication campaigns often employ a wide range of message strategies and communication channels (such as interpersonal counseling, support groups, lectures, workshops, newspaper and magazine articles, pamphlets, self-help approaches, computer-based information systems, school- and primary care–based educational programs, billboards, posters, radio/television programs, and public service announcements) to target high-risk populations with information designed to educate, motivate, and empower risk reduction behaviors. Modern campaigns have become increasingly dependent upon integrating interpersonal, group, organizational, and mediated communication to effectively disseminate relevant health information to specific high-risk populations.

Research performs a central role in strategic health communication campaigns. Data are gathered in the planning stage to identify consumer needs and orientations and in the communication analysis stage to target specific audiences, evaluate audience message behaviors, field-test messages to guide message conceptualization and development, and identify communication channels with high audience reach, specificity, and influence. In the implementation stage, research is used to monitor the progress of campaign messages and products and to determine the extent to which campaign objectives are being

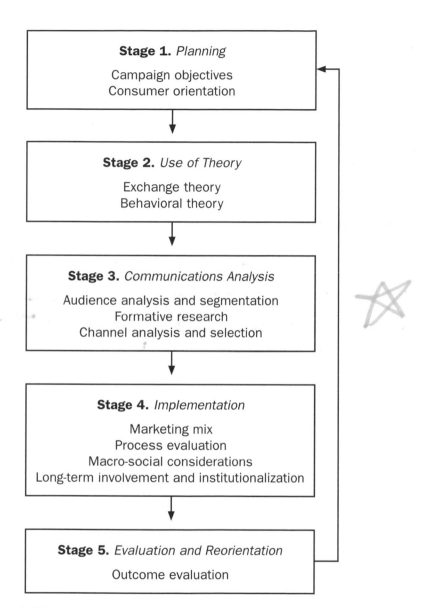

Figure 4-1 The Strategic Health Communication Campaign Model

achieved. Finally, in the evaluation and reorientation stage, evaluation research is conducted to determine the overall effects of the campaign on target audiences and public health. Note that the results of outcome evaluation research often identify new health promotion objectives and may initiate the planning of new health communication campaigns. This model suggests that to maximize the effectiveness of health promotion efforts, health communication research must be used to guide the development, implementation, and evaluation of strategic health communication campaigns.

Developing and implementing effective health communication campaigns is a deceptively simple enterprise. Health promotion campaign planners must recognize that mere exposure to relevant health information will rarely lead directly to desired health behavior changes. The Strategic Health Communication Campaign Model identifies five major stages and numerous key issues that health promotion campaign planners should consider in developing and implementing health promotion programs.

Stage 1: Planning

The planning stage of the Strategic Health Communication Campaign Model addresses two major issues: setting clear and realistic campaign objectives, and establishing a clear consumer orientation to make sure the campaign reflects the target audience's specific concerns and cultural perspectives. In setting clear and realistic campaign objectives, the campaign planner evaluates community health needs and deficits, as well as examines the opportunity to introduce specific health promotion programs to improve public health. What are the objectives of the campaign? Do you want to raise consciousness about a health issue, promote health education, change entrenched health behaviors, or maintain behavioral changes over time? Based on the campaign goals, different communication strategies will be needed. How realistic is it to introduce different health promotion programs within specific communities? What strategies are likely to be most effective within these communities? These are important planning questions that must be addressed before developing health promotion interventions. A consumer orientation means that the whole campaign is designed from the unique cultural perspective of the target audience and that members of the audience are involved as much as possible in campaign planning and implementation. It is important for campaign planners to fully understand the unique characteristics and needs of target audiences, as well as the best strategies for helping these audiences live healthy and fulfilling lives.

A crucial first step in the development of effective health communication campaigns is the identification and clear conceptualization of an important public health threat or issue that can be effectively addressed by a communication effort. This means that the threat addressed is genuine and of significant danger to warrant communication intervention. It also means that the campaign planner understands the potential causes and solutions to these threats. There must be clearly identified and proven strategies for addressing these health threats that can be promoted with the campaign.

A primary goal of the campaign is to influence the way the audience thinks about the health-targeted threat. If the target audience already believes this issue is very serious and of great relevance to their lives, this will lead the campaign planner to craft health promotion messages that will support these preconceptions. If, on the other hand, members of the target audience barely recognize this health threat and are not at all concerned about it, the campaign planner must design communication strategies to raise the audience's consciousness and concern about this topic.

Generally, campaign planners want to convince target audiences to recognize and take the identified health threat seriously. They want to influence the audience's beliefs, values, and attitudes about this issue to support the goals of the campaign. Only after a communication campaign raises audience consciousness and concern about the threat can they begin to influence (persuade) the target audience to adopt specific recommendations for resisting and treating the identified health threat. The communication strategies used to raise consciousness and the strategies used to motivate action may be quite different. It is imperative that the campaign planner clearly understands the orientation and predispositions of the intended campaign audience to the targeted health threats to craft the most appropriate and effective health promotion messages for this audience.

In this stage the campaign planner carefully evaluates the nature of the health problem and considers possible messages and techniques that will influence the affected audience(s). Identifying the health problem involves articulating the health problem and identifying why it is a problem. There are many ways to approach this task. For example, it is possible to describe the death and disability associated with the health problem (e.g., health indicators, health behaviors), past and projected trends associated with the problem, costs associated with the problem (e.g., economic, social, environmental), or how the problem compares with other important health problems (e.g., why it is a priority health problem). Defining and describing the problem also requires identifying factors that directly or indirectly contribute to the problem. A direct cause is a behavioral, biological, or psychological factor that leads directly to the health problem. An indirect cause is a social, environmental, or political factor that exerts an effect on a direct cause (e.g., poverty, crime, lack of education).[10]

Stage 2: Theory

The second stage of the Strategic Health Communication Campaign Model uses relevant theories and models to direct health promotion efforts. Theories provide campaign planners with strategies for designing, implementing, and evaluating communication campaigns. It is recommended that a wide range of different theories be used to direct health promotion campaigns. Exchange theories,[18] behavioral theories,[19,20] and readiness-to-change theories (such as the Transtheoretical Model)[21] have been used most effectively in directing health promotion efforts at multiple levels (individual, network, organizational, and societal levels). For example, the Transtheoretical Model developed by Prochaska and DiClemente[21] assesses the readiness for change of targeted audience members; based on the members' current stage of readiness for change on any given campaign topic, the campaign planner can design the most effective campaign messages to influence movement through the stages of change to the adoption and maintenance of recommended health behaviors. Audience members can vary on their readiness for change along a continuum of stages of change, ranging from precontemplation of change, to contemplation of change, to preparation to engage in change, to action to engage in the change, and finally to the maintenance of change. This theoretical model provides campaign planners with important information about the most effective communication strategies to use with different audiences to influence their adoption of specific campaign recommendations.

Stage 3: Communication Analysis

The third stage of the Strategic Health Communication Campaign Model examines three critical communication issues in designing health promotion campaigns: (1) audience analysis and segmentation, (2) formative research, and (3) channel analysis and selection.

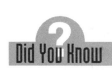
Did You Know

Health communication played a primary or contributing role in the completion of 219 of 300 objectives in Healthy People 2010.

After the problem has been defined and properly described, it is important to identify a primary, or specific, target audience that will receive the health communication. An analogy to define this process of narrowing a large population is the "shotgun and rifle" comparison. The shotgun approach represents a strategy that is widely implemented to everyone in a population. The hope is that enough of the population will become engaged in interventions and make the desired changes. In contrast, a rifle approach involves being more focused on a specific target. The term used to describe this approach in health communication is segmentation, which is the task of breaking a large population into manageable segments. Segmentation has been defined as a process of dividing a population into distinct segments based on characteristics that influence their responsiveness to interventions, such as the product benefits they find most attractive or the spokespersons they trust the most. Programs that target a population segment are generally more effective because program efforts and resources can be focused directly on the specific wants and needs of that particular segment.

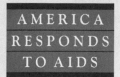

Community connections 1

Alice, the director of health education at an urban county health department, was assigned by her supervisor to assess the major health problems in her county and establish a priority health problem and focus. She and her staff began the task by reviewing all available mortality and morbidity data from the county. They collected and examined Behavioral Risk Factor Surveillance System data and other lifestyle risk factor data provided by the state health department, and visited the five hospitals in the county and collected discharge data. After isolating what Alice and her staff believed were the ten most significant health problems in the county, they calculated several epidemiological rates, including years of potential life lost. They also assessed total economic costs and evaluated the general level of suffering, pain, and disability associated with each problem.

After applying their data to the Basic Priority Rating Model, HIV/AIDS was identified as the most significant health problem in the county. Alice proceeded to write a problem statement that defined and described the HIV/AIDS problem in her county. It was determined that adolescent heterosexuals aged 15 to 24 were at highest risk for infection. Factors that led directly to the problem included unprotected sexual activity and an attitude of invulnerability among the target audience. Indirect factors included a lack of political and public health commitment to address the root causes of the health problem.

Audience segmentation involves breaking down large, culturally heterogeneous populations into smaller, more manageable and more homogenous target audiences for health promotion campaigns.[22–24] Segmentation requires the identification of a primary target audience that shares common characteristics (e.g., levels of readiness for change, health beliefs) and that seems to be at highest risk for the health problem. Generally, demographics (e.g., age, sex, race, education, income), geographics (e.g., residence, place of work, cultural characteristics), or psychographics (e.g., attitudes, opinions, intentions, beliefs, values) are used to make initial decisions. Segmenting a population also requires identifying the following: the size of the subgroup or segment within the population; where members of the segment live, work, or go to school; how the health problem directly affects the segment; and the level of involvement the segment has with risk factors related to the health problem. Gathering this information will allow a health educator to compare the relative merits of targeting different segments and to eventually decide on a final target audience. The target audience should be large enough and different enough from the general population to justify exclusive attention. The greater the cultural homogeneity of a target audience (i.e., the more they share cultural attributes and backgrounds), the better able campaign planners are to design health promotion messages specifically for them.[25]

Campaign planners must identify specific (well-segmented) focus populations who are most at risk for the identified health threats to be addressed in the health campaign. These populations of individuals become the primary audiences to receive strategic campaign messages. Too often health promotion campaigns are used with audiences that are too broad and have different segments of people with very different attitudes and beliefs about the topic of the campaign. When this occurs it is very difficult to generate uniform reactions to campaign messages. In fact, the campaign messages may work well with some segments of the population, but have negative (boomerang) effects on other segments of the audience. This can result in negative campaign effects, where the campaign actually increases the negative health attitudes and behaviors it is designed to curtail. Sometimes the health promotion messages are so broad that they are not very effective at influencing segments of the population. It may be better to focus campaigns on a targeted, smaller, and more homogenous (similar) audience with messages that these audience members are likely to pay attention to and be influenced by.

Health communication campaign research focuses on the effective dissemination of relevant health information to promote public health. To strategically develop and design persuasive health promotion messages that will be most influential with the specific target audiences, campaign planners must conduct audience analysis research to gather relevant information about the health behaviors and orientations of target audiences. Audience analysis also helps campaign planners learn about the communication characteristics and predispositions of target audiences.

After segmenting the target audience into the most culturally homogenous group possible, the campaign planner should gather as much information as possible about the group's relevant cultural norms, beliefs, values, and attitudes to guide the design of the campaign.[26] The more complete the audience analysis process is, the more prepared the campaign planner is to tailor the health promotion messages to the specific needs and predilections of the target audience.

It is necessary to gather input from the audience and perform assessments to better understand that audience. This process is known as **formative research**, which involves identifying the wants and needs of an audience as well as factors that influence their behaviors, including benefits, barriers, and readiness to change. Only after a target audience has been segmented does the bulk of formative research really occur. Common formative research assessments include surveys, focus groups, in-depth interviews, expert interviews, opinion polls, and case studies. Formative research is used to guide the design and development of the campaign by gathering relevant information about the

Community connections 2

Once Alice had identified a priority health problem, a target audience, and direct and indirect contributing factors, she and her staff were ready for audience input through formative research. After consulting with her supervisor and marketing specialists at the state health department, Alice decided that in order to collect information from 15- to 24-year-olds, she would contract with a local market research firm to conduct three focus groups at each of the six high schools in the county. It was decided that her staff would also perform intercept surveys in the food court at the local community college. Alice also discovered that one year ago, the state health department, in conjunction with the education department, conducted a statewide telephone survey of high school seniors and their parents to determine how to best address teen pregnancy, sexually transmitted diseases, and premature sexual behavior.

Because the survey report presented data by county, Alice decided that many of the findings could be used to assist her and her staff in their formative research process.

The focus groups and intercept surveys were designed to help Alice and her staff understand the barriers, challenges, and concerns, as well as the wants, needs, hopes, and aspirations, of the target audience related to factors associated with HIV/AIDS. Formative research also addressed issues related to the marketing mix (e.g., what programs or products would most effectively reduce HIV infection, what the costs associated with abstinence or adopting safer sexual practices were, where and how the programs or products should be delivered, and how the programs or interventions could be communicated most effectively). With this information, Alice and her staff were positioned to develop appropriate interventions for the target audience.

target audience and their likely reactions to campaign messages. Formative research should also help campaign planners make knowledgeable choices about which communication channels to use in the campaign because they are most likely to reach and influence specific target audiences.

Audience analyses are conducted to identify target audiences' unique information needs, cultural characteristics, communication preferences and competencies, and any social/environmental factors that can either support or inhibit campaign implementation and success. The data gathered through audience analysis are crucial to identifying the most relevant target audiences for communication campaigns, as well as the most appropriate and effective communication media, messages, and delivery strategies to use with these audiences.

Formative research also involves audience, market, and channel analysis. **Audience analysis** focuses on the distinct characteristics of the target audience, including wants; needs; motivational and resistance points; general attitudes, behaviors, and preferences related to the health problem; what they know; what they fear; and how they will likely react to specific methods related to the health problem. Audience analysis is an attempt to get inside the head and heart of the target audience and understand how they think and feel. Health education efforts that routinely include audience analysis as part of formative research are generally more likely to develop interventions that ring true with consumers and produce the intended effects.[27]

Market analysis examines the fit between the focus of interest (e.g., desired behavior change) and important market variables within the target audience. The term used in consumer-oriented communication and marketing for these variables is the *marketing mix*. The marketing mix is composed of four components: product, price, place, and promotion, also known as the four Ps. The *product* may be a behavior, a service or product desired for target audience use (e.g., a mammogram), or even an idea to be adopted. *Price* is the cost the consumer must pay to adopt the new behavior. It may include money, time, energy, or convenience, to name a few. For example, exercise requires that a person exert a certain amount of energy and time to perform the behavior correctly. If those costs are too high for a consumer, the behavior will not be performed. *Place* is where the product is accessed or obtained. It is important to determine if the product is best provided in a setting that allows for social support (e.g., a class or group process) or if it is more appropriately distributed over the Internet, through the mail, or some other channel. Finally, *promotion* involves the methods used to communicate with the target audience and is very similar to channel analysis (described next). All of the factors in the market mix are analyzed in the context of the target audience and provide additional information to be incorporated in the development of settings, channels, and methods.

Channel analysis is a process that helps determine which communication settings, channels, and methods will most likely appeal to the target audience. This includes an analysis of where the target audience is most easily reached (settings), how they receive most of their information (**channels**), and their preferences for communication methods. Channel analysis is concerned with television, radio, and newspaper usage patterns; perceptions of who the target audience sees as credible spokespersons; and computer literacy. For example, if the target audience is young males aged 12 to 17 years, channel analysis may reveal that a significant percentage listens to a particular radio station most, if not all, days of the week. It may be suitable to direct a portion of available communication resources to this particular communication channel. In most cases, using multiple channels and methods increases the likelihood that the message will be heard and acted upon. If, however, the message is not consumer-oriented and is not adequately supported by an effective market

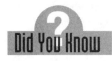

Did You Know

Health communication constitutes a separate major chapter in *Healthy People 2010* and is related to 18 other focus areas in Healthy People 2010.

Community connections 3

Formative research indicated, among other things, that although members of the target audience understood HIV transmission, they did not believe they were at risk or vulnerable. Furthermore, engaging in sexual activity was viewed as an adult behavior and a display of independence. Interest was expressed in learning more about the "actual" risks of heterosexual HIV transmission and the relative risks and benefits of abstinence, monogamy, and safe sex. It was discovered that the target audience would make changes in sexual behavior if they thought the risks of getting infected outweighed perceived benefits. Their preferred communication channel was receiving information from local professionals in a safe and confidential manner. Both high school students and young adults indicated they would prefer television and radio ads that referred them to either a hotline or clinic for more information. High school students indicated they would be interested in a school-based curriculum that dealt with the risks of HIV transmission and how to be safe.

With formative research in the forefront, Alice and her staff performed literature reviews and specific searches for best practices in HIV prevention that were consistent with what they had learned about their target audience. Alice ascertained that while several strategies had been shown to be appropriate and effective in reducing HIV infection among similar target audiences, health communication was generally the focal point. With this in mind, Alice decided to begin her campaign with health communication as the primary strategy.

mix, the channel itself is relatively unimportant. That is why all these factors are analyzed in unison.[18]

Using the audience perspectives obtained through formative research, the health communication process focuses on identifying the messages, settings, channels, and methods that will compose the intervention strategy. Despite the additional work and resources necessary to obtain inputs such as proper segmentation and formative research, the payoff in terms of quality of interventions and successful outcomes is worth the investment. Note, however, that there are circumstances in which identifying audience inputs is not feasible because of time or resources. In those rare cases, health professionals should consider all that is known about the audience, as well as theoretical and best-practice perspectives, to select the best combination of intervention strategies.

Stage 4: Implementation

The fourth stage of the Strategic Health Communication Campaign Model involves establishing effective strategies for implementing health promotion interventions. Successful health education practice involves much more than simple health fairs, media campaigns, and educational seminars. Although these techniques are valuable and widely used, leading health promotion experts have long advocated for the use of strategies that encompass education and awareness along with other key activities. **Strategy** may be defined as a general plan of action that may encompass several activities and considers the characteristics of the focus population.[10] Strategy options help shape the selection of methods.

Strategic communication interventions often use **social marketing** principles to guide implementation of campaigns. The social marketing mix for the campaign involves evaluating the campaign process, identifying macro-social conditions that may influence accomplishment of the campaign goals, and designing strategies for promoting long-term involvement and institutionalization of campaign activities with the target audience.[26] Marketing mix (the four Ps: product, price, placement, and promotion) refers to establishing a clear set of campaign activities and media (products) that promote objectives audience members can adopt with minimal economic or psychological costs (price) that are presented in an attractive manner likely to reach the target audience (placement) and provide audience members with information about how, when, and where they can access campaign information and programs (promotion).[25]

Campaign planners identify appropriate intervention strategies (education, policy, health services, engineering, community mobilization) needed to modify the health problem. This includes determining whether communication is a primary or supporting strategy. For example, a media campaign intended to raise awareness about breast cancer (primary strategy) will use different methods from a health communication strategy designed to support passage of tobacco legislation (supporting strategy). It also involves creating messages necessary to support the selected intervention strategies. Selecting the appropriate setting—the place where the target audience can be reached most effectively—is also very important. Settings are determined, in part, from input received in stage 2 and usually include schools, health care centers, worksites, neighborhoods, homes, and organizations. The best communication channels are selected (such as interpersonal, small group, organizational, mass media, community, technology) to reach the audience. The best health communication media (such as press releases or conferences, presentations, counseling, Web pages, print material, or films) are also selected.

Did You Know

There are several journals dedicated exclusively to health communication (the *Journal of Health Communication, Health Communication,* and the *Journal of Media and Health Communication*). (The lead author of this chapter is a founding member of the editorial boards for all three of these journals.)

Once a strategy option or options are carefully selected, consider the messages needing to be communicated to the target audience. The strategy selected will influence the type of message the target audience will receive. For example, a water fluoridation campaign that focuses on building aware-

Community connections 4

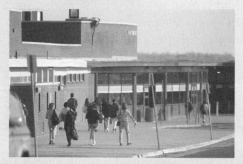

Based on the process that had unfolded to this point, Alice and her staff were now faced with the task of developing television and radio ads that served two purposes: (1) to decrease sexual behavior that placed those in the target population at risk, and (2) to motivate those in the target population to access services provided in the clinics. As Alice and her staff reviewed data from the formative research, they realized that several issues needed to be addressed in the design of messages. The main issues were that members of the target audience felt invulnerable because they believed HIV infection couldn't happen to them and that heterosexuals were relatively safe; that the target audience felt that sexual activity represented adulthood or independence; and that the target audience believed the risks of unprotected sexual activity must outweigh the perceived benefits in order to modify current behavior.

In considering the quality of messages, it was determined that messages should re-flect similar attitudes to those expressed in the formative research among HIV-positive adolescents and young adults. Messages would be fact or evidence based and would portray the ease with which infection can occur among heterosexuals (i.e., just one exposure). The source for the messages would be members of the target audience or peer spokespersons. Internal factors influencing the design of the messages included the concept that sexual activity should be associated more closely with concepts such as commitment and responsibility than with perceived issues of adulthood and independence. The concept of invulnerability would also be addressed as an internal factor. Finally, external factors to be developed in message design included exposure and risk to sexual partners; social norms that encourage abstinence, monogamy, and safe sex; and support from and access to clinic services.

Once the television and radio ads were developed, they were pretested with the target audience. Again, three focus groups were conducted at each of the six local high schools. Storyboards of the television ads and an audio copy of the radio ads were presented. At the food court of the local community college, intercept interviews were conducted that presented the same storyboards and radio ads. Based on feedback received from the target audience, the messages were modified accordingly.

ness through health communication may have the following messages: "Water fluoridation is safe and effective for all, and will reduce dental decay by 38 percent. Contact your legislators and tell them that you support improved dental health through water fluoridation." A policy/enforcement message could be as follows: "Water fluoridation is the most cost-effective approach to improve dental health among all citizens." A message to support engineering may be: "The monitoring and regulation of water fluoride in culinary water systems is the most sure way to decrease dental disease." A message supporting community mobilization may be: "Your elected legislator chooses not to support water fluoridation, despite the fact that his or her constituents overwhelmingly support this essential community priority. Your voice counts in making your elected official listen. Call 555-2222 to join your voice with others." Clearly, a well-designed health communication message is an important component of any type of strategy.

Effective messages are based on how the method will bring about change and appeal to its intended audience. Messages involve key points that will prompt the audience to an intended reaction. A message is more likely to be effective if it possesses specific characteristics that appeal and relate to its audience. Four characteristics should be considered when designing a message. The first characteristic is *quality,* which is often measured through appeals to emotion. Common emotional appeals include messages that are sad, funny, fear inducing, foreboding, one or two sided, fact or evidence based, implicit, or explicit. The second characteristic is *source.* A well-contrived message may be disregarded if it is not disseminated through an appropriate or credible source. Example message sources include celebrities, peers, government officials, physicians, counselors, nurses, scientists, news broadcasters, parents, teachers, religious leaders, administrators, and politicians. The third characteristic involves *internal factors* related to the audience, such as attitudes, knowledge, values, behavioral intentions, behaviors, literacy level, race or ethnicity, psychological disposition, experience with recommended actions, skills, perceived susceptibility to and severity of health problems, readiness to change, concerns about approval of others, life goals, and self-standards. The final characteristic involves *external factors,* such as social support from family and friends, support from institutions, local media, social norms, socioeconomic status, political climate, laws, worksite policies, and access to health-relevant community services.

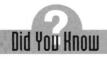

Did You Know

According to the National Communication Association, 71 universities or colleges in the United States offer a degree in health communication.

The implementation of many health communication messages includes the development of **supportive material**, which is defined as tangible items needed to support the health communication methods or messages. This supportive material helps enhance the message, improve its acceptance, strengthen its appeal, summarize its main points, and complement a message communicated through a channel within a given setting. Examples include media press kits, videos, posters, advertisements, thank-you notes, fact sheets, place mats, curricula, and program coordinator's guides (Table 4-1).

Table 4-1	Supportive Materials for Health Communication Methods	
Brochures	Moderator guides	PSA tapes
Handouts	Overhead transparencies	Scripts for oral presentations
Curricula	Advertisements	Talking points
Fact sheets	Bookmarks	Hotline telephone numbers
Radio PSAs	Stickers	Answers to frequently asked questions
Media press kits	Banners	
Videos	T-shirts	Storyboards for television PSAs
Posters	Pens/pencils with inscriptions	Billboard layouts
Thank-you notes	Log books	Activities calendars
Place mats	"How To" handbooks	
Program coordinator kits		
CD-ROMs		

PSA, public service announcement.

An essential component of any health communication activity is determining the setting for communicating the message. *Setting* refers to the place or places where messages are best received or preferred to be received by the audience. It also refers to places where the audience can be reached and influenced to think about the message. Common settings for message delivery include homes, schools, workplaces, health care centers, retail businesses, community sites, churches, government agencies, libraries, malls, health fairs, coalitions, transportation devices, PTA meetings, and neighborhoods. Setting selection is clearly related to both the message to be communicated and the strategy selected.

The setting influences the types of ways, or channels, that can be used to reach a given audience. *Channel* refers to the means through which a message is communicated to a given audience. Selecting appropriate channels for an audience is often related to, or in some cases limited by, the setting or settings selected. The selection of appropriate channels is also based on audience feedback through formative research activities. For example, if the home is identified as the prime setting, appropriate channels could include one-on-one home visits, technology via the telephone, or mass media via television or radio. The settings where messages are to be delivered directly influence the types of channels needed to reach the target audience. Many channel options exist, including the following:

- *Interpersonal channels.* Face-to-face or one-on-one interactions. For example, provider-to-patient sessions, peer counseling, and professional counseling are common ways to communicate health messages.

Community connections 5

With the pretested messages for the high school and community college students, Alice and her colleagues were able to determine the preferred places, or settings, in which these students wished to hear the messages. Because the target audience wished to receive confidential information from local professionals in a safe and comfortable place, settings that included private health clinic offices and counselor offices at the schools were selected. Further, because television and radio ad messages designed to give reasons for making wise sexual behavior decisions were preferred, the home (or apartment) setting was also chosen. Finally, the target audience stated that many would respond to a hotline referral from television or radio ads. Because the calls might be placed from a cell phone from one's vehicle, this setting was also considered. Alice's next task was to determine how and through whom the messages would be delivered to the target audience.

- *Small group channels.* Small numbers of persons, often organized to receive educational messages or to interact with other members within that small group. Examples of specific channels include support groups, seminars, and classes.

- *Organizational channels.* Institutions or agencies that communicate messages to their members or that collaborate or communicate with each other, and professional associations.

- *Mass media channels.* Mass-reach media, including messages communicated via radio, television, school cable networks, newspapers, magazines, billboards, public transportation displays, and community newsletters.

- *Community channels.* A catchall category for channels that are not organizational in nature, such as community messengers; community events; services or activities sponsored through malls, schools, hospitals, churches, libraries, or worksites; and open houses.

- *Technology channels.* The Internet, interactive Web sites, kiosks, video technology, and email.

Most health communication campaigns utilize mass communication channels (e.g., newspapers, radio, television) to convey health promotion messages to large, and sometimes diverse, audiences. These channels for communication often have the ability to reach many people over vast geographic distances. There is a trade-off, however, with the use of different communication channels. Some channels are more personal and dramatic than other channels; some are likely to be more trusted than others. It is important for campaigns to match the use of communication channels and messages to the demands of the campaign and the message/channel preferences of targeted audiences.

Community connections 6

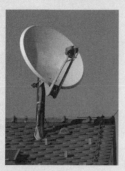

Through the formative research process, Alice and her staff found that local country and pop rock radio stations and the syndicated Fox Network were the preferred mass media channels. The time of day and day of the week when most target audience viewers listened to these channels were determined, and paid ads were created to air on these prime-time stations. Additional channels determined to be important included print material, specifically brochures, and the Internet. These channels were believed to be important because target audience callers to the hotline would likely prefer hands-on information. Once the previously developed messages were integrated into an attractive brochure and Internet site, they were pretested and refined to reflect the preferences of the target audience. The channels used in the health clinic and school counselor offices included trained professionals in a one-to-one communication. Additionally, these trained counselors provided further resources, including the brochure and Internet site, as channels for message delivery.

Stage 5: Evaluation and Reorientation

The fifth and final stage of the Strategic Health Communication Campaign Model is when a summative evaluation (evaluation of campaign outcomes) is conducted to determine the relative success of the campaign in achieving its goals at an acceptable cost, as well as to identify areas for future health promotion interventions. The information gathered through such outcome evaluations reorients campaign planners to the unmet health needs of the target audience, inevitably leading campaign planners back to the first stage of the model (planning), where they identify new health promotion goals for future communication campaigns.

Process evaluation is used to keep track of and assess campaign activities to identify areas for fine-tuning campaign communication efforts. Since target audiences reside within and are interdependent with the larger society, campaign planners must attempt to involve these larger social systems (such as business organizations and government agencies) in supporting and participating in campaign activities. Furthermore, to make sure that the campaign's health promotion goals and activities are fully implemented and established into the life of the target audience, the campaign planner should design strategies for the audience's long-term involvement and the institutionalization of these activities as a regular part of the consumer's daily life. An excellent strategy for such institutionalization is to empower target audience members to get personally involved with implementing and manag-

Community connections 7

Alice discovered that television and radio campaigns designed to present abstinence-based messages along with referral for contraceptive and related counseling were generally effective in helping adolescents and young adults make informed decisions. Alice also learned that messages on radio stations, in particular, that focused on responsible and mature decision making played well to youth who were sexually active or contemplating sexual activity. Staff indicated to Alice that while print material such as pamphlets had little reported effect on the sexual practices of adolescents and young adults, Web pages on the Internet that provided factual education and resources were well received. Staff also identified an abstinence-based curriculum with options for those who were sexually active as another effective health communication method. With this information, Alice and her staff made initial decisions on preferred health communication methods.

ing campaign programs. In doing so, they have a greater stake in achieving campaign goals, and the campaign activities become part of the audience's normative cultural activities.

Practical Application of the Health Communication Process

This section provides practical, real-life examples of health communication in community health promotion, including primary strategies and supportive strategies.

Health Communication as a Primary Strategy

Health communication as a primary strategy is most appropriate when the goal is to increase awareness or knowledge about a particular health issue among members of a certain population.

Ready. Set. It's Everywhere You Go!

The "Ready. Set. It's Everywhere You Go!" campaign, developed by the CDC, is an example of health communication as a primary strategy. This media campaign was developed to increase awareness of the new physical activity guidelines outlined in the 1996 *Surgeon General's Report on Physical Activity and Health*. The message was that physical activity did not have to be a planned, structured exercise but could become part of a person's daily routine, since opportunities for physical activity are all around.

The setting—where the target audience could be reached and where messages could be received—was the home. The channel through which the message was communicated was mass media, including radio, television, and newspaper. The health communication methods included television ads, radio spots, posters, and print ads. The CDC developed a packet of health communication materials for health professionals to use in their own communities.

Great American Smokeout

Another example of health communication as a primary strategy is the Great American Smokeout (GAS), sponsored by the American Cancer Society. The GAS is an annual event held the third Thursday of November, with the purpose of encouraging smokers to quit tobacco use for just one day, in anticipation that they will become permanently smoke free.

Health educators in local communities can sponsor events to support the GAS. For example, adults can be reached through worksite settings. The channels used to communicate messages include organizational, technology, and small group channels. Specifically, a health communication method could include a health fair or a display in a main gathering area, such as a lobby or cafeteria. Supportive materials, including educational pamphlets or brochures that highlight the risks of smoking and tips for quitting tobacco use, could be provided. Employees could sign pledge cards, promising to be smoke free for the day. They could also be provided with the opportunity to register for smoking cessation classes either on-site or at a nearby location. Another health communication method could be classes or presentations, such as a lunchtime seminar on smoking cessation or a related topic. Using technology and organizational channels prior to the event, employees could receive smoking prevention messages on their paycheck stubs or through the company email or voicemail systems.

Did You Know

The Centers for Disease Control and Prevention (CDC), the National Institute of Occupational Safety and Health (NIOSH), and the National Cancer Institute (NCI) each has created health communication research branches in their organizations to focus on the role of communication in health care and health promotion.

Another setting for communication during the GAS could be neighborhoods. Channels could include small group, mass media, and community channels. For instance, health communication methods used in one community during a recent GAS included holding a community "Tobacco Free Night" (a type of health fair) at a local elementary school. Print educational materials were provided on the benefits of quitting smoking and remaining smoke free. Other health communication methods included presentations on tobacco use, and participants had the opportunity to register for smoking cessation classes.

In another community, a partnership was created between the schools and a supermarket. Communication about tobacco and health included community channels. Students drew pictures relating to smoking and health on paper grocery sacks. On the day of the GAS, store patron's groceries were placed in these bags.

Mass media channels can also be used in an event such as the GAS. The health communication method could include a press conference held at a local elementary school, with a press release being the supporting material. The news story could highlight students who have pledged to be smoke free and not use tobacco during the GAS. It could also emphasize the health risks of smoking and the reasons to quit.

Health Communication Supporting Other Strategies

As mentioned previously, health communication is rarely used as an independent strategy to address a public health need. In a multicomponent approach, however, a health communication strategy is an integral part of all other health promotion strategies, whether policy, engineering, health services, or community mobilization. The successful implementation of these strategies relies, in part, on effective health communication. The following scenarios are illustrations of cases in which strategies other than health communication were the primary focus, but in which health communication was relied on to fully and effectively implement the strategies.

Walk Our Children to School Day

Walk Our Children to School Day (WOCS) is an example of health communication methods used to support three strategies: community mobilization, policy, and engineering. WOCS was developed to increase awareness of the option of children walking and bicycling to school with their parents as a way to promote healthy lifestyles, as well as of the need for safe, pedestrian-friendly communities.

Did You Know

Standards for quality health promotion and public health information on the Web are monitored by the Office of Disease Prevention and Health Promotion, the Scientific Panel on Interactive Communication and Health, and subunits of the Federal Trade Commission.

Community mobilization is one strategy used in WOCS. In each community, a WOCS event was organized, involving parents, school administrators, teachers, public safety officers, and businesses. The settings to reach parents included neighborhoods; to reach teachers and school administrators, the school; and to reach partners (e.g., police, businesses), local organizations.

Several channels were used to communicate the message. These included small group, one-on-one, and mass media channels. The channel selected to communicate the message depended on the purpose of the message or communication. For instance, small group (e.g., PTA) and one-on-one (e.g., friends talking to friends) channels were used to recruit parents to lead a walking group and to recruit community partners to join the project. Mass media channels were used to increase awareness and inform community members about WOCS.

The specific materials for WOCS included flyers, brochures, and press releases about the event. Additionally, print materials on safe walking, safe routes to a particular school, and the benefits of physical activity were provided to schoolteachers.

Although WOCS began as a one-day event, it became the catalyst for additional policy and engineering methods. Some communities developed permanent walking groups led by parents (sometimes called "walking school buses"). Other communities identified the need to improve the quality of sidewalks in the neighborhood and to improve the safety of walking or biking routes to school.

The implementation of community mobilization, policy, and engineering strategies relied on the support of health communication. For example, the target audience for these policy and engineering strategies was local policy and decision makers. The setting to reach the target population was in organizations, such as local planning commissions and city councils. To implement these strategies, mass media and small group channels were used. Press releases were sent to the media that highlighted WOCS and the need for improving the sidewalks and increasing safety along walking paths to and from school. Health communication methods included presentations at county commission or city council meetings. One-on-one communication was used as citizens spoke directly with the city mayor or commission members, encouraging them to support the initiative to provide sidewalks in the community.

5 a Day for Better Health

The national 5 a Day campaign is an example of a multicomponent program that incorporates several strategies, reaches target audiences in several settings, communicates messages through a variety of channels, and uses several methods and materials to communicate its messages. The following is an illustration of projects that occurred during several years of community health interventions at the Utah Department of Health.

The goal of the 5 a Day initiative was to increase the proportion of people who ate the recommended five servings of fruit and vegetables each day. To address this issue, the Utah Department of Health developed a strategic plan that focused on a primary target audience of children, with adults as a secondary target audience. Health communication, policy, and community mobilization strategies were used.

A community mobilization strategy was a critical component of the 5 a Day intervention. The organizational setting was used, and through community, small group, and one-on-one channels, individuals and organizations were recruited to become members of the 5 a Day coalition. The coalition was instrumental in the successful implementation of all other strategies.

Health communication was used both as a primary strategy and to support or complement other program components. For the health communication strategy, homes and neighborhoods were the primary settings. Mass media channels included press kits for various community events. These events included the annual 5 a Day Week and the 5 a Day Across the USA event held in spring 2000. Messages were also communicated by billboards and by posters displayed on the local bus transportation system; one bus was shrink-wrapped with photographs of fruit and vegetables.

Small group channels were used statewide as schools implemented a 5 a Day curriculum and provided tours of grocery stores for third-grade students. For the curriculum, a specific 5 a Day toolkit that included lesson plans and activities was developed. The purpose of the grocery store tours was to increase awareness among students about the variety of fruit and vegetables available and how to select produce.

Technology channels included a Web page on the Internet (http://www. hearthighway.org). This interactive health communication method included materials such as resources, ideas, and recipes for healthy eating for parents, children, and schoolteachers.

Community channels were used when a fruit and vegetable display was held at the annual state fair. Fair attendees obtained information about adequate servings of fruit and vegetables. Children also voted for their favorite fruit and vegetable.

Policy strategies were critical to increasing fruit and vegetable consumption among school-aged children. By working in the school setting and collaborating with school food service personnel at the school and district level, policies regarding the type, amount, and variety of fruit and vegetables served in school cafeterias were modified. For example, salad bar carts were purchased and deployed, and vegetable pizza was served in addition to traditional varieties. Successful implementation of this method required one-on-one and small group communication between 5 a Day coalition members and school personnel.

Strategies for Overcoming Challenges to Effective Health Communication

Perhaps the most common barriers encountered in implementing the health communication process include limited or no audience input and the subsequent lack of audience feedback and pretesting. Why are these components often overlooked? The simple and most common cause is a lack of time or resources. It is true that seeking such consumer input and feedback takes time and costs money. To improve the odds of an effective program and maximize long-term impact, these barriers should be hurdled in whatever way possible.

Certain legitimate circumstances may warrant not seeking an audience's perspectives. One example is risk communication, which involves the immediate need to notify key officials and audiences that may be affected by a health danger. In cases such as these—when the urgency of the message is more important than how the message will be received and accepted by the audience—there are justifiable reasons to avoid audience perspectives. Fortunately, most messages are not designed for these kinds of conditions.

Barring a nonsupportive administrator, having few resources, or having nonresponsive target audiences, many of these barriers can be overcome. Perhaps the most effective way to jump the hurdle of lack of audience input and feedback may be to plan for it when budgets are created, discuss its importance to key stakeholders and administrators, and learn as much as possible about it. From the authors' perspectives, some of the most enjoyable community health projects we have engaged in were due to the direct involvement we had with our audiences.

Conclusion

Health behaviors and health status are influenced by a variety of factors; therefore, the use of strategic communication intervention to address these health problems must also be multifaceted. Knowledge and awareness about health, disease, wellness, or risk factors within a focus population are generally not enough to significantly improve the health of a community. A system or environment that facilitates, encourages, and supports healthy lifestyles must exist. Consequently, health communication is rarely used as an independent strategy in community health. Rather, health educators use several strategies to address a particular health issue within the community.

The process presented in this chapter is useful in planning effective messages that link a combination of strategies. This process also is important in helping the reader obtain essential audience perspectives to select appropriate methods for the health problem faced by a focus population. By considering the unique health problems of a community, the most important health information needs of an audience can be identified and campaign goals can be established. Campaign messages needed to reach and influence target audiences must be strategically developed from the audience perspective. These strategies include strategic message design, selecting the settings where the audience can best be reached, and determining the best channels for reaching the intended audience. Relevant theory and research are used to guide strategic health communication interventions as well as to evaluate their effectiveness and future directions for intervention.

KEY TERMS

audience analysis: A method used to identify the distinct characteristics of the target audience, including wants; needs; motivational and resistance points; general attitudes, behaviors, and preferences related to the health problem; what they know; what they fear; and how they will likely react to specific methods related to the health problem.

channel analysis: A process that helps determine which communication settings, channels, and methods will most likely appeal to the target audience.

channels: Routes through which communication or message delivery occurs (e.g., interpersonal, small group, organizational, mass media, community, technology).

formative research: Gathering inputs from a target audience and performing assessments to better understand that audience. Formative research involves audience, market, and channel analyses.

health communication interventions: The crafting and delivery of messages and strategies, based on consumer research, to inform and influence individual and community decisions that enhance health.

market analysis: Examines the fit between the focus of interest and important market variables within the target audience.

pretesting: Evaluating the impact of communication strategies on targeted audiences before implementing these strategies within health promotion campaigns.

segmentation: The process of dividing a population into distinct segments based on characteristics that influence their responsiveness to interventions such as products, services, or messages.

setting: The place where the target audience can be reached most effectively.

social marketing: The application of marketing principles (product, price, placement, and promotion) to establish a clear set of campaign activities and media (products) that promote objectives audience members can adopt with minimal economic or psychological costs (price) that are presented in an attractive manner likely to reach the target audience (placement) and provide audience members with information about how, when, and where they can access campaign information and programs (promotion).

strategy: A general plan of action that may encompass several activities and that considers the characteristics of the target population.

supportive material: Tangible items needed to support the communication methods or messages by enhancing the message, improving its acceptance, strengthening its appeal, summarizing its main points, and complementing the message.

target audience: Distinct groups that are like each other in key ways and have a high likelihood of responding to a given message, service, or product in similar or predictable ways.

REFERENCES

1. Department of Health and Human Services. (1998). *Healthy People 2010 objectives: Draft for public comment.* Washington, DC: Office of Public Health and Science.

2. Kreps, G. L., Query, J. L., & Bonaguro, E. W. (2007). The interdisciplinary study of health communication and its relationship to communication science. In L. Lederman (Ed.), *Beyond these walls: Readings in health communication* (pp. 2–13). Los Angeles: Roxbury.

3. Maibach, E. W., Kreps, G. L., & Bonaguro, E. W. (1993). Developing strategic communication campaigns for HIV/AIDS prevention. In S. Ratzan (Ed.), *AIDS: Effective health communication for the 90s* (pp. 15–35). Washington, DC: Taylor and Francis.

4. Department of Health and Human Services. (2001). *Making health communication programs work: A planner's guide* (2nd ed.) (NIH Publication No. T-068). Washington, DC: Office of Cancer Communications, National Cancer Institute, National Institutes of Health.

5. Clift, E. C., & Freimuth, V. (1995). Health communication: What is it and what can it do for you? *Journal of Health Education, 26,* 68–74.

6. Rogers, E. M. (1996). The field of health communication today: An up-to-date report. *Journal of Health Communication, 1,* 15–23.

7. Kreps, G. L., Bonaguro, E. W., & Query, J. L. (1998). The history and development of the field of health communication. In L. D. Jackson & B. K. Duffy (Eds.), *Health communication research: A guide to developments and direction* (pp. 1–15). Westport, CT: Greenwood Press.

8. Kreps, G. L. (2002). Public health campaigns. In J. R. Schement (Ed.), *Encyclopedia of communication and information,* Vol. 3 (pp. 773–778). New York: Macmillan Reference.

9. Kreps, G. L. (2006). One size does not fit all: Adapting communication to the needs and literacy levels of individuals. *Annals of Family Medicine* (online, invited commentary). Available: http://www.annfammed.org/cgi/eletters/4/3/205.

10. U.S Department of Health and Human Services, Healthy People 2010. *Health communication (Chapter 11).* Available: http://www.healthypeople.gov/document/HTML/Volume1/11HealthCom.htm.

11. National Prevention Information Network, Centers for Disease Control and Prevention. (n.d.). *Campaigns and initiatives: Health communication strategies.* Available: http://www.cdcnpin.org/scripts/campaign/strategy.asp.

12. Maibach, E., & Holtgrave, D. R. (1995). Advances in public health communication. *Annual Review of Public Health, 16,* 219–238.

13. Ratzan, S. C. (1999). Strategic health communication and social marketing on risk issues. *Journal of Health Communication, 4,* 1–6.

14. Centers for Disease Control and Prevention. (1999). *CDCynergy* [CD-ROM]. Atlanta, GA: U.S. Department of Health and Human Services, Office of Communication, Office of the Director.

15. Centers for Disease Control and Prevention. (1999). *CDCynergy content and framework workbook*. Atlanta, GA: U.S. Department of Health and Human Services, Office of Communication, Office of the Director.

16. Roper, W. L. (1993). Health communication takes on new dimensions at CDC. *Public Health Reports, 108,* 179–183.

17. Center for Communication Programs. (1998). *Strategic communication: Making a difference*. Baltimore, MD: School of Hygiene and Public Health, Johns Hopkins University.

18. Lefebvre, C., & Flora, J. (1988). Social marketing and public health intervention. *Health Education Quarterly, 15,* 299–315.

19. Bandura, A. (1986). *Social foundations of thought and action: A social cognitive approach*. Englewood Cliffs, NJ: Prentice Hall.

20. Rogers, E. M. (1983). *Diffusion of innovations*. New York: Free Press.

21. Prochaska, J., & DiClemente, C. (1984). *The transtheoretical approach: Crossing traditional boundaries of therapy*. Homewood, IL: Dow Jones-Irwin.

22. Forthofer, M. S., & Bryant, C. A. (2000). Using audience-segmentation techniques to tailor health behavior change strategies. *American Journal of Health Behavior, 24,* 36–43.

23. Slater, M. D. (1996). Theory and method in health audience segmentation. *Journal of Health Communication, 1,* 267–284.

24. Slater, M. D., Kelly, K. J., & Thackeray, R. (2006). Segmentation on a shoestring: Health audience segmentation in limited-budget and local social marketing interventions. *Health Promotion Practice, 7,* 170–173.

25. Kotler, P., & Roberto, E. (1989). *Social marketing: Strategies for changing public behavior*. New York: Free Press.

26. Bryant, C. (1998, June). *Social marketing: A tool for excellence*. Paper presented at the eighth annual conference on social marketing in public health, Clearwater Beach, FL.

27. Neiger, B. L., Thackeray, R., Merrill, R. M., Miner, K. M., Larsen, L., & Chalkley, C. M. (2001). The impact of social marketing on fruit and vegetable consumption and physical activity among public health employees at the Utah Department of Health. *Social Marketing Quarterly, 7,* 9–28.

5

Social Marketing Concepts

Karen Denard Goldman, Ph.D., CHES

Author Comments

Years ago I attended a continuing education course on marketing, and my approach to health education forever changed. The use and promotion of social marketing has been an integral part of my career as a health education practitioner and college professor ever since.

Both health education and social marketing are about planning, implementing, and evaluating offerings to voluntarily change behavior. Social marketing principles and practices complement health education priorities and processes. Their interaction is synergistic.

The purpose of this chapter is to help students and practitioners begin to think like marketers. After defining social marketing and placing it in its historical context, the chapter outlines and highlights the differences and similarities between the health education and social marketing processes and then discusses key marketing concepts and their implications for practitioners. It presents predictable social marketing pitfalls, along with suggestions of how to avoid or overcome them. The chapter concludes with a discussion of realistic outcomes one can expect from social marketing efforts.

Introduction

Marketing. People in the health field seem to either like it or dislike it. People who dislike marketing claim that it wastes money, is intrusive, manipulates clients or patients, lowers the quality of care as a result of deceptive advertising or advertising by incompetent providers, forces health care facilities to compete, and creates an unnecessary demand for care. With equal passion, those who believe in the importance of marketing praise its ability to increase the satisfaction of the target audience, attract more marketing resources, and improve organizational efficiency. What is the difference between these two groups? Usually, it is the fact that those who like marketing understand what it *really* is. Those who dislike it tend to think "marketing" means "selling."

Regardless of one's views, there is a niche for marketing in health education. Marketing can be defined as the "analysis, planning, implementation, and control of carefully formulated programs based on consumer research designed to bring about voluntary exchanges of values with target markets for the purpose of achieving organizations' goals and objectives."[1] It can be said that when there is only a hammer, every problem is treated as if it were a nail. The wide variety of problems with which health practitioners are faced requires the use of an equally broad array of tools and techniques. Expanding the repertoire of problem-solving, intervention-designing, and program-planning strategies to include a marketing orientation, marketing concepts, and marketing tools can help health practitioners achieve their health education goals.

Marketing is a deliberately planned, orchestrated, and implemented *process* of mutually satisfying exchange facilitation. In product marketing, a company succeeds (makes money) by accurately identifying the needs and wants of target markets and offering products or services that satisfy those needs and wants more effectively and efficiently than competitors' offerings.[1] Marketing cannot be successful if potential consumers do not attach greater value to what a company has to offer than what they, the consumers, already have or do.

Marketing first became popular in the mid-1950s among consumer packaged-goods businesses, such as General Electric, Procter & Gamble, General Motors, and Coca-Cola. Its orientation toward satisfying consumers' needs differed from other commercial approaches that focused on getting a consumer's business either by offering low prices (made possible by low production costs), making the best possible product, or focusing on product promotion.[1]

Marketing's appeal and success spread from packaged-goods firms to companies producing durable goods (furniture, automobiles) for individual consumers and to industrial equipment companies. Soon after, service organizations, such as airlines, banks, insurance companies, stock brokerage firms, colleges and universities, and hospitals, were adopting a marketing approach—or at least claiming to adopt it. Next, business professionals, including lawyers, accountants, and physicians, became interested in marketing their services and professions. In time, more professions began applying marketing principles to their organizational development plans and program and service strategies. Eventually, marketing experts began to see the value of using commercial principles and strategies to address social issues.[2]

Social marketing, which differs from, yet is based on, marketing, is the "process for influencing human behavior on a large scale, using marketing principles for the purpose of societal benefit rather than commercial profit."[3] The key features of social marketing are taken directly from commercial marketing. *Social marketing* is a generic term: It is not specifically about using marketing techniques to change health behavior. For example, social marketing campaigns have been used to influence behaviors related to public transportation, solar energy, conservation, military recruitment, urban planning, voter registration, and adopting children, as well as health behaviors.[4]

Social marketing is *not* another term for media advocacy, health communication, social advertising campaigns, or social communication. *Media advocacy* is the strategic use of mass media to advance public policy by applying pressure to policy matters.[5] *Health communication* is the crafting and delivery of messages and strategies based on consumer research in order to promote the health of individuals and communities.[6] *Social advertising campaigns* are advertising tools that attempt to influence attitudes and behavior related to social causes without any tie-in with accessible, affordable products and services. The limitation of social advertising campaigns led to the evolution of *social communication*, which expands promotional efforts beyond the mass media approach and incorporates a network of appropriate people to assist in the "selling" of a particular cause. Thus, a social communication campaign for good nutrition could include the participation of local hospital and spiritual healers. In order for the message to take hold, however, and to actually influence behavior change, additional programmatic elements must be added—elements that add up to social marketing.

Over the past 30 years, social marketing has been used successfully to increase health care and health education program use, improve client satisfaction, and achieve social and individual health behavior change. It has been effective in increasing contraceptive use, reducing blood pressure, increasing consumption of fruits and vegetables, and increasing public awareness of the association between certain risk factors and particular health conditions.[7–9] Three notable long-term social marketing successes based in the United States are the National High Blood Pressure Education Program, the Pawtucket Heart Health Program, and the Stanford Five-City Project Smokers' Challenge. Another example of a social marketing program is the Washington Heights low-fat milk campaign in New York City.[10]

This chapter is not designed to address the social marketing process; the scope of the marketing process merits a book itself. Rather, it introduces the social marketing process, emphasizing concepts associated with a social marketing approach.

The Social Marketing Process: An Overview

The social marketing process is a program-planning process with some major similarities and differences when compared with traditional health education program-planning models. Though the jargon is different, the planning processes of health education and social marketing are similar. Both include assessing potential consumers and the intervening organization(s); setting clear goals and objectives; and planning, implementing, evaluating, and modifying offerings. Key differences are that marketers routinely segment the market of potential customers into smaller groups based on key buying characteristics; analyze market segments in terms of values, motivations, attitudes, opinions, media habits, preferred information channels, and, most especially, benefits sought; consider the competition; develop separate offerings for each market segment; develop a personality for each offering to distinguish it from the competition; design each offering with equal attention to product design, price, distribution outlets, and promotion; formally pretest each offering; and conduct a wide range of research activities, such as advertising research, business economics and corporate research, corporate responsibility research, product research, and sales and market research.

Because success in marketing depends on achieving desired exchanges by satisfying the needs and wants of members of target populations, the majority of steps in the marketing process are research related. The first step is to identify the problem. When there is a difference between the ideal or desired state and the actual state of a situation or circumstance, a problem exists or is perceived to exist. There is no foundation for a marketing plan without a problem. Problems are identified through observation, interviews, and surveys of target population members, other people or organizations providing similar or competitive services or unhealthy behavior, and topical experts. Second, an overall, general goal is set. Third, a market analysis is conducted. A market analysis is the process of identifying and evaluating a potential market—people with an immediate or potential interest in seeking a solution to the problem at hand.

At this point, market segmentation occurs. Market segmentation is the process of dividing a heterogeneous market into homogeneous target groups by demographic, psychographic (e.g., attitudes, interests, values, lifestyles, and opinions), or behavioristic variables (e.g., benefits sought, user status, use rate, loyalty status, and readiness to change). Once the market is subdivided into homogeneous segments based on the most appropriate variable, the next step, a consumer analysis, is implemented. In a consumer analysis, each of the segments to be pursued is studied thoroughly in terms of knowledge, attitudes, skills, referent group relationships, media preferences, and related behaviors. The goal is to know potential audiences so well that services, products, and programs are developed, priced, promoted, and distributed in ways specifically designed to meet their preferences.

Influence channel analysis is then done to determine the most effective way to make services, products, and programs accessible to a target population. People are influenced in many different ways (e.g., by what they read, with whom they speak regularly, by role models, by films they see). The channels themselves vary according to the particular issue, service, or physical product being offered. The challenge is to identify all the channels of influence that are relevant, analyze them to determine their relative degree of influence, and then coordinate outreach efforts that use the most appropriate channels.

The goal of all up-front research is for health educators to know and understand members of each key market segment so well that they are able, in the next phase, to develop a marketing mix for each key market segment that meets or satisfies their needs. Marketing mix development is basically a two-step process of initial design and test marketing. To make certain that the marketing mix is appropriate, a pilot test or test marketing is essential. Though time-consuming, sometimes expensive, and often perceived as impractical, pilot testing reduces the risk of product failure, corporate embarrassment, and financial loss if any of the marketing mix components are off-target. The resulting tailor-made product, program, or service should, if based on accurate information, sell itself. The final steps in the marketing process are generic to all good program planning: program (marketing mix) implementation, evaluation, and modification.

Table 5-1 is a condensed step-by-step outline of the social marketing process with an emphasis on the up-front research steps.[9] Key marketing concepts fundamental to both a general marketing approach and the specific marketing process are discussed in the next section.

Marketing Concepts

A thorough understanding of how social marketing can be used requires an understanding of how traditional marketing concepts such as consumer orientation, exchange, market segmentation and consumer analysis, demand, competition, marketing mix, positioning, consumer satisfaction, and brand loyalty can be applied to health-related issues.

Consumer Orientation

To be a consumer-driven health educator, one must adopt a mindset of "the customer is king." **Consumer orientation** is the basic concept that an organization's mission is to bring about behavior change by meeting the target market's needs and wants. It is recognizing that customers have unique perceptions, needs, and wants that the marketer must learn about and adapt to. It means conducting

Table 5-1   Social Marketing Process

I. Plan

  1. Analyze the problem and situation

    a. Problem to be addressed

- What aspects of the problem will be addressed?
- What is the epidemiology of the problem at the individual, group, organizational, community, and policy levels?
- Which of these risk factors are important and changeable?
- Which of these can be addressed, and how can the problem be prevented from occurring or spreading?
- What are the consequences of the problem?
- What has been done in the past? How well has that worked?

    b. The environment in which the program will be implemented

- Social, economic, or demographic factors at work in the community
- Political climate in relation to this problem
- Current policies or pending legislation that might affect the target audience's response
- Other organizations' activities regarding this issue
- Competition for this audience's attention
- Outlets or channels for services, messages, and products

    c. Resources available

- Budget
- Staff and consultants: numbers and skills
- Time
- Equipment
- Facilities
- Access

  2. Segment the target audience

    a. Define segments

- Primary audiences: The people whose behavior is to be changed
- Secondary audiences: Groups that influence the behavior of intended audiences

    b. Research the segments

  3. Develop strategy

    a. Set goals and objectives

    b. Allocate resources

II. Develop a Preliminary Social Marketing Mix for a Particular Market Segment

  Address all Ps: product, price, place, promotion

III. Pretest the Marketing Mix

  1. Conduct the pretest

Table 5-1	Social Marketing Process (Continued)

2. Analyze results

3. Modify marketing mix based on pretest results.

IV. Implement the Marketing Mix

  1. Develop an implementation plan with tasks, time frames, and people responsible

  2. Monitor implementation

V. Evaluate

  1. Identify evaluation measures and all possible indicators: satisfaction; loyalty; demand levels; organizational or institutional resources, conditions, facilities, and policies; community changes; and policy and regulation changes

  2. Plan evaluation

  3. Implement evaluation

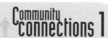

Community connections 1

Harold, a health educator working at a local health department, was asked to design a childhood lead poisoning prevention program. An effective health educator, Harold has always been sensitive to the needs and interests of many stakeholders: his supervisors, staff, the agency, program funders, community members, local political leaders, and other actual and potential supporters. Thinking like a marketer, Harold realized he must also approach his latest challenge from the perspective of his potential clients. He realized that in order to design a program that would help reduce lead poisoning among children in the community, he needed to know all he could about the people whose behavior he would be trying to change. He realized that before he could jump in and announce any initiatives, he needed to see his clients as consumers whose wants and needs his offerings would have to satisfy if he wanted to be successful.

consumer research, because the most important activity in marketing-oriented health education is learning as much as possible about the people whose behavior is to be influenced. It means recognizing that consumers have their choice among competing ideas, services, and products and, for whatever reasons, are more satisfied by the current offering. It means believing that the organization most knowledgeable about and responsive to consumer needs will "win."

Exchange

The objective of the commercial marketing specialist is to facilitate mutually satisfying **exchanges** between consumers and companies. The consumer receives a product or service he or she values, and the company makes money.

Exchange theory, the linchpin of the marketing approach, indicates that by using the right promotion techniques to offer the right product at the right price, through the right distribution channels, potential buyers will exchange or give up what they currently have, use, or believe for what is offered. If a more desirable alternative is not offered, there will be no exchange.

The essence of marketing-oriented health education is thinking, "For my target population, how can I facilitate a voluntary exchange of what they are currently doing for the behavior I have in mind that will leave us both satisfied?" The difference between commercial and social marketing is that in social marketing, the marketer's objective for exchange is behavior change, whereas in commercial marketing the objective is financial profit.

Community connections 2

While thinking about devising a home-cleaning campaign to reduce lead poisoning, Harold asked himself, "What benefits can I build into my program that my clients would value and be willing and able to pay for in terms of their time, energy, and money? If I want parents to clean their homes more thoroughly to reduce their children's exposure to lead, what kind of a clean-up system are they actually able and willing to engage in that will reduce their children's exposure?" In thinking about his parental population, Harold realized these parents were young, juggling childrearing and a job. They did not have much time and money to invest in the cleaning process. Given who they were, Harold contemplated what would be the least time-consuming cleanup he could ask them to do that would reduce their children's exposure to lead. Harold's question became "What can I ask them to do that they can and will do?"

Market Segmentation and Consumer Analysis

Because no single offering will please everyone, offerings are designed for and promoted to subgroups of the universe of all the people to be reached (the market). These subgroups, or market segments, are composed of members of the population united by a distinctive feature—a feature that becomes the focus of the marketing plan. For example, the market for smoking cessation offerings might be segmented by (1) a demographic characteristic (age, gender, education level, occupation, ethnicity, or religion), (2) a behavior (experimenting with smoking, social smoking only, smoking one pack a day every day), (3) an attitude ("my health is my business," "I wouldn't do anything to hurt anyone else," "I need to set a good example for my children"), (4) an opinion (smoking is not harmful, smoking can be harmful in some ways, smoking kills), or (5) a value (family, excitement, professional development, control, independence, looking good). In comparison, the market for weight-reduction programs might be segmented by possible perceived benefits sought by different market segments, such as sex appeal, fitness level, pleasure, image, or social connection.

A more complex, research-based attribute by which to segment a market is lifestyle. For example, the public relations firm Porter/Novelli identified seven health styles of target markets: decent dolittles (24%), active attractives (13%), hard-living hedonists (6%), tense but trying (10%), noninterested nihilists (7%), physical fanatics (24%), and passively healthy (15%).[9] The study of the market-at-large provides a framework for categorizing potential clients into groups based on key characteristics that then become the driving force behind the development of marketing mixes.

Market research techniques include interviews with intended audience representatives and experts (e.g., one-on-one interviews, meetings, panels, brainstorming, community forums, nominal group process, and focus groups), telephone surveys, mailed surveys and questionnaires, literature reviews, report reviews, and observations.

Community connections 3

Harold knew he did not have much money to work with but needed to find a way to divide his potential clients into categories based on some key defining characteristics. Based on his past experiences, he knew there were at least two types of families in his community—those with roots in the community and those who had recently moved in or were temporary residents. He knew that he would need to modify his initiatives based on whether they were designed for people who were long-term members of the community with roots, connections, and ties to local community organizations, or if they were for people with less community connection. Harold planned to use what he learned about these two different groups to design different interventions for each. He knew that each group would respond best to the strategy designed specifically for it.

Demand

Though the goal of marketing is to facilitate exchanges through the satisfaction of client needs, the frequency with which these exchanges or transactions occur varies depending on the market segment. In short, **demand** for services varies; everyone in a given market does not desire a particular service, program, or product all the time and at the same level. It would be ideal to have full demand for one's products, meaning that an organization or company has precisely the amount of business it wants. However, because demands are human needs shaped by culture and personality and backed by purchasing power, they vary.

Community connections 4

In considering how to design his different interventions for the different market segments, Harold realized that for each of the market segments he identified, he was going to have to determine the level of demand for a home-cleaning program. When he discovered that parents were interested in cleaning, but more so in the winter when the children were in the house, he used his knowledge of irregular demand to change what he asked parents to do at different times of the year. In the winter, he would stress cleaning, and in the summer he would stress other activities, like running the water before using it for drinking, cooking, or washing children's hands.

There are eight demand states, or levels, that health educators as marketers need to know about, recognize, and respond to in order to be effective.

- *Negative demand* exists when a large segment of a market dislikes a product and would even pay to avoid it. A marketer needs to find out the reasons for the resistance and plan strategies to counteract resistance.

- *No demand* occurs when customers are unmotivated by or are indifferent to a product. The marketer's job is to connect potential product benefits with the needs and interests of prospective customers.

- *Latent demand* exists when customers cannot find an existing product that meets a need they want satisfied. Marketers need to find out just how large the unsatisfied market is and decide if it is enough to warrant developing new products.

- *Falling demand* reflects a significant drop in the level of demand for a product. The job of the marketer in this case is to identify the causes for the dropoff and plan strategies to reverse the trend.

- *Irregular demand* is characterized by fluctuation in the use of a product based on the season, the day of the week, or even the time of day. The marketer can increase demand during those seasons, days, or times of day by modifying the price, distribution, promotion, and features of the product.

- *Full demand* exists when a company has all the business it needs. The marketer must then focus on the competition and possible changes in customer needs to make sure demand does not drop.

- *Overall demand* exists when the demand is higher than the organization can or wants to handle. The marketer is in the position of needing to raise prices, change product features, decrease access to the product, or cut back on promotion activities to reduce the demand level.

- *Unwholesome demand* for dangerous or harmful products distributed by competitors requires marketers in other companies to come up with price, product, distribution, and promotion strategies to persuade people to give up those products.

Competition

No matter what the topic or who is in the market segment, competition must be expected and dealt with. **Competition** is any alternative to an offering. Sometimes it is the same program or product offered by someone else (but who, perhaps, has more credibility), such as two smoking cessation patches offered by two different companies or agencies. Sometimes it is another (somehow more appealing) version of what is being offered—a prettier patch, a shorter series of cessation classes, or a more user-friendly self-help book. Often it is a different and more appealing way of achieving the same benefits sought—a smoking cessation gum versus a patch. And sometimes, it is something more compelling the consumer wants to accomplish before engaging in an activity, such as losing 20 pounds before trying to quit smoking.

Community Connections 5

Harold's marketing knowledge triggered a key question when he realized that parents were not cleaning even in the winter months as often as or in the way he had taught them. "What," he asked himself, "are people doing instead of what I want them to do? What are they doing besides cleaning? Why are they doing that instead of cleaning? And, if they are cleaning, what is the other method, which is less effective than what I taught, that they persist in using and why?" In essence, Harold was asking himself the all-important question, "What is the competition?"

His next step was to find out what people were doing instead of cleaning and why. His staff interviewed parents, who freely shared information. He found out that some parents did not have the right soap or the mops and buckets needed to clean as thoroughly as needed. Harold started providing that equipment as part of his program. For others who claimed they did not have the time for certain strategies, Harold devised cleaning shortcuts or offered exposure-control alternatives so that lead source areas were covered, thus reducing the need to clean. In some cases, he found that the competition was the landlord, who was threatening to evict tenants who complained about lead exposure. Harold suggested that the parents work through community organizations rather than directly with their landlords to bring pressure to bear and, in the meantime, to focus on careful cleaning and other strategies within their control.

The Marketing Mix

A **marketing mix** is a combination of factors put together, based on an understanding of the wants and needs of the target market segment, to make the target market segment want to exchange what they currently do or believe for the product, service, or idea being offered.

A marketing mix can have anywhere from four to eight components. Traditionally, a commercial marketing mix is described as having four components, commonly known as the four Ps of marketing. The four Ps are interdependent and fundamental to a marketing approach; they are the four dimensions of the offering that influence clients' decisions about whether to make an exchange. For further input on utilizing the four Ps, see Table 5-2.

- *Product.* The product is a physical good, service, or idea that satisfies a need. *Physical goods* are tangible bundles of attributes that can be offered to a market segment for attention, acquisition, use, or consumption in order to satisfy a want or need. A *service* is a largely intangible activity or benefit one party can offer to another to meet certain needs and wants. Its production and delivery may or may not be tied to a physical product. An *idea* is a more abstract bundle of attributes that satisfies certain needs and wants or solves problems.

  Ideally, every offering should have three dimensions: (1) a core product that has a value-satisfying component (e.g., getting a blood test for lead poisoning for a 2-year-old child should give parents peace of mind or equal opportunity for their child, who may now escape a major handicap), (2) tangibles (e.g., physical components of the blood-lead test that clients can see, such as a kind person drawing blood, clean equipment, and attractive bandages to place on the child's arm), and (3) added-value components, which are extras that clients receive after the exchange has been made to reinforce their adoption or purchase decisions (e.g., making certain that mothers whose children have had blood-lead tests are fast-tracked to a service they value or get a discount on another product or service).

- *Price.* The price is a financial, temporal, emotional, or energy cost the population can pay. Ideally, an offering should not take any more time, money, energy, or emotion than clients are willing to exchange. Marketers should anticipate and eliminate or reduce these cost barriers. An example is clients who are interested in obtaining prenatal care but are faced with barriers, such as the cost of transportation, babysitters, or the prenatal care service; the emotional cost of asking for a day off from work; the emotional cost of undressing before a care provider and answering personal questions; the time cost of taking an afternoon or day off from work; the energy cost involved in making the appointment, arranging to get to the provider, waiting to see the provider, and worrying about what will be learned from the provider; and the price of taking the risk of giving up the "bliss" of ignorance about pregnancy health care

Table 5-2	**Thinking Like a Marketer**

Product

What is the *core* product?

- What benefit valued by clients should be offered (e.g., hope, more time with family, equal opportunity, peace of mind)?

What is the *tangible* product?

- How is the offering packaged?
- What are the offering's features?
- What kind of style does the offering have?
- What is the quality level of the offering?
- What is the brand name (i.e., symbol, sign, or word that identifies the offering of one seller and differentiates it from those of competitors)?

What is the *augmented* product?

- How can value be added to the offering (e.g., services, purchase options)?
- What else do clients receive after they buy the product or use the service?

Price

What does it cost someone in the market segment in terms of money, time, energy, or emotions to adopt, use, or buy the offering?

Place

Where is the offering currently available?

Is there any stigma, in the eyes of the target population, in going to that place?

Is there any reason they would be hesitant to go to that place?

Are there places the people in the target group cannot or will not go to for the offering?

Where do these people go on a regular basis that has positive connotations?

Are these places where the offering can occur, no matter how untraditional it is?

Promotion Mix

What percentage of the promotion mix is devoted to the following items?

- *Advertising.* A paid form of nonpersonal communication about an organization and its products that is transmitted to a target audience through a mass medium
- *Personal selling.* A process of informing customers and persuading them to purchase products through personal communication in an exchange situation
- *Publicity.* Nonpersonal communication regarding an organization and its products that is transmitted through a mass medium in news story form at no charge
- *Sales promotion.* An activity or material that acts as a direct inducement, offering added value or incentive for the offering to resellers, salespersons, or consumers

Next Steps

Have all four Ps been addressed?

What gaps exist?

What might be done to complete the mix?

issues. These costs are often far more than a client is willing to pay to do something for which, in the client's eyes, there is no tangible benefit.

- *Place.* Place in the marketing mix consists of convenient distribution or outlet channels for getting a physical offering, service, or idea to consumers. Offerings should be available through places that are convenient, comfortable, credible, and prepared to properly respond to clients. A setting that is dirty, in an unfamiliar neighborhood, hard to reach, staffed with untrained or culturally insensitive personnel, not set up properly for the services, or located too close to home for comfort among the people to be reached will jeopardize the exchange.

- *Promotion.* Promotion involves a product promotion campaign appropriate for the market segment. A promotion mix usually includes advertising, incentives, face-to-face selling, and public relations. The ideal is to develop a promotion mix that uses the media, spokespersons, incentives, language, and tone best suited to appeal to the market segment.

Social marketing experts have expanded the four core commercial components of the marketing mix to address the social and usually nonprofit part of social marketing. Additional components include publics, partnership, policy, and purse strings. *Publics* are the primary and secondary external and internal stakeholders in the program that must be considered throughout the planning process. *Partnership* refers to the importance of teaming up with other organizations to deal with problems so complex that no single organization could hope to solve them alone. *Policy* refers to the need to address environmental and contextual changes, such as laws and public policies, that have to be made to support behavior change. *Purse strings* are the variety of funding sources (e.g., foundations, government, private donors) needed to support social marketing efforts.[9]

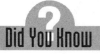

Did You Know

Positioning

Positioning is about creating a personality for an offering based on its key attributes. A well-positioned offering holds a unique place, or niche, in the consumer's mind. For example, imagine a consumer considering the purchase of an over-the-counter medication. One medication is designed to be and is promoted as "strong on pain, but soft on your stomach." This product was created for people who want something that fixes the problem but does not cause uncomfortable gastric side effects. It differs from a second medication for the same purpose that was designed for people who need to know their medication is actively working on their problem. Each medication has a different personality and was designed to meet the needs of consumers with different needs.

Another example of positioning is the long product line of different types of toothpastes. Different market segments want different benefits from their toothpaste. For example, there are toothpastes for people who want brighter, whiter smiles; toothpastes for people who want to prevent cavities; toothpastes that taste like candy and sparkle or are multicolored to entice children who otherwise would not brush; and toothpastes made without additives for people who prefer all-natural products. Each is a different product with a different personality, is sold in different ways (e.g., stores, catalogues, Web sites, warehouses or discount stores, elite boutiques) and at different prices, and has different promotion campaigns.

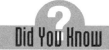

Did You Know

The United States hosts two annual social marketing conferences: Innovations in Social Marketing, held in Washington, DC (www.social-marketing.org); and Social Marketing in Public Health (dstewart@hsc.usf.edu or www.hsc.usf.edu/publichealth/conted/).

Consumer Satisfaction

The goal of marketing is **consumer satisfaction**—giving people what they expect, or more than they expected. Some dissatisfied customers will do nothing about being dissatisfied, but a marketer should not count on it. Research has shown that a satisfied customer will tell 3 people of his or her positive

Community connections 7

Harold discovered that when it came to reducing children's exposure to lead in the home, parents in one market segment wanted a strategy that would not take much time and was not unnecessarily burdensome (e.g., involving a lot of equipment and using products that had strong odors). He realized he might get more people to adopt cleaning if he dropped his earlier push for the use of a special HEPA vacuum cleaner and focused on damp mopping. When that still did not work in a few cases, he realized he was going to have to sit down and devise an approach with those clients' input, to determine what they would be willing and able to do. He had to change the product, rather than hammer away at new promotion strategies for an unsatisfying product.

experience, while a dissatisfied customer will tell 11.[1] A full range of actions and reactions by dissatisfied customers are possible: Some will seek redress directly from whoever offered the product or service, including taking legal action to obtain redress, complaining, deciding to stop buying the product or brand or to boycott the seller, and warning friends about the product or the seller.

The more tangible the offering, the easier it is to satisfy a customer. For example, clients who purchase toothbrushes are more easily satisfied than clients receiving routine dental checkups and cleanings. Those who are being educated about the importance of dental cavity prevention and early detection are even harder to satisfy. The reason for this is that physical goods are more tangible than services, and services are less vague than ideas. One can examine a bottle of mouthwash, a toothbrush, or alternative cleaning tools. They can be picked up, tried out, and, if bought (e.g., an electric toothbrush or pick), can be returned if they do not work properly or if one is dissatisfied with how they handle. Services, on the other hand, are far less tangible. A dental cleaning cannot be "handled," and dental hygienists cannot be tested out in advance. The quality of physical offerings can be counted on because they may have to meet legal standards, be inspected, and the like. If one brand of toothbrush is bought, the odds are that the next purchase of that brand will be very similar, if not identical. A dental cleaning, however, is much harder to control. It is experiential, and experiences can vary dramatically depending on factors that customers cannot control, such as their own mood; the functioning, features, and arrangements of the machinery involved; the music being piped into the room; the chair; the lighting; the mood, training, and experience of the hygienist; the receptionist's attitude; and the day of the week.

Community connections 8

Harold knew people would be satisfied with their home-cleaning experience if it met their expectations. Therefore, Harold's job was to control client expectations by giving them information about home cleaning that would lead to realistic expectations and a reduced sense of risk and uncertainty. He then must make sure that the home-cleaning solution—the method and the people who taught it—met client expectations. Harold focused on the tangible aspects of the cleaning services he would offer, including an initial house cleaning and a demonstration of routine (twice a week) cleaning and exposure control (damp mopping and dusting). He put time and energy into allaying client anxieties by providing testimonials about the service from past users. He prepared the client for the service by thoroughly describing it, and developed a mechanism for client feedback. He informed his staff to observe clients' reactions, and empowered them to do all they could within the guidelines of the agency to satisfy the customer. Before launching the cleaning services, Harold double-checked to make sure his services, procedures, and materials were user friendly. He knew how important it was to try to see everything his agency offered through his clients' eyes. He learned a key marketing principle: The more he anticipated and satisfied clients' needs, the more loyal they would become.

Brand Loyalty

A brand is a name, term, sign, symbol, design, or combination of these intended to differentiate products of one company from competitors' products. **Brand loyalty**, a consistent preference for and choice of one particular company's product or service, develops among customers over time as a result of consistently satisfactory experiences with a particular company and its products. Every time consumers consider a purchase, they have the opportunity to weigh the advantages and disadvantages of thousands of brands of products. Though many are willing and eager to try out new products, most appreciate being able to rely on a product that has "proven itself satisfactory" and can be readily identified. Many get psychological satisfaction from knowing they are using well-known branded products. Brand names can help stimulate demand, provide protection against substitution, give the brander a chance to identify a market segment of loyal consumers, and make it easier to introduce new products.

Did You Know

The term *social marketing* was first introduced in 1971 to describe the use of marketing principles and techniques to advance a social cause, idea, or behavior.

Source: Kotler, P., & Zaltman, G. (1971). Social marketing: An approach to planned social change. *Journal of Marketing, 35*, 3–12.

There are three levels of brand familiarity. *Brand recognition* occurs when a customer remembers having seen or heard of the brand. *Brand preference* is when customers choose a brand out of habit or past experience, but will accept a substitute if the preferred brand is not readily available. When customers would rather fight than switch to another brand and go out of their way to search for it, marketers have achieved the highest level of brand familiarity: *brand insistence*.

Community connections 9

As a marketer, Harold knew that he could foster loyalty to his agency by satisfying his customers and by reducing any sense of risk they might experience related to his agency's programs, services, or messages. If, for example, he was able to cultivate a positive feeling toward his agency as a result of his consumer-friendly approach to making clients' homes lead safe, if not actually lead free, then those same customers, when faced with a different health problem, were likely to either come to him or his agency for help or to respond well to his agency's offer to help. Because his agency at this point had not earned the loyalty of the clients he needed to reach regarding childhood lead poisoning, Harold considered partnering with an agency that had a very loyal following of clients who would be more inclined to adopt its lead poisoning prevention program than the program offered by Harold's agency.

Overcoming Challenges to Social Marketing

Although there are many positive rewards to the social marketing process, it is not without its challenges. Possible challenges to effective social marketing include limiting its scope to program or product promotion, attempting full-scale social marketing versus a step-by-step implementation process, failing to evaluate the social marketing effort or campaign, and encountering problems associated with marketing functions.

Do Not Limit the Marketing Process

Marketing is frequently misinterpreted as the effective use of communication strategies to successfully influence or change attitudes and behavior. Much of today's talk about marketing health care programs and services, marketing patient compliance strategies, marketing physicians, or, most recently, marketing health messages reveals a misguided common tendency among health professionals to use the word *marketing* to mean "using persuasive communication strategies." For example, people often say they are "marketing programs and services" when they mean they are "trying to get people to come participate in programs and use agency services." Service marketing programs frequently only address promotional strategies to generate and maintain service participants. "Marketing health education" is often someone's well-intentioned shorthand for getting good media placements for public service announcements.

The effective use of communication strategies to successfully influence or change attitudes and behavior is only one aspect of marketing. Communication strategies, usually promotion or advertising, are substituted frequently for the word *marketing*. The fact is, advertising is one of *many* kinds of communication or promotion strategies, and communication or promotion, in turn, constitutes only one of about a dozen fundamental concepts of marketing and only one component of a marketing mix. This basic misperception of marketing may contribute to both skepticism about the value of marketing in health education and to health educator resistance to adopting a marketing approach.

Take a Step-by-Step Approach

There is no law that says everything has to be done the marketing way or not at all. The fun of adopting a new perspective like marketing is that one can begin by integrating a few of the ideas discussed here over time. Alan Andreasen suggests ten steps for integrating a marketing approach into an organization:[7]

1. *Know oneself.* Recognize that not every individual has a marketing orientation.

2. *Start at the top.* Discuss marketing with the power brokers in the organization and get their support.

3. *Start doing research.* Learn all that is possible about current and prospective clients and competitors.

4. *Rub shoulders with real marketers.* Attend marketing conferences or enter into partnerships with qualified marketing firms and spend time with their marketing staff.

5. *Hire marketing specialists.* Do not limit staff to topic specialists (e.g., experts on child health, injury prevention, heart disease, or tuberculosis). If marketing expertise is needed, hire a marketer.

6. *Reward risk-taking and experimentation.* Support staff and volunteers who are willing to try something new. Remember, one definition of insanity is "continuing to do things the same old way and expecting them to turn out differently."

7. *Look for consumer barriers to dismantle.* Expect resistance. Address the client's perceived product, price, place, or promotion barriers—not necessarily barriers that are anticipated.

8. *Continually reassess all four Ps.* When in doubt, check out the product, price, place, and promotion aspects of an offering.

9. *Conduct routine "marketing audits" of the agency's philosophy and practice.* With time, one will ask, "If this is not working, what is it about the client that was not known or that was ignored and now needs to be addressed?"

10. *Go about tasks in a different way.* Take a chance. Commit to trying one or two marketing techniques and watching the results. The most important concept is being client or consumer centered, that is, designing offerings that address client values, needs, wants, and perceptions.

Devise an Evaluation Plan

Even with consumer research and market testing of appropriate marketing mixes, it is still very difficult to evaluate social marketing programs. In a classic paper written to explore reasons for the lack of evaluation activity in social marketing, Paul Bloom reviewed the problems confronting the evaluator:

> The most fundamental, overriding problem facing the evaluator of a social marketing program is that evaluations tend to be expensive, bothersome, risky (i.e., budgets can be cut if results are poor), and capable of detecting only weak program effects. This makes it difficult to obtain cooperation and support for evaluations from program administrators. . . . Even if cooperation and support are available from program administrators, problems can arise in developing measures of effectiveness and choosing a research design.[11]

As in health education, social marketing evaluations are based on program goals and objectives. In the case of social marketing program evaluation, the evaluator must be clear about whether the program was designed to effect cognitive change, action change, behavioral change, or value change—each of which is increasingly difficult to perform and to evaluate. Constructs and variables must be identified and monitored throughout program execution to see if the objectives are being met. Pencil-and-paper scales, interview questions, and record-keeping systems need to be developed that reflect operational definitions of those constructs and are valid, reliable, and relatively easy to implement. One must also, as in any good research project, be on the lookout for any secondary effects that may need to be analyzed.

Overcome Social Marketing Concerns

Besides evaluation, social marketers should expect other frustrations that are specific to particular marketing functions and that commercial marketers do not face.[12]

- *Market analysis problems.* Social marketers have less secondary data available about their customers and have more difficulty obtaining valid, reliable measures of salient variables; sorting out the relative influence of identified determinants of consumer behavior; and getting consumer research studies funded, approved, and completed in a timely fashion.

- *Market segmentation problems.* Social marketers face pressure against segmentation, in general, and especially against segmentation that leads to the ignoring of certain segments. They frequently do not have accurate behavioral data to use in identifying segments, and their target segments must often consist of those consumers who are most negatively predisposed to their offerings.

- *Product strategy problems.* Social marketers tend to have less flexibility in shaping their products or offerings, more difficulty formulating product concepts, and more difficulty selecting and implementing long-term positioning strategies.

- *Pricing strategy problems.* Social marketers find that the development of a pricing strategy primarily involves trying to reduce the monetary, psychic, energy, and time cost incurred by consumers when engaging in a desired social behavior. They have difficulties measuring their prices, and they tend to have less control over consumer costs.

- *Channel strategy problems.* Social marketers have more difficulty utilizing and controlling desired intermediaries.

- *Communications strategy problems.* Social marketers usually find paid advertising difficult to use. They often face pressure not to use certain types of appeals in their messages, they usually must communicate relatively large amounts of information in their messages, and they have difficulty conducting meaningful pretests of messages.

- *Organizational design and planning problems.* Social marketers must function in organizations in which marketing activities are poorly understood, weakly appreciated, and inappropriately located; they must function in organizations in which plans (if any are developed) are treated as archival rather than action documents; they must function in organizations that suffer from institutional amnesia; and they must predict how both friendly and unfriendly competitors will behave.

- *Evaluation problems.* Social marketers frequently face difficulties trying to define effectiveness measures, and they often find it difficult to estimate the contribution their marketing program has made toward the achievement of certain objectives.

Expected Outcomes

The positive outcomes that can be expected from social marketing are many and encouraging. The social marketing process is very similar to health education program planning, and so health educators can expect to feel very comfortable while integrating new tools into a largely familiar process. As in the health education program planning process, health educators should expect to spend most of the time on up-front research. In addition, as the result of intensified research efforts, health educators can expect greater and stronger ties to and understanding of the communities and populations that become target market segments. The extensive research effort will result in fewer but more tailored interventions. One will no longer be looking for the "magic bullet" program that solves everyone's problems with a single event or service.

Creating more tailored interventions also means creating more interventions to be tailored. As practitioners become more involved in social marketing, they can expect to see their organizations develop a veritable product line of programs, services, products, and messages (like commercial campaigns) for particular audiences. Does a clothing company sell one type of outfit at one price to one age group at one store? Of course not. In addition to their premier clothes line, they have a division that offers "teen clothes" to teens in teen-friendlier settings and through catalogues. Can the same be said of our smoking cessation efforts? A social marketing approach results in a wide variety of smoking cessation products for seniors, newly diagnosed patients who need to quit, teens, pregnant women or women expecting to become pregnant, husbands of pregnant women, health professionals, and employees in high-pressure jobs. Offerings may take the form of gums, patches, self-help books, audiotapes, videotapes, compact disc and e-learning programs, regularly scheduled classes, support or maintenance groups, quitting supplies, and kits. Yes, it will take longer to get the interventions up and going. They will be more effective, however, because products will match market segments' personal needs, support their values, have the attributes and benefits they want, and include behavior changes they are willing and able to make.

An extended product line may well lead to extended partnerships and a more diverse and part-time staff. No one organization can provide all the products and services needed by all the possible market segments. Forming alliances among service providers is a practical step that benefits the consumers and all organizations involved. For example, lung associations, cancer societies, and heart associations work closely together to provide a full range of services that none could provide alone. One may want to evaluate staff and consider their responsibilities and how to recruit consultants or part-time workers who are similar to target markets to increase the authenticity of the research and marketing mix design.

The research that leads to more tailored interventions should also lead to more rapid behavior change. If health educators design offerings of appropriate services, products, or new behaviors at a cost the market segment can afford; make these offerings accessible through convenient, familiar channels; and create awareness of the offerings through messages and media that resonate with the market segment, clients can be expected to more quickly make the desired change.

Having tailored interventions will mean spending less money on service or program promotion activities. The up-front research will obviate the need to mobilize any massive promotion campaigns. Instead, efforts only need to be expended to make the target market segment aware of a product or service and to demonstrate how what they want has been incorporated.

Finally, because salespeople or selling strategies will not be relied upon, staff will be available to spend more time monitoring the implementation of and response to programs and services while evaluating impact. More client feedback can be expected because clients will realize it is wanted and utilized. This will ultimately lead to higher levels of consumer involvement within targeted market segments and to greater commitment to programs and services (i.e., customer satisfaction and loyalty).

Conclusion

"Marketing is a social and managerial process by which individuals and groups obtain what they need and want through creating and exchanging products and value with others."[1] In health terms, marketing is the process of planning and carrying out the development, pricing, promotion, and distribution of offerings. Social marketing is the application of commercial marketing principles to social issues. Social marketing offerings may be health related and can be physical goods such as nutritious lunches, services such as stress management workshops, or ideas and concepts such as encouraging safer sex or preventing heart disease.

Marketing is much more than promotion. Marketing is a process that involves planning, implementing, and managing the design, price, place, and promotion of offerings to satisfy the needs of clients and meet organizational goals. It is also a program-planning tool that can enhance offerings and increase the likelihood of their success. It can be used with other planning models.

Marketing is not a panacea. No one method is a magic bullet. Marketing's principles and practices, however, offer new ways to look at new and old problems—they trigger creativity. Social marketing efforts will be more successful if one partners with the marketing departments of colleges and universities and with real marketing firms (not just advertising agencies). When possible, hire professional marketers as staff or consultants, or recruit marketers to the board.

Lastly, when in doubt about what to do about a health challenge, or when wondering why what one is doing is not working, look at the offering from the client's perspective. The answer is usually in one or more of the four Ps: product, price, place, and promotion.

KEY TERMS

brand loyalty: A consistent preference for and choice of one particular company's product or service.

competition: Alternatives to an offering.

consumer orientation: Focusing on the needs and wants of consumers.

consumer satisfaction: The extent to which consumers' expectations of a product, service, or idea are met.

demand: The degree to which a transaction is wanted.

exchange: The process of consumers giving up what they currently have, use, or believe for what is being offered.

marketing mix: A combination of factors (product, price, promotion, place), based on an understanding of the wants and needs of the target market segment, to offer to the target market in exchange for what they currently do or believe.

positioning: Creating a personality for an offering based on its key attributes.

social marketing: The application of commercial marketing principles to social issues.

REFERENCES

1. Kotler, P., & Armstrong, G. (1998). *Principles of marketing* (8th ed.). Englewood Cliffs, NJ: Prentice-Hall.

2. Fine, S. (1981). *The marketing of ideas and social issues.* New York: Praeger.

3. Smith, W. A. (2000). Social marketing: An evolving definition. *American Journal of Health Behavior, 24,* 11–17.

4. Fine, S. H. (1992). *Marketing the public sector: Promoting the causes of public and nonprofit agencies.* New Brunswick, NJ: Transaction.

5. Wallack, L. (1990). Media advocacy: Promoting health through mass communication. In K. Glanz, F. M. Lewis, & B. K. Rimer (Eds.), *Health behavior and health education: Theory, research, and practice.* San Francisco: Jossey-Bass.

6. Roper, W. L. (1993). Health communication takes on new dimensions at CDC. *Public Health Reports, 108*(2), 179–183.

7. Andreasen, A. A. (1995). *Marketing social change: Changing behavior to promote health, social development, and the environment.* San Francisco: Jossey-Bass.

8. Goldberg, M. E., Fishbein, M., & Middlestadt, S. E. (Eds.). (1997). *Social marketing: Theoretical and practical perspectives.* Mahwah, NJ: Lawrence Erlbaum Associates.

9. Weinreich, N. K. (1999). *Hands-on social marketing: A step-by-step guide.* Thousand Oaks, CA: Sage Publications.

10. Wechsler, H., & Wernick, S. M. (1992). A social marketing campaign to promote low-fat milk consumption in an inner-city Latino community. *Public Health Reports, 107*(2), 202–207.

11. Bloom, P. N. (1980). Evaluating social marketing programs: Problems and prospects. In R. Bagozzi, K. L. Bernhardt, P. D. Busch, D. W. Cravens, J. F. Hair, Jr., & C. A. Scott (Eds.), *Marketing in the 1980's: Changes and challenges* (pp. 460–463). Chicago: American Marketing Association.

12. Bloom, P., & Novelli, W. D. (1981). Problems and challenges in social marketing. *Journal of Marketing, 45,* 79–88.

ADDITIONAL RESOURCES

Print

Backer, T., Rogers, E., & Sopory, P. (1992). *Designing health communication campaigns: What works?* Newbury Park, CA: Sage.

Center for Substance Abuse Prevention. (1994). *Technical assistance bulletins: Guides for planning and developing your ATOD prevention materials.* Rockville, MD: U.S. Department of Health and Human Services, Public Health Service, Substance Abuse and Mental Health Services Administration. (Free from the National Clearinghouse for Alcohol and Drug Information, 1-800-729-6686.)

Frederiksen, L., Solomon, L., & Brehony, K. (Eds.). (1984). *Marketing health behavior: Principles, techniques, and applications.* New York: Plenum.

Kotler, P., & Roberto, E. (1989). *Social marketing: Strategies for changing public behavior.* New York: Free Press.

National Cancer Institute. (1992). *Making health communication programs that work: A planner's guide.* Washington, DC: U.S. Department of Health and Human Services. (Free from the Cancer Information Service, 1-800-4-CANCER, or online at http://rex.nci.nih.gov/nci_pub_interface/hcpw/home.html.)

National Center on Child Abuse and Neglect. (1996). *Marketing matters: Building an effective communications program.* Washington, DC: U.S. Department of Health and Human Services. (Free from the National Clearinghouse on Child Abuse and Neglect Information, 1-800-394-3366.)

Ogden, L., Shepherd, M., & Smith, W. A. (1996). *Applying prevention marketing.* Atlanta, GA: Centers for Disease Control and Prevention, Public Health Service. (Free from the National AIDS Clearinghouse, 1-800-458-5231.)

Internet

Academy for Educational Development. *The ABCs of human behavior for disease prevention.* Available: http://www.aed.org/publications/news/fall95/disease_prev.html.

Centers for Disease Control and Prevention. *Marketing strategies for physical activity.* Available: http://www.cdc.gov/nccdphp/dnpa/readyset/market.htm.

Health Canada. *The social marketing network.* Available: http://www.hc-sc.gc.ca/hppb/socialmarketing.

Indiana Prevention Resource Center. *Prevention newsline.* Available: http://www.drugs.indiana.edu/publications/iprc/newsline/winter92.html.

Johns Hopkins University. *Center for Communication Programs website.* Available: http://www.jhuccp.org.

Population Health Social Marketing. Available: http://www.health.gov.au/pubhlth/strateg/educat/index.htm.

Social Marketing Institute. Available: http://www.social-marketing.org.

II

Implementing Methods and Strategies at the Individual Level

6

Facilitating Support Groups

Lynne Durrant, Ph.D.
Traci Rieckmann, Ph.D.

Author Comments

Traci: Group processes have always fascinated me both professionally and person-ally. In different settings the dynamics of teams, classroom groups, even social groups, volunteer groups, and supervision or training groups, have left me more curious and aware of the intense, multifaceted process. This interest expanded with my graduate education in health education and psychology. Simultaneously, I attended group behavior change courses and then facilitated groups with incar-cerated youth. In each experience I was amazed at how the group members did everything that group theory said they would and how both university graduate students and 13-year-old youth expressed some anxiety and adjusted their behavior as they joined the group. In all group experiences, the members set up formal and informal norms, they storm and then re-norm, and there are personal and group goals. In my class and in the youth treatment groups, there were established com-munication patterns; we dealt with problem members, and we all gained insight into our own behavior. Two diverse settings and yet the similarities and application of group theory and behavior change through group work were powerful. As my career evolves, my training and experience with groups continue to reinforce to me their energy and influence on human interaction and growth. In the classroom, while leading therapy groups, in teaching veterans about sleep disturbance, and even in my research teams for clinical trials, group dynamics influence our experiences, the outcomes, and each individual's development.

My coauthor, Lynne Durrant, and I have similar backgrounds in health education and psychology. Drawing on our combined knowledge and experience, our purpose with this chapter is to give you information on how to set up a support group, to acquaint you with all the processes that occur when a group meets, and to teach you how to use these processes to help facilitate community groups or even to become a more productive member of a group. Nicole Stettler, my research assistant, also helped with this chapter. Her experiences include group membership in social, academic, extracurricular, and work settings. She noted that as a psychology major in college, she began to learn about and understand group processes through her coursework in social psychology. She then had the opportunity to facilitate playgroups for families with young children, which allowed her to examine group dynamics as a leader and direct service provider.

Finally I will end this section with one caveat: Work within your training and scope of practice. As you work with community groups, remember that you are a talented and important health educator, but not a counselor or a licensed psychologist. You must recognize the limits to your expertise and be prepared to refer individuals who need therapy or professional counseling to an appropriate mental health provider. You cannot be all things to all people, and it is critical that you know how to seek consultation, help, and outside support.

Introduction

Group work is a powerful tool in modifying or changing human behavior. For a group member the strength of this intervention lies in two areas: being able to gain objective insight into personal behavior, and realizing that one is not alone in trying to cope with life's problems. Insight comes from the power of group feedback. People who have similar concerns or problems are able to share their perspective and experiences to help each other cope with their situation. And as group members share those experiences, they realize that their feelings and behavior are not unique. The author C. S. Lewis once said that people "read to know that we are not alone." The same is true of groups. Individuals join groups to know that they are not alone; groups give people a sense of community.

Throughout history, human beings have found it beneficial in terms of survival and prosperity to work in groups rather than alone. From the time a person is born, group membership is important. People belong to family, community, and cultural groups; economic, geographic, and demographic groups; and social, religious, and professional groups. Some belong to groups because of shared characteristics or shared objectives, and others join groups to achieve goals that could not be achieved on their own. This is especially true of support groups.

What Is a Support Group?

A group is defined as two or more individuals who meet face-to-face to achieve agreed-upon goals.[1] The Association for Specialists in Group Work has further defined group work as "a broad professional practice that refers to the giving of help or the accomplishment of tasks in a group setting."[2] Thus, there are a wide range of groups, including psychoeducational/guidance groups, counseling/interpersonal groups, psychotherapy/personality-oriented groups, task/work groups, self-help groups, and support groups. The focus of this chapter is the support group, which is sometimes called a therapeutic group. **Support groups** are structured groups that focus on a specific problem, task, or theme and incorporate both interpersonal and educational gains.[2] They function to provide information, comfort, and connectedness with others who are experiencing similar circumstances.[3] Support groups also offer advantages to the agencies that sponsor them. They are economical in that people receive services in groups rather than individually. Members of support groups often use other services offered by the sponsoring agency, and members may be more likely than nonmembers to feel that the agency is supportive of their needs.

The purpose of a support group is to increase knowledge, clarify changes an individual may want to make in order to reduce a variety of symptoms, and assist in the development of skills necessary for making these changes. In terms of health promotion, the support group offers a safe community or environment in which the participating members may learn from listening, observing, trying out new behaviors, receiving feedback, and experiencing support from others. Examples of topics that might be addressed by a health education support group include stress management, weight management, eating disorders, smoking cessation, anger management, and cancer or cardiovascular disease prevention or recovery.

Types of Support Groups

Support groups come in many forms, varying in terms of size, cohesiveness, and target population. Facilitating a support group requires knowledge of the unique needs of the target population. For instance, an adolescent smoking cessation group would vary greatly from a smoking cessation group for older adults. A facilitator would need to be aware of the social, cognitive, and moral developmental stages and needs of each of these populations. The adolescent smoking group would probably focus on adolescent needs of belonging to a group, being seen as cool, and being independent. The older adult group would be more concerned with issues of addiction and health. So in order for the support group to bring about behavioral change, the facilitator must develop an appropriate and effective social culture.

Support group facilitators need to understand the nature of group process. It takes more than knowledge of healthful practices to run a successful group. For example, the director of a small nonprofit agency decided to improve employee morale and health by hiring a health behavior change consultant to help staff learn how to eat more nutritionally. Staff were paid while attending the group, which met one hour each week for 12 weeks. The group started out with 18 enthusiastic members. However, by week 4 or 5, there were only three regular attendees. The group facilitator had made a fatal mistake in conducting this group—she set the goals and tasks to meet her needs, not the group's. She had members keep a daily food diary in which they wrote how they felt before and after eating. This may be an effective tool in monitoring eating habits, but this technique, which involved a tremendous amount of writing, did not work well with a staff who already spent a tremendous amount of time writing as part of their jobs. Group members became frustrated and stressed when they could not keep up with the daily writing and so they chose to work rather than attend group meetings.

Support groups also vary in terms of structure and eligibility for membership. Some groups are **time-limited** and open only to selected participants. Most of these groups range from six to ten sessions and are based on a prepared curriculum or facilitator guides. Others are **ongoing** and open to new members. These types of support groups tend to be more free-flowing and less structured. Groups may also differ in the length of meeting time and how often the sessions are held. For example, groups for children may last only 40 minutes, whereas those for adults may meet for 90 minutes. The majority of groups are time limited and aimed at symptom relief, problem solving, development of interpersonal skills, or patient education. Ongoing support groups for individuals are increasing in popularity, specifically with clients who have chronic illnesses or addictions. These open-ended support groups are becoming common in local hospitals, mental health agencies, and community meeting places.

Support Groups for Children and Adolescents

Groups for children and adolescents, though similar in many ways to other groups, warrant special consideration. Groups for children are typically for those younger than 14 years, and groups for adolescents tend to have participants who range in age from 13 to 19 years. During these years youth face many changes, which can increase apprehension when it comes to group interactions. Again, it is important to consider the unique needs and developmental

Community
connections 1

Ricardo and Kendra are both employed at the state department of health, which has just begun a statewide tobacco-prevention program. As part of the program, they have been asked to facilitate a smoking cessation group at a local high school. Eleven students—seven males and four females—have volunteered to be part of this group. The principal has given the students released time for one and a half hours every Monday morning at 10:00 A.M. for a period of eight weeks. Ricardo and Kendra have decided to bring treats to each group meeting as a way of encouraging attendance and promoting cohesion.

During the first meeting, members were asked to share with the others what the biggest obstacle was in trying to stop smoking. As members shared their fears, the facilitators pointed out how many of them had the same concerns—such as weight gain, boredom, and withdrawal. Jennifer, a shy, nervous-looking member, seemed to be debating what to say when her turn came. When Ricardo finally called on her, she blurted out that her father was an abusive alcoholic and that smoking was the only way she could relieve the stress of her chaotic home life. Ricardo gave Kendra a "wow, what do we do with this" look as Jennifer continued to describe her home situation. Ricardo's first impulse was to jump in and start helping Jennifer deal with her problem. However, he quickly realized that abuse was beyond the scope of the smoking cessation group and his own expertise. Ricardo, very wisely, empathized with Jennifer and then told her he could refer her to professionals who could help her cope with her situation. He then moved on to talk about alternative ways to manage stress. By handling the situation in this way, Ricardo acknowledged Jennifer's emotional pain and offered help, but also kept the group focused on the main issue of smoking cessation.

levels of the focus population. When organizing a support group for children and adolescents, a concrete explanation of the purpose of the group and the expectations of the members is important. Issues such as parental involvement, confidentiality, and termination become significant. Health educators who are interested in developing support groups for youth must be aware of the unique circumstances related to issues such as age and gender, the coping skills of the child and his or her family, and the nature of the problem. Choice of activities should be influenced by the needs and abilities of the participants. In a study of a support group for traumatized children, the developers' goals were to rebuild trust, counteract isolation, and acknowledge community resources. They achieved this through a basic structure of four parts: opening/greeting, physical activity, main activity, and closing/goodbye.[4] The setting and atmosphere as well as the style of leadership are also important in working with children and adolescents. For example, a community-based group related to depression and anxiety is more likely to be successful when the facilitators are focused on the positive outcomes of the group. It should be called a Life Skills group rather than a Depression Management group.

Support Groups for Adults

Support groups for adults cover the period of life from ages 20 to 60, which is full of transitions, growth, and concerns of identity, intimacy, and generativity (the nurture and guidance of the next generation). In terms of health promotion, groups for adults may focus on wellness issues such as fitness and nutrition, smoking cessation, parenting skills, and coping with chronic illness. Because this part of the lifespan is so large, the range of experiences and needs varies considerably. Some adults may be looking for support in changing specific behaviors, whereas others are looking for help with increasing spirituality and balance in their lives. Health educators who want to facilitate a group for adults should explore the needs of this specific population and be aware of other community resources set up to meet these needs.

Support Groups for Older Adults

As the number of elderly individuals in the United States has increased, so have the efforts to offer appropriate services. Health educators and administrators developing support programs for elderly individuals must be aware of their unique concerns and potential. With this population there is a strong link between mental and physical health. For example, physical problems such as chronic pain, hypertension, cancer, and asthma may be positively affected by addressing the mental problems of loneliness, isolation, and loss of meaningful productivity. Group work offers the opportunity for new friendships, personal growth, and increased knowledge related to health care advancements.

One issue to keep in mind when working with the elderly is the social prejudice toward older adults. Facilitators need to be prepared for this issue and should be open to discussion of this concern. Time of day for group meetings is another issue to consider. Nighttime meetings are not recommended because of safety issues and also because many elderly individuals have early bedtimes. Travel may also be an issue for those who do not drive or who need to schedule their trips through a care facility. Finally, process and content materials should be prepared appropriately in a larger font size, and there should be accommodation for hearing limitations.

Support Groups for Substance Abuse Issues

Substance abuse is a major public health problem that is often addressed in support groups and group therapy. One of the most well-established peer-based support groups is Alcoholics Anonymous (AA), a group dedicated to recovery from alcohol use disorders. Indeed, most group work within the field of substance abuse treatment is facilitated by peers or paraprofessionals specializing in the area.[5]

A review by Weiss and colleagues looked at the effectiveness of groups in the treatment of substance abuse. They found that adding special group therapy to treatment as usual seems to improve outcomes for some participants. Group therapy in addition to individual therapy also showed better outcomes for substance abuse versus individual therapy alone. Additionally, group therapy alone showed similar outcomes to group therapy combined with individual therapy. There was little support for any differences between particular types of group interventions.[6]

Group work is often considered the primary form of treatment for substance abuse; however, there are still important issues to consider in the formation and maintenance of such a group. First, the population of potential participants is incredibly diverse, making it useful to draw on different treatment modalities to address the needs of the entire group. This may include combining psychoeducational and therapeutic elements (i.e., motivational interviewing and cognitive-behavioral work) in group sessions. Leaders also need to be prepared for a demand for more self-disclosure, particularly in relation to their substance use background, as well as a potentially difficult and transitional membership base. Educating members on the norms and expectations early on may help alleviate potential conflicts. Finally, it is important to pay particular attention to the size of groups and the length and location of sessions to be sure that they meet the needs of the group as a whole as well as individual members.[5]

Peer-Led Support Groups

One emerging topic in the field of group work is peer-led, or self-help, support groups. These are community groups that are not led by any sort of health professional or paraprofessional, but rather are led by mutual consensus or peer facilitation.[7] The most common participants are those with substance use or mental health concerns; however, groups may also focus on chronic physical illnesses, disabilities, stigmatized statuses, and other health and social concerns.

There are specific benefits to a peer-led support group. It can be a more accessible route to illness management and health promotion because of its low cost and community base. It can also enhance the effects of professionally led programs.[7] Involvement in these groups can help members develop a wider support network. They also provide not only emotional but also practical support for a long-term period. For example, a study on self-help support groups for young men found that the participants reported several benefits, including emotional support, a supportive atmosphere, practical advice from people with similar experiences and/or backgrounds, and a sense of connection. The opportunity to participate allowed them to develop friendships and also served as a reminder of their past and the importance of self-care in maintaining their new life.[8]

Web-Based Support Groups

The increasing use of the Internet has provided a new forum for support groups. There are several advantages to online groups: accessibility by a wide range of people, including those who are homebound or lack transportation; broader interaction by a larger, more heterogeneous membership base; greater convenience for members' schedules; and an ability to reach not only active members, but also those who "lurk" (i.e., read messages but do not actively participate). There are also limitations to this type of interaction. These include a potential lack of consensus on how to handle negative or hostile comments, inaccessibility by those who do not have computer skills or Internet access, a loss of nonverbal interaction and cues from participants, and limited outcome data supporting their use.[9–12]

Several variables must be considered when forming and maintaining an online support group. One is synchronous versus asynchronous groups. **Synchronous** groups join together in some type of text- or audio-based session at the same time, much as a face-to-face group would meet. Although this allows for a more conventional type of session, with a leader facilitating planned activities or topics, it can require advanced technology skills, which may be a barrier for some members. In contrast, an **asynchronous** group does not meet at planned times; rather, members may post by email via a listserv or on a bulletin board–type program.[13] This structure has greater flexibility for participants. A large proportion of online support seems to occur between 7:00 p.m. and 1:00 a.m.[10] It also allows for more people to access information without direct participation by lurking.

Some other important considerations to recognize are concerns about leadership and safety. Groups will need to address what type of content will be deemed acceptable and how to deal with members expressing hostility or negativity. Because membership may constantly change over time, a group facilitator may want to introduce a set of norms from the beginning and have them available for all new members. Another issue is the paucity of research on the development and outcomes of online groups.[12] This area is still developing, although rapidly, and continued attention by group leaders and researchers will be important.

Steps for Conducting Effective Support Groups

Support groups are effective if the facilitator or facilitators have taken the time beforehand to lay the groundwork. Careful planning will eliminate many of the common problems that plague community groups. The facilitator should think about the group he or she is going to facilitate. Careful consideration should be given to the selection of the target audience; where the meetings will be held; what the goals, objectives, and activities of the group will be; and what materials will be needed. Only after the groundwork has been laid can effective facilitation occur.

Define the Audience

Defining the group, or audience, to reach is critical in support group development. Consideration must be given to the unique needs of the potential members. Determining the target audience sets the stage for planning group content, selecting an appropriate facilitator, and determining what should happen to achieve desired outcomes. For example, when developing a support group for smoking cessation, first complete a brief assessment to determine what resources exist in the community. This provides an idea of what services are available and where the gaps in services might be (i.e., what populations are not being served). Next, decide if the group will be heterogeneous or homogeneous. There are advantages to facilitating homogenous groups because members share common characteristics and goals and group activities can be tailored to their specific needs. In comparison, heterogeneous groups offer members differing perspectives in terms of life experiences that are sometimes very beneficial.

The next step involves recruiting group members. Keep in mind that people join groups because they perceive they will be better off than if they had not joined the group. It is important to educate prospective members on the benefits of being part of the group. This can be done in a variety of ways, including flyers, presentations, referrals from health educators or medical providers, public service announcements, newspaper articles, and company newsletters. Personal contact with potential group members is also helpful for recruitment. This allows for information concerning dates and location to be shared and questions to be answered. Finally, it is easier to recruit members when the focus of the group, in terms of goals, objectives, and activities, is clear.

Select a Facilitator

The leader, or group **facilitator**, plays a significant role in the success of support groups. The facilitator is an individual who has experience, expertise, and an interest in the focus of the support group. Ideally this individual will have been involved with the group from the beginning—from the conceptualization of the project to the recruitment of members. The facilitator must be skilled at creating an environment where group members can discuss their fears and experiences while educating one another through these interactions. Leaders who are open, aware of cultural influences, and nondefensive, who have courage and self-awareness, and who attend to ethical issues are likely to find the experience successful and rewarding. Selecting a group leader who has both training and experience is helpful. Facilitators should be able to demonstrate skills such as active listening, reflecting, summarizing, questioning, confronting, empathizing, supporting, and suggesting.

Co-facilitation may be beneficial in some support groups; indeed, one comprehensive review found that 45% of therapeutic groups were co-led.[13] Advantages of co-leading a group include decreased leader burnout, support in processing intense feelings, and more flexible scheduling (if one leader is ill or unavailable). Advantages of co-facilitations for group members include an objective perspective, information from more than one leader, and increased facilitation for all members. On the other hand, co-leading can be difficult if the facilitators do not agree on leadership styles or ethical issues, or if there is a lack of respect or trust between the leaders.[2] In co-facilitating a group, the facilitators must work collaboratively and negotiate issues that may arise. This type of close working relationship is best accomplished if both leaders are involved from the beginning.

Some groups have used co-facilitation as a way to bring in a peer facilitator in addition to a health professional. In one analysis of a chronic illness peer support (CHIP) program, the role of a peer facilitator was described as three-fold: to share his or her own experiences to encourage other group members to do the same, to act as a positive role model, and to provide a link between the participants and the health professional to minimize any perception of the professional as a "teacher" or "therapist."[14]

There are several types of group leaders, depending on the task to be accomplished. Tasks can be generally grouped into two categories: goal-oriented tasks and relationship-oriented tasks. *Goal-oriented tasks* include imparting of information, development of skills, and completion of a project. A leader in this situation needs to be directive and task-oriented. *Relationship-oriented tasks* include the development of a strong supportive emotional or social atmosphere that fosters personal growth. A leader in this situation needs to demonstrate good listening skills and the ability to create an empathetic group atmosphere. Overall, a support group leader generally provides stability, enforces norms, and provides a caring, supportive, and nonjudgmental atmosphere. Leadership effectiveness seems to be based on the ability to assess the needs and goals of the group and to adjust approaches to meet them. Table 6-1 lists general characteristics of effective leaders.[15]

Select a Site

There are several items to consider in selecting a site, or meeting place, for the group. The location must provide privacy and be free of distractions.[2] Settings should provide an atmosphere that is inviting and physically comfortable. Most facilitators prefer to have participants sit in a circle where

| Table 6-1 | Qualities of a Good Leader |

- *Believes in the group process:* Feels that the group process is valuable in helping people change and communicates that enthusiasm
- *Creates an open, caring atmosphere:* Makes members feel valued and understood
- *Facilitates communication among members:* Encourages open communication patterns and discourages destructive patterns
- *Values creativity:* Helps the group explore and appreciate new ideas and experiences different from his or her own
- *Clarifies individual ideas or suggestions:* Makes sure the group members are "on the same page"
- *Facilitates the group process:* Describes what is happening in the group; provides insight
- *Keeps the group focused on the present:* Emphasizes the "here and now" to promote interpersonal awareness
- *Helps the group set standards and goals:* Creates awareness of direction and progress
- *Summarizes group ideas or suggestions after a discussion:* Provides a conclusion that the group can accept or reject

they are able to see one another. This type of arrangement allows for verbal and nonverbal communication. It is also helpful to have the leaders sitting across from each other to avoid a "we-versus-them" atmosphere. Group facilitators should also consider the special needs of groups, such as those who are differently abled or those who may need regular medical attention. Options for meeting locations may include office buildings, local health departments, churches, schools, community or nonprofit agencies, universities, mental health agencies, hospitals, or medical clinics or physicians' office space.

Define Goals, Objectives, and Activities

A detailed proposal, or game plan, is the driving force behind a successful support group. Facilitators must be very clear regarding the purpose of the group and the goals they hope to accomplish through group meetings. Activities should be outlined for each session so that members have a clear sense of direction. There are five key areas to cover in a group proposal:[3]

- *Rationale or overall goal.* This involves determining why the group is necessary.
- *Objectives.* Objectives should include what needs to be accomplished and how it is intended to be accomplished. Objectives should be specific, measurable, and attainable and are often supported by specific activities or procedures.

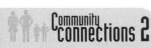

Because Kendra and Ricardo were asked to conduct a support group with adolescents, they had to consider several issues as they set up the group. In recruiting for the group, Ricardo designed a flier advertising a positive Lifelong Learning Skills Group that included smoking cessation. Prospective members were self-referred or referred by the school counselor, but each one had to have expressed a desire to quit smoking. The facilitators signed up 15 members, knowing that through natural attrition, the group would be smaller.

Perhaps the most important ethical issue for the facilitators was parent notification and informed consent. Even though students had volunteered for this group, parents were notified and received clear and accurate information as to the purpose and structure of the group. Kendra and Ricardo made sure each student had a signed consent form before the group began. Kendra commented to Ricardo that even though obtaining these forms was an added burden, in the long run it would be beneficial to have the parents involved. In fact, Kendra designed several specific homework assignments that had to be shared with parents. For example, students were taught stress management techniques and then were required to teach at least one of these techniques to one of their parents or guardians. This assignment not only reinforced the skill, but also added the involvement and support of the parent.

Kendra and Ricardo also interviewed each prospective member before the group began. During this interview, the students were assured they could withdraw from the group at any time, and that everything said in group meetings would be confidential. By conducting these initial interviews, the facilitators began establishing trust and understanding with the group members.

- *Practical considerations.* Group developers should address issues of site selection; membership recruitment; whether the group will be open or closed, time limited or ongoing; and how often meetings will be held.
- *Procedures.* These include activities the health educator or facilitator has selected to meet the stated goals.
- *Evaluation.* All groups need some type of evaluation to determine if the goals have been met, such as pre- and post-tests on knowledge, or satisfaction inventories.

Prepare Content and Process Materials

The last preparation step recommended for group development is the creation of content and process materials. This includes choosing a theoretical basis for the group interaction. *Theories* are explanations of the ways or processes by which health behavior is changed. Tenets from health behavior change theories, such as the Health Belief Model, the Theory of Reasoned Action, the Theory of Planned Behavior, or the Transtheoretical Model of Stages of Change, can be used to determine what information and activities will be implemented and what skills will be taught in the group.

For example, the tenet behind the Health Belief Model states that people will change behaviors if they think they are susceptible to harmful and severe consequences and if they think that by changing their behavior they will reduce or eliminate these harmful and severe consequences. In using this theoretical basis for a smoking cessation group, a facilitator might want to use content materials that demonstrate the negative consequences of smoking and the positive benefits of quitting. The group members would then process their own experiences with negative effects of smoking and what they perceive as the benefits of quitting. There are several health behavior and education books on the market that describe in detail how to educate or facilitate change using these models.

Facilitate the Support Group

Up to this point, information has been provided on how to set up a support group. It is equally important to understand the underlying processes that occur when individual members evolve into group members and the group actually becomes a "group." The following subsections explain what processes take place as the group develops, including a discussion of the various stages that characterize group development.

Form the Group

Seven general processes are involved in group development. A knowledge of these processes will provide a greater understanding of what is going on in the group and how these processes can be used to move the group forward in an insightful and beneficial way.

Selective perception. Anxiety is the dominant emotion that occurs when people first attend a group meeting. This anxiety alters behavior because people have conscious or unconscious feelings of danger and self-doubt. There is a role shift from individual to group member and a wish to belong—to be accepted by the group. People are uncomfortable because they do not know what to expect. To deal with this anxiety, group members relate to that which makes them most comfortable—that is, **selective perception**. They may choose to participate or not participate. They tend to gravitate to other members they perceive as more like themselves, and they form stereotypes of other group members. They also act in a way to preserve their own sense of self. An example of this is an adolescent in a group who assumes a bored, unconcerned attitude

Did You Know

It has been estimated that 6.25 million people, or 3.7% of the population over the age of 17, attended 500,000 support groups in the 1980s. This number probably increased to over 10 million by 1999, indicating that support groups have become a major force in delivering mental health care in America.

Source: Yalom, I. D. (1975). *The theory and practice of group psychotherapy* (2nd ed.). New York: Basic Books.

and makes fun of what is happening. The adolescent is anxious and afraid, and this is how she deals with it. The facilitator's job is to not take this personally, to understand the feelings that are driving the behavior, and to try to reduce the anxiety. This can be accomplished by immediately involving the group in a meaningful activity.

Always begin every group with an icebreaker or group activity that relates to the purpose of the group and starts to build cohesion. For example, with a stress management group, one could use a bowl of colored candy and have members select a piece of candy and then, depending on the color, share a type of stress in their lives (e.g., if the candy is red, share a major stressor in school life; if the candy is green, share a major stressor in family life). Another approach might focus on having members say why they are there and what they hope to get out of the group. There are many books available on icebreakers and group activities that can provide creative ideas on how to get a group started. The important concept to remember is to start building group cohesion immediately: Get the members talking to each other and sharing experiences.

Communication.   Communication in a group is influenced by four needs: (1) the need to survive without a loss of personal integrity; (2) the need for identity (who am I in this group?); (3) the need for power, influence, and control; and (4) the need for acceptance by others. The facilitator's role is to encourage the group to provide realistic feedback to each speaker in a non-judgmental, nonthreatening manner. Members will stop sharing if they feel they are being criticized, diagnosed, ordered, or threatened, or if they feel their concerns are not being addressed. Facilitators can model good listening skills, such as making eye contact with someone as they speak, rephrasing what the member has said to ensure understanding, and responding to comments in an empathetic manner. As members of the group begin to feel more comfortable and as they begin to see that the group is nonjudgmental and supportive, they will begin to become more open and communicative. The facilitator models this nonjudgmental acceptance in order to create a safe environment.

Group size and structure.   The ideal group size is five to eight members. This size makes it easier for all group members to be heard. If the group is much larger, some members may not participate; if it is much smaller, it becomes more of an individual intervention. An open structure that encourages participation from all members results in higher morale, but less efficiency in getting tasks accomplished. A central leader who emerges and takes control and directs the group will create a more stable, efficient group, but the group member morale will be lower. In general, if the group members are more incompatible in terms of presenting problems or personalities, structure will help minimize the potential negative effects on the therapeutic outcome.[13]

Membership.   People join groups to get certain needs met; they believe the group will be helpful. Factors that increase the attractiveness of a group include a cooperative group attitude, a great deal of member interaction, and the feeling that people want to belong. Factors that decrease attractiveness include inability to agree on a group goal; fighting and arguing among members; dominating, self-oriented members; and a feeling that the group is not attractive to others. The facilitator plays a large role in creating the cooperative attitude and member interaction and in decreasing dissension among the members.

Norms.   **Norms** are ideas in the minds of the individual members about what should or should not be done by themselves or other group members (i.e., expectations of behavior). Norms serve to regulate the group's behavior and to keep it on track. They are formed by the acceptance or rejection of certain behaviors by the majority of the group members. Four types of norms exist. *Formal norms*, or rules, are usually written down. *Explicitly stated norms* are either stated verbally or are easily recognized by all members. Examples might include not interrupting a member who is speaking, or arriving on time. *Nonexplicit*, or *informal*, *norms* are rules of behavior that are accepted but not stated. Examples might be members sitting in the same seat every time or the way they dress for group. *Unconscious norms* are sometimes called *taboos*. These are the norms that are not voiced but are very rarely violated, such as uttering racial slurs and telling off-color jokes. If these norms are ever violated, there is usually a negative group reaction, such as members getting up and leaving, becoming silent, or becoming angry.

It is the role of the facilitator to model group norms, which are usually set in the first few sessions. Members tend to emulate group leaders. For instance, members are more likely to be on time if the facilitator is also on time. Delaying the beginning of group until tardy members arrive will result in others coming late. If the facilitator talks to a group member when someone else is talking, then members will feel free to do the same. Group facilitators have a powerful role here and should keep in mind that once group norms are set, they are very hard to change.

Goals.   Goals are what the group wants to accomplish. They are the desirable outcomes that provide motivation for joining a group. These goals may be short or long term, and they may be individual or group goals. Individual and group goals need to be compatible if the group is to be effective. Measurable goals are most effective because individuals can track their progress. It is helpful to agree upon group goals, through consensus, during the first meeting. Goals imposed by a leader or a dominant member are rarely successful. The group facilitator should help members develop reachable individual and group goals, and then serve as a motivator in reaching those goals.

Leadership.   Leadership is usually established through a working relationship among the group members. A group member may become a leader by being an active participant and by demonstrating leadership qualities. Members will follow a group leader if they think the leader is competent and knowledgeable and shares their goals. Group leaders can be democratic, which leads to high morale among group members but is often inefficient in quickly accomplishing tasks; or they can be authoritarian, which is very efficient in accomplishing tasks but often leads to low morale. A laissez-faire leader is one who does not lead but allows the group to stumble around on its own until another leader emerges. Leaders lead by challenging the status quo, by inspiring a clear mutual vision, by empowering members through cooperative teamwork, or by leading by example.[16] In a support group, the facilitator is usually seen as the leader in the beginning. As the group progresses, however, other members may assume leadership roles; the facilitator then becomes more of a true facilitator—someone who helps members process the progress of the group.[17]

Ongoing Stages of Group Development

As part of their interactional process, groups tend to move through stages, including the initial, transition, working, and ending stages. Although many ongoing support groups never move to the ending phase because they are structured to continue, it is still significant to examine this portion of the process in order to understand group development.

Initial stage.   During the first stage of the group process, the focus is on creating a group structure, orienting members, and dealing with group expectations. This phase, known as the **initial** or **forming stage**, tends to be marked by members cautiously observing others and deciding whether or not they fit in the group. Trust may or may not begin to be established, and there may be periods of silence or nervous laughter. During this stage the participants turn to the group leader or leaders for direction. It is during this phase that members decide whether this is an attractive group or not and whether they will continue to be participants. The group facilitator has a dominant role at this point and should model basic norms of open communication, caring, and acceptance.

Transition stage.   As the group begins to move forward toward the working phase, a period of "storming" or transition occurs. The **transition stage** is significant because anxiety and conflict emerge and groups will either move through the phase successfully or become stuck in the turmoil of storming.[2] Support groups in the transition stage are marked by members who are shifting from maintaining their best image to risking the expression of their real concerns and issues. Communication styles are tested as members begin to share more intimate details and perceive others as attending to or ignoring them. The transition stage may also involve testing of the leader and struggles for control and power. Even time-limited, educationally focused support groups may experience a type of storming in which members increase or decrease their participation and modify their communication patterns. The facilitator's role during this period is to maintain objectivity and continue to model acceptance, interest, and support.

Working stage. The third stage in the group process is often referred to as the **working** or **performing stage**. This period tends to be marked by productivity in addressing personal change and education. When groups function well in the working stage, significant growth may be achieved. A sign that the group has moved into this phase is when both leaders and members feel relaxed in taking action and trying out personal expressions or new behaviors. Enough trust must exist between group members for this to be accomplished, which means that power and control conflicts must have been adequately addressed.

During the performing stage, there is an increase in self-disclosure, confrontation, feedback, and humor. Participants are more at ease with each other. For example, during the third session of a support group for adults with sleep disturbance, one member began teasing the facilitator about looking tired. The other participants then joined in and began to tease one another, asking, "Why were you late, Dean, did you sleep through group?" Another joked, "Maybe he didn't get enough REM sleep so he couldn't concentrate on where he was driving and missed the turn." The members enjoyed laughter and a type of bonding during this interaction that suggested they were retaining the material and were more comfortable with each other. This is also the stage where new activities such as homework or role playing may be incorporated.

Ending stage. The final stage in all groups is the **ending stage**, or termination. Some groups may last for several weeks and some for several years, but all groups will face closure or termination at some point. Some groups are set up in the beginning to meet for a specified period of time (e.g., an eight-week smoking cessation group). Other groups are ongoing and may end when group tasks are completed, when there is significant attrition, or when there is a structural change, such as a facility closing or a facilitator retiring. The health educator who is facilitating a group facing termination must be prepared for the emotions and behavior of group members as this shift occurs. Reactions to termination may vary depending on the length of the group, the trust and the cohesiveness of the group, and how the previous stages and sessions were handled. Some individuals may feel especially sad if they are not ready to function without the support of the group. Others may experience anxiety or

Community connections 3

Kendra and Ricardo were talking one afternoon about the progress of their smoking cessation group. The group had been meeting for five weeks, and several interesting group processes had occurred. Kendra pointed out how Jennifer had changed over the five weeks, becoming more relaxed and confident in group. In fact, Ricardo added that the group itself seemed more cohesive and trustful. "Remember in the beginning," said Kendra, "when everyone looked at you or at me when they talked. There seemed to be a lot of nervous giggling and posturing during those first meetings as the kids tried to figure out how they fit into the group." "Or even," added Ricardo, "if this was a group that they wanted to be a part of."

"Maybe feeding them made this an attractive group," joked Kendra. "We've had pretty consistent attendance. We always have eight or nine who show up, which is a nice size group. Although one of the norms seems to be to wander in a few minutes late, it doesn't bother me because it really isn't disruptive, and kids do have to be cool. Anyway, they seem to respect each other, they never make derogatory comments, and they are genuinely trying to help each other quit smoking. These are probably more important issues than getting to group on time."

"I think starting every group with some sort of icebreaker really helped lower the anxiety and got the kids interacting with each other," commented Ricardo. "I especially liked the activity where the group created a tobacco-prevention curriculum for elementary school kids. They got pretty creative and I think it also helped them think about why they, too, should avoid tobacco." "Right," agreed Kendra. "I think at this point we really do have a cohesive group, and the kids are progressing toward their goal of smoking cessation."

concern because they are afraid they will not interact with these individuals again. Still others may express some disappointment or anger as the group closes because they did not accomplish their goals.[1]

To set the stage for a successful termination, it is recommended that facilitators begin discussing the ending several weeks prior to the final session. As the date of the last meeting draws near, time should be allotted to discuss individual reactions and thoughts regarding termination. This is a stressful time, but being able to share feelings of anxiety and sadness with others in the same situation can be very helpful for group members. For example, one health educator facilitating a loss group for elderly widowers noted that the participants were avoiding discussions of termination. She finally asked the group members to each take a turn and comment on their emotions and thoughts related to closure. Each member was able to share feelings of sadness and anxiety related to the impending event, and members expressed a desire to continue to meet. With this group and others, members may set up informal meetings on their own to delay the ending process. Offering a follow-up or booster session a month or so after ending the group is also helpful in reducing termination anxiety.

It should be noted that there are other models of group development. Bennis and Shepard were among the first to develop a series of stages to describe the changes in groups over time. They noted two general phases: dependence, when the group is focused on structure, order, and authority relations; and interdependence, when they are more concerned with interpersonal relations. Within these stages, they also noted subphases: dependence-submission, counterdependence, and resolution during the first stage; and enchantment-flight, disenchantment-flight, and consensual validation during the second.[13] Tuckman, in 1965, offered a five-stage model similar to the one just discussed. The stages he originally proposed included forming, storming, norming, and performing. He later added the adjourning stage.[13] More recently, MacKenzie proposed a four-stage model of group development based on Tuckman's work, collapsing the norming and performing stages on the theory that therapeutic groups tend not to separate focusing on developing norms from focusing on individual adjustment. His four stages are engagement, differentiation, interpersonal work, and termination.[13] Although all three models have been supported by research, it is important to note that group development can follow any or none of these models. Indeed, some groups may skip certain stages or move through them out of the proposed order.[13] One important theme concerning this development is the recurrence of issues related to conflict and authority. Group facilitators should take care to help the group negotiate these matters.

Tips and Techniques for Successful Support Group Facilitation

The most successful support groups are so because of careful planning and preparation. There are several strategies that facilitators can implement beforehand in order to minimize potential problems and increase the effectiveness of groups. Facilitators should also be aware of several issues that may affect the success of the group, such as community buy-in and the availability of community resources. Additionally, all facilitators should be very aware of the ethical issues involved with working with vulnerable populations. This section offers suggestions on how to maximize the effectiveness of the group process.

Plan in Advance

One of the greatest mistakes made by program developers and health educators is cutting the group preparation time too short. Generating a proposal, selecting group members, and selecting a site to meet can take several months. In groups where the leader is well prepared, participants experience a sense of commitment and the facilitator tends to be more confident and reassuring. This allows for rapid development of group cohesion. Preparing a proposal and content materials in advance also allows the health educator time to communicate with supervisors and referral sources in the community. Communicating with representatives from the department or team allows the health educator the chance to educate them about what the group can and cannot do, as well as what administrative support is necessary. Planning in advance increases the support for the project and allows others to feel that they were considered in the process.

Over-Recruit Members

Another suggestion for successful community-based support groups is over-recruiting of members. Most people lead busy lives or have little experience with support programs, which can lead to problems with attrition. At the onset or early phases of the group, individuals may express sincere interest, but when it comes to actually making the effort to attend the group, they may change their minds. Support groups compete with other activities or distractions that demand their attention. With this in mind, decide on an appropriate number of participants based on the type of group and the space available, and then try to enroll more members than are ideally desired. Thus, if aiming for a group of 10 members, enroll at least 15 or more, knowing that as the group progresses probably 10 will be consistent attendees.

Support the Facilitator

Supporting the facilitator(s) will aid in maintaining a cohesive and effective group. Resolving conflict and attending to the needs of several individuals takes a lot of energy. At times, facilitators may feel pulled in many directions and may find themselves drained from trying to follow and retain information presented by six or seven different participants. There is also a good deal of pressure not to cancel or reschedule a group. Co-facilitation is one way to avoid the burnout experienced by some facilitators. Another idea is to schedule breaks or weeks when the group will not meet or when a special speaker will replace the current leader. This may allow the leader time for rejuvenation, as well as give group members an opportunity to hear from someone new.

When appropriate, facilitators should also work to encourage the group members to manage and direct their discussions independently. For example, group leaders may offer topics or educational materials, or start the session. Once participants begin to express their needs and concerns, the facilitator may encourage group members to help one another by saying, "That's a great point to share. What do others think?" Participants may even be encouraged to rank their need to address a specific issue on a scale of 1 to 5 so that topics may be prioritized. When facilitators have the opportunity to ask for assistance and support, they are more likely to remain enthusiastic and committed to the group.

Know What Is Available in the Community

A community needs assessment is crucial to the successful development and implementation of a support group. Every community is different in terms of available resources and the needs of community members. The group facilitator should contact local medical care providers, county and city health departments, school programs, and other community-based agencies to determine what services are currently available. The individuals at these sites may also offer helpful suggestions regarding what health needs or gaps exist in community health services.

Generate Initial Buy-In

Support groups are more successful if they get off to a strong start. Getting group members to buy into the process at the first meeting sets the stage for continued participation and commitment to the group. Encouraging this connection can often be accomplished by providing food, interesting conversation, and goal-centered activities. Group members may appreciate the chance to introduce themselves, share a brief background, and then visit with other group members. Planning an interactive activity for the first session encourages individuals to develop a brief connection with other people, which increases the likelihood they will return. Providing light refreshments communicates to members that the facilitators think it is important to make the group experience a pleasant one. It expresses a kind of preparation and caring that is especially important in the early stages of the group process.

Be Aware of Ethical Issues

Support group facilitators are sometimes faced with ethical dilemmas. The Code of Ethics for the Health Education Profession outlines six ethical areas of general concern for all health educators: (1) responsibility to the public, (2) responsibility to the profession, (3) responsibility to employers, (4) responsibility in the delivery of health education, (5) responsibility in research and evaluation, and (6) responsibility in professional preparation. Those health educators that also act as support group facilitators must also be aware of the ethical, professional, and legal issues relevant to group work.

Many ethical issues come up unexpectedly and must be dealt with immediately. Group facilitators should prepare carefully for this group experience, including getting to know the clients and being sensitive to their unique needs. Facilitators should be aware of the guidelines for ethical behavior in two areas: the rights of group participants, and the ethics of group leaders' actions. The following is a list of ethical issues concerning the rights of group participants.

- *Informed consent.* Most people participate in a group because they want to. Prospective members should be provided with clear and accurate information about the group in order to make an educated decision about becoming a group member. If the participants are underaged or mentally unable to understand what the group is about, consent to participate must be obtained from a parent or legal guardian.

- *Freedom to withdraw from the group.* It should be clear to all group members that they may withdraw from the group at any time without repercussion. It is the member's responsibility, however, to inform the group and the facilitator of his or her impending departure. If possible, it is beneficial to the group and the member to discuss why he or she is leaving.

- *Psychological risk for members.* Members should be informed that there are risks of potential life changes because of group participation. Even though these changes are beneficial, there are sometimes negative repercussions. Group members may be exposed to group pressure, scapegoating, loss of confidentiality, and confrontation. These risks should be discussed with group members, and the facilitator and the group should discuss how to avoid these dangers.

- *Confidentiality.* It is very important that whatever is said in-group, stays in-group. This is probably the first rule that should be established. The facilitator should discuss this issue in the first meeting and gain assurance from each member that they, and the facilitator, will keep each other's confidences.

- *Multicultural awareness.* The group leader has a powerful role in influencing the values of the group process. It is imperative that group facilitators be aware of the cultural backgrounds of their members and ensure that the group process respects those backgrounds.[2]

  With regard to ethics concerning group leaders' actions, perhaps the most important issue is that of blending social or personal relationships with professional ones. In this realm, there are three major issues to consider:

- *Personal relationships between leaders and members.* Personal or social relationships are not appropriate with group members if the relationship interferes with the group process. These relationships are harmful if they interfere with the facilitator's objectivity or professional judgment, or if they affect the group member's ability to fully participate in the group. Facilitators should not use their leadership role to meet their personal needs.

- *Socializing among group members.* Members meeting outside of the group often interferes with the group process and can be counterproductive. The work of the group often stops if cliques form or members gossip outside of the group. A group facilitator can prevent this by bringing up the issue in the first meeting and exploring the negative impact this type of socializing might have. If, in fact, members do meet outside of the group, the facilitator must make them aware of their responsibility to bring the information from that meeting to the group.

- *Leaders' values and their impact on the group.* Group facilitators must be aware of how their values influence their behavior, and, in group, their leadership style. Group facilitators should not use the group to advance their own personal agenda or impose their views on members. Support groups should be a forum for members to explore their own cultural values and beliefs. Facilitators should also be aware of and monitor how their personal reactions to members might affect the group process.[18]

Other ethical issues might arise. If the facilitator is not sure how to handle these situations, he or she should seek advice from a professional counselor or a legal advisor and adhere to the health education professional code of ethics.

Overcoming Challenges to Effective Support Groups

Support group facilitators will almost always face two major barriers—problem members and attrition (loss of group members). The success of the group depends on how well the facilitators handle these potential barriers and others that may emerge. Facilitators should think about these barriers and prepare for them in advance to ensure an effective group process.

Deal with Problem Members

All groups have problem members. The following subsections describe three of the most common types of problem members and suggest how a facilitator might handle their disruptive behavior.[19]

The Monopolist

This member is the biggest problem in most groups and the most difficult with which to deal. This person is motivated by anxiety and a need for attention and control. Monopolists are anxious if they are silent, so they tend to respond to every statement.

Effect on group. At first the group welcomes and encourages the monopolist. Later they experience anger and frustration.

Facilitator role. Begin by asking the group why they allow one member to carry the burden of the whole group, which may encourage more passive members to participate. Keep the monopolist on task and encourage others to talk. This can be accomplished by reframing what the monopolist has said to make it more meaningful to the discussion or by asking other members for their reaction to what the monopolist has said. The facilitator may also be very direct and thank the monopolist for his or her contribution, but state that others also need to be heard. The point is not to silence the monopolist, but to make the interaction more meaningful.

The Silent Member

This member is less disruptive than the monopolist, but equally challenging. This person is motivated by fears of disclosure, not being perfect, confrontation, and other members.

Effect on group.   The silent member is not valued by the group and may be accepted, ignored, or resented.

Facilitator role.   Do not unduly pressure a silent member to speak, but comment on nonverbal cues and ask him or her for verification. Also ask the group for their perception of the effect on the group of the silent member's behavior. It is important that the group and the facilitators do not negatively judge the silent member's lack of participation. Many times silent members begin participating when they see they will not be judged and begin to feel safe in the group.

The Help-Rejecting Complainer

This member requests help from the group and then rejects it. This person tends to take pride in insurmountable problems and feels that his or her problems are the most important and the most difficult. Motivation stems from feelings of dependency and a need for attention.

Effect on group.   The group generally becomes bored, frustrated, and impatient. They feel if the group is not working for this person, the person should drop out.

Facilitator role.   This member is looking to validate a sense of self-worth and is not really interested in solutions to his or her problems. Listening and empathizing with this member, rather than offering solutions, is sometimes helpful. Facilitators may also reframe the member's rejection of help and ask the group for other suggestions that might be considered at a later date.

Maintain Attendance

Dealing with attendance and attrition issues is an important challenge for facilitators. These issues include members dropping out of group, attending group sporadically, or attending group but not participating. When attendance becomes a problem, group leaders should address the issue by asking participants what barriers have disrupted their attendance. This may be done in-group with those who attend intermittently, or with a call or letter to those who no longer participate. There are many reasons why people miss or stop attending group meetings. They may have experienced critical life incidents or felt they did not connect with other group members. Tracking this type of information provides feedback for group facilitators that may enable them to modify the group to better meet member expectations. When ongoing, open support groups struggle to retain members, there is also the option of discontinuing the group or changing the focus, depending on the needs of the participants. Excessive absenteeism or attrition will cause discomfort among group members, so these problems must be dealt with in an open and honest way.

Did You Know

The Alcoholics Anonymous movement that began in the 1930s has become one of the most successful of all community support groups. Its success rate in keeping members sober is based on members sharing experiences, offering support, and learning from each other.

Expected Outcomes

Human beings are social, interdependent individuals. Although the extent of interdependence varies from culture to culture and from family to family, people generally assist one another in obtaining their most basic needs. Structured groups are an example of this interdependence. Psychological and interpersonal needs for affiliation, power, affection, and social support can all be achieved through group interaction.[20] Irvin Yalom, the well-known group theorist and practitioner, cited 11 therapeutic or **curative factors** that may result from group work, including instillation of hope, universality, imparting information, altruism, the corrective recapitulation of the primary family group, development of socializing techniques, imitative behaviors, interpersonal learning, group cohesiveness, catharsis, and existential factors.[21] These aspects of group experience vary from group to group depending on the group's topic, structure, and overall dynamics. Not all curative factors are appropriate for every group. For example, a group may be successful without ever expressing strong emotional feelings.

Although the focus of Yalom's work is psychotherapy groups, several of the curative factors are significant in community-based support groups as well. Health educators who are facilitating support groups may want to focus on instilling hope in their members. When participants have hope that they can improve, their confidence level increases and they are more likely to try new behaviors. The role of the facilitator is to point out the positive changes being made by group members and to encourage group members to support each other as they begin to progress toward their goals.

Universality is another curative factor that is especially powerful in a group experience. The role of the facilitator is to help members see the commonality of their problems. As Yalom stated, "There is no human deed or thought which is fully outside the experience of others."[21] Members feel a sense of worth and interrelatedness when they feel that others share their same obstacles and concerns.

Community connections 4

Kendra and Ricardo met before their last group session. Many of the members had expressed a sadness that the group was ending because they felt they would lose the peer support they had learned to rely on. "Well," said Kendra, "maybe we could plan a social get-together some Friday night and get together for pizza." "That's a great idea. We could have each student talk about what benefited them most from this group," added Ricardo, "and perhaps strategize about things they could do on their own to keep them smoke free."

"Well, from my own perspective," said Kendra, "I think the most important things they seemed to have gotten from group were a belief that they really could quit smoking and the realization that they were all in the same boat. Most of their reasons for smoking and the problems they had in trying to quit were similar. Based on that commonality, they really did reach out and support each other in their attempt to stop smoking."

"Plus," added Ricardo, "I think we gave them a lot of valuable information, especially the idea that if they stop now, they can reverse much of the damage smoking has done to their bodies. Even though not all of them have quit completely, they seem motivated to keep trying."

"You know," said Kendra, "even though we had some problems with some of the members, like Jennifer, the group handled them well. Jennifer seemed to have the most and the biggest problems, which for a while seemed insurmountable. But, I think, after listening to the others and realizing that maybe some of their suggestions would work for her, she actually started to try to take responsibility for solving some of her issues."

"We were lucky. The group became pretty cohesive and I think they learned a lot about themselves from this experience," commented Ricardo. "Let's schedule a follow-up meeting in about a month to see how well they are doing. They probably won't feel so abandoned if they know we will get together again."

"Good idea," said Kendra. "Now let's go meet with them and wrap this up."

Imparting information is probably the foundation of most health education support groups. The facilitator and the group members are able to share their combined knowledge and experience with each other. Group satisfaction, insight, and behavioral change often occur when people have new knowledge, combined with opportunities for social interaction. For example, a health educator leading a group for partners of HIV-positive people found that dedicating time for advice and information about medical developments and community services, as well as providing time for communicating with providers, increased the level of satisfaction and expression within the group. Additionally, studies of women diagnosed with cancer who attended support groups have shown they were less depressed and anxious, had more knowledge about their illness and treatment, had a more positive view of health care providers, and were better adjusted to their illness than those who did not attend such groups.[22]

One other curative factor important in support groups is that of interpersonal learning. Participating in a group provides members with the unique opportunity to see themselves through the eyes of others in a safe environment. The facilitator should encourage members to give realistic feedback to each other as they share experiences or emotions. It is also the role of the facilitator to ensure that the environment is safe for such sharing. A safe environment can be created from the beginning by establishing norms that forbid personal attacks or derogatory comments.

Interpersonal learning also takes place when the facilitator works to keep members focused on the present. Working within the here and now increases the effectiveness and power of the group so that members are able to experience new levels of awareness in the group and in their present lives. By reminding participants that they cannot change the past but that they can learn in the moment and move forward in the future, facilitators are more likely to contribute to successful outcomes for group members.

Conclusion

Learning to facilitate effective health-centered support groups is a valuable skill for all health educators. Regardless of the health education setting or the health-related topic, most clients benefit from a group experience. Group members create a miniature society in which they feel a sense of belonging. They are able to share common problems and receive feedback and support that may not be available in their real lives. Members broaden their views of themselves and are able to observe and imitate new coping behaviors. Groups enhance self-exploration and introspection and increase self-confidence. And, from an agency point of view, groups are economically advantageous. More people can be helped for less time and money. Health educators should consider group work as a cornerstone in creating healthy communities.

KEY TERMS

asynchronous: Exchanges occurring in non-real time, such as bulletin boards and discussion groups.

curative factors: Factors that contribute to the acquisition of knowledge, skills, and greater interpersonal insight as a result of interaction in a group experience.

ending stage: The stage in which members face the issues of anxiety regarding the ending of the group experience. Also known as termination.

facilitator: Group leader who keeps the group on task and acts as a catalyst to move the group forward toward its goal.

informed consent: Voluntary participation in a group based on clear and accurate information as to the purpose and the structure of the group.

initial (forming) stage: The first stage in the group process, in which members evaluate each other and the group and begin establishing norms. Also known as the forming stage.

norms: Ideas that members have about what behaviors are appropriate in group for themselves and for other members.

ongoing groups: Groups that have no specified ending date. These groups continue until the task is completed, members drop out, or the program is discontinued. These groups generally address chronic mental or physical illnesses or addictions.

selective perception: A strategy that new group members use to help them deal with the fear and anxiety that usually occur as a new group meets.

support group: A structured group that focuses on a specific problem, task, or theme.

synchronous: Real-time exchanges, such as an online chat.

time-limited groups: Groups that have predetermined beginning and ending dates. These are groups that generally address symptom relief, problem solving, development of interpersonal skills, or patient education.

transition stage: The "storming" stage of the group process, in which members begin to raise issues, challenge each other and the facilitators, and perhaps struggle for control and power.

working (performing) stage: Occurs after the "storming" stage has been resolved. In this stage members begin to work productively in addressing personal change, skills development, and knowledge gain in order to accomplish the goals of the group. Also known as the performing stage.

universality: An important curative factor whereby members feel a sense of interconnectedness by seeing that others share the same obstacles and concerns.

REFERENCES

1. Gladding, S. T. (1995). *Group work: A counseling specialty* (2nd ed.). Englewood Cliffs, NJ: Prentice-Hall.

2. Corey, M. S., & Corey, G. (1997). *Groups: Process and practice* (5th ed.). Pacific Grove, CA: Brooks/Cole.

3. Peterson, J. V., & Nisenholz, B. (1995). *Orientation to counseling* (3rd ed.). Boston: Allyn and Bacon.

4. Stewart, D., & Thomson, K. The Face Your Fear club: Therapeutic group work with young children as a response to community trauma in Northern Ireland. *Child Care in Practice, 11*(2), 191–209.

5. Kominars, K., & Dornheim, L. (2004). Group approaches in substance abuse treatment. In J. L. DeLucia-Waack, D. A. Gerrity, C. R. Kalodner, & M. T. Riva (Eds.), *Handbook of group counseling and psychotherapy.* Thousand Oaks, CA: Sage Publications.

6. Weiss, R. D., Jaffee, W. B., de Menil, V. P., & Cogley, C. B. (2004). Group therapy for substance use disorders: What do we know? *Harvard Review of Psychiatry, 12*, 339–350.

7. Klaw, E., & Humphreys, K. (2004). The role of peer-led mutual help groups in promoting health and well-being. In J. L. DeLucia-Waack, D. A. Gerrity, C. R. Kalodner, & M. T. Riva (Eds.), *Handbook of group counseling and psychotherapy*. Thousand Oaks, CA: Sage Publications.

8. Dadich, A. (2006). Self-help support groups: Adding to the toolbox of mental health care options for young men. *Youth Studies Australia, 25*, 33–41.

9. Lieberman, M. A., & Goldstein, B. A. (2005). Self-help on-line: An outcome evaluation of breast cancer bulletin boards. *Journal of Health Psychology, 10*, 855–862.

10. Coulson, N. S. (2005). Receiving social support online: An analysis of a computer-mediated support group for individuals living with irritable bowel syndrome. *CyberPsychology & Behavior, 8*, 580–584.

11. Beder, J. (2005). Cybersolace: Technology built on emotion. *Social Work, 50*, 355–358.

12. Page, B. J. (2004). Online group counseling. In J. L. DeLucia-Waack, D. A. Gerrity, C. R. Kalodner, & M. T. Riva (Eds.), *Handbook of group counseling and psychotherapy*. Thousand Oaks, CA: Sage Publications.

13. Forsyth, D. R. (2004). Therapeutic groups. In M. Brewer (Ed.), *Applied social psychology*. Oxford, England: Blackwell Publishing.

14. Olsson, C. A., Boyce, M. F., Toumbourou, J. W., & Sawyer, S. M. (2005). The role of peer support in facilitating psychosocial adjustment to chronic illness in adolescence. *Clinical Child Psychology and Psychiatry, 10*, 78–87.

15. Bennis, W., & Nanus, B. (1985). *Leaders: The strategies for taking charge*. New York: Harper & Row.

16. Johnson, D., & Johnson, F. (1997). *Joining together: Group theory and group skills*. Boston: Allyn and Bacon.

17. Napier, R., & Gershenfeld, M. (1993). *Groups: Theory and experience* (5th ed.). Boston: Houghton Mifflin.

18. Corey, G. (2000). *Theory and practice of group counseling* (5th ed.). Pacific Grove, CA: Brooks/Cole.

19. Yalom, I. D. (1975). *The theory and practice of group psychotherapy* (2nd ed.). New York: Basic Books.

20. Forsyth, D. R. (1990). *Group dynamics* (2nd ed.). Pacific Grove, CA: Brooks/Cole.

21. Yalom, I. D. (2005). *The theory and practice of group psychotherapy* (5th ed). New York: Basic Books.

22. Ahlberg, K., & Nordner, A. (2006). The importance of participation in support groups for women with ovarian cancer. *Oncology Nursing Forum, 33*(4), 52–61.

ADDITIONAL RESOURCES

Internet

American Psychological Association. Available: http://www.apa.org. (Provides extensive material for group work within group therapy and support group venues.)

International Association for Facilitators. Available: http://www.iaf-world/org. (Provides a journal titled *Group Facilitation: A Research and Applications Journal*.)

Center for Continuing Education in the Health Sciences. Available: http://www.hitchcock.org/pages/ceb/cce.html. (Provides information about a collaborative effort with Dartmouth-Hitchcock Medical Center.)

Local county and state Web sites. (These often offer information such as different local support groups and facilitator training opportunities.)

7

Selecting Presentation Methods

Keely S. Rees, Ph.D., CHES
Malcolm Goldsmith, Ph.D., CHES

Author Comments

Having polished presentation skills is of utmost importance; however, over the years, we have found that the preparation steps and methods chosen are what enhance a presentation. As educators, we often teach students public speaking skills as well as health content. We then ask them to give presentations in a variety of settings, and we emphasize the importance of planning, organizing, and preparing methods to use for the presentation. This is a difficult process, at times, even for seasoned professionals. In the diverse school and community settings in which we have worked, we have found that the combination of changing populations and emerging educational technologies challenges us to spend more time in the preparation of meaningful presentations.

Introduction

Health educators utilize presentations for imparting information in almost every setting in which they work. How they go about presenting the information is known as the **method**, which is traditionally defined as a systematic approach or procedure that is specifically carried out or conducted by teachers, presenters, and speakers to disseminate information, objectives, and lesson materials.[1] A method can also refer to a specific part of the intervention, lesson, or presentation.[2] In essence, it is the methods of the presentation that dictate how well information is received and retained. Over the years, the education field has studied and determined what types of methods are successful and appropriate based on content, settings, and audiences. These findings have become essential for health educators in terms of choosing appropriate methods for their presentations.

Community connections 1

Natalie, a new health educator for a rural county health department, was hired to work with local public school teachers and to provide a series of mandatory in-service trainings on a number of health topics throughout the school year. Approximately 150 teachers would be attending the in-services every nine weeks. Her first presentation was to be about at-risk youth in the local community and what teachers should be aware of regarding substance abuse and violent behaviors.

Six months ago, Natalie had presented to high school coaches on substance abuse and athletic performance, so she felt she already had most of the material prepared. She did, however, search the Internet for additional resources dealing with high-risk youth that could be shared with the teachers. The night before the presentation, she frantically pulled together the presentation, telling herself she was the type who "worked best under pressure." She assumed she would be able to divide the participants into small groups to create an informal workshop environment. Upon arrival, however, she found that all 150 of the teachers were in the school's auditorium. She was to speak on a stage, with a microphone, with the teachers seated theater style in the darkened room.

Needless to say, Natalie's first in-service training did not go well. Teachers were daydreaming, engaging in small talking circles, and grading papers. Her evaluations consisted of many negative comments, some of which were constructive criticism. What a disappointment! Natalie knew the audience was not engaged due to the type of presentation method she used—formal lecture. Thus, the teachers left feeling bored and frustrated, not having learned any new skills or information. How could Natalie better prepare for the next teacher in-service, which was designed to focus on stress management and coping mechanisms?

Whether presentations are delivered in a school or community setting, in small or large groups, or across diverse content areas, health educators should first address what information is to be disseminated and then how it can best be presented. The methods chosen should be congruent with the objectives and overall goal of the lesson plan, agenda, or workshop. This component of the preparation stage of health education presentations is often overlooked. Content or information can be delivered in a polished manner by a competent and dynamic speaker, but if the health material presented is not given in a meaningful and insightful manner, the audience will be less engaged in the learning process. The health educator can transfer information in hopes the audience or students will *learn* it, but it is much more likely that participants will turn this knowledge into actual *skills* if they are engaged in the process. This chapter addresses how to choose appropriate methods based on the target audience; the content area, setting, and objectives of a presentation; the importance of choosing methods from a theoretical perspective; and what health educators can expect from using certain methods.

Steps for Selecting and Implementing Presentation Methods

In many health education programs, there are situations in which limited learning occurs, yet the educator is very popular simply because of the way he or she teaches. Selecting fun or popular teaching methods, however, is not always in the best interest of the target audience. Selecting appropriate teaching methods is first and foremost about utilizing processes that will help achieve desired program goals and objectives. This is not to say that methods cannot be fun, but rather that their selection should be part of a planning process that reflects both theoretical and ethical elements. The following steps are essential in helping health educators select presentation methods that can enhance program goals, achieve targeted objectives, and ensure that ethical codes of conduct are followed.

Understand the Assets and Needs of the Focus Population

The significance of assessing assets and needs for health education and promotion program planning has been well documented.[3–6] As one of the major areas of responsibility for health education professionals, needs assessment provides the foundation for program planning, including presentation planning.

Needs assessments can be used in several ways to aid the selection of appropriate presentation methods. First and foremost, they can provide direction for matching objectives to the selection of methods. For example, data gathered during a needs assessment may reveal a problem with asthma among children and adolescents in the community. The data may also reveal that many working parents are sending their sick children, who often lack self-care skills, to school. Presentation methods that allow children and parents to learn together, such as computer-based and experiential problem solving, could accomplish several objectives.

Assessments can also be utilized to better understand the learning styles of a given population, such as those measured by the Multiple Intelligences of Learning (MIL).[7] This type of assessment helps presenters understand how individuals prefer to learn (e.g., visual, kinesthetic, verbal, interpersonal, intrapersonal, logical-mathematical, musical, or naturalistic). Methods suitable to identified learning styles can then be incorporated into the presentation plan. Focusing on the

Did You Know

Learners retain

5% from lecture

10% from reading

20% from audiovisual materials

30% from demonstration

50% from discussion

75% from practice by doing

90% by teaching others or some other immediate use of the learning

Source: Cohen, M. (1991). A comprehensive approach to effective staff development: Essential components. Presented at Education Development Center, meeting for Comprehensive School Health Education Training Centers, Cambridge, MA.

audience's assets, or what they understand or engage in already, can provide the educator with key insights when planning the methods and presentations. For example, today's adolescents are adept and competent with technology, so incorporating the use of Web-enhanced activities, video streaming, or handheld computers could enhance the overall seminar, lesson, or training. Educators can also use assessments to select methods more suitably matched to other needs of the target audience. For example, proper use of appraisal scales and inventories helps both participants and educators gain insights about learning, as well as plays a role in both motivating learners and guiding program direction. Surveys and appraisals may also reveal cultural, geographic, religious, or other preferences that can affect the selection of appropriate methods.

The identification of the environmental, social, and cultural factors that influence participant health behaviors is often part of a formal assets and needs assessment, but this information may also be found by reviewing the literature associated with a target population. Specific social, cultural, and environmental factors that can be examined include social and peer influences, support systems, available resources, knowledge and education, health history, accessibility, affordability, cultural and subcultural norms, and environmental influences. Knowledge of these factors along with other needs assessment data should be used to develop meaningful goals and objectives and guide method selection.

For example, in a community with a very high and growing incidence of sexually transmitted infections (STIs), one of the targeted populations might be youth and young adults ages 12 to 24. An examination of social, cultural, and environmental factors may reveal an environment in which there is a lack of supervision of young children, dating pressure and exposure to older youth, abstinence-only education programs in schools, limited access to condoms, and poor access to clinics and treatment. Further assessment could reveal that most of the target population does not perceive a risk of getting an STI from their behavior or see severe health consequences. Many may be engaging only in oral sex and believe that STIs can only be acquired from intercourse. Some know about the dangers of STIs but believe that you can tell who has them. In this instance, it is clear that simple educational messages about the dangers of STIs will not be enough to influence behavior. Presentations developed to deal with this issue need to incorporate multiple presentation methods that target myths, lesser-known facts, and insights. Presentations that highlight real case studies, examine epidemiological data, and help develop skills in reducing exposure to STIs could be employed. Hands-on methods to make people comfortable and knowledgeable about seeking treatment and discussing contacts could also be helpful.

Develop Meaningful Goals and Objectives to Guide Selection of Methods

Goals are general statements of the desired outcomes of a program. They are primarily long term and provide the ultimate direction to which all objectives should be targeted. The creation of goals and **objectives** allows the presenter to determine exactly what it is he or she wants participants to take away from the session. Without a plan of where one wants to go, it is highly unlikely a presenter will systematically affect a group. Failure to develop meaningful goals and objectives also creates an environment in which presenters will be unable to effectively evaluate a presentation's impact.

The connection between objectives and presentation methods requires the health educator to assess the relevant content (information) and skills that are part of the presentation. Well-written objectives make it clear to both the target

Community connections 2

In reflecting on her negative experience from her first teacher training, Natalie concluded that for her second training she would communicate with school officials on what objectives the in-service was designed to meet and assess what the teachers already knew about stress and coping skills. In addition, she would assess the cultural and social factors affecting teachers, instead of making assumptions. Because she was a county health department worker, she would have easy access to county morbidity and mortality rates. She would also speak with school administrators regarding the school's social atmosphere, and would spend time with teachers to better determine the types of stresses they were specifically experiencing in their classrooms. This background information would better prepare her for identifying information about stress that would be beneficial for the teachers, as well as the types of coping skills they could be taught.

audience and the presenter exactly what is expected. Once these are developed, the health educator needs to know how to successfully achieve objectives. In theory, the task of the presenter becomes relatively simple: How does a health educator provide the needed components to enable participants to achieve the desired objective? In reality, the task is very complex because of a multitude of variables, including (1) ownership of the objective (participants or educators), (2) length of the program (one time versus ongoing), (3) complexity of the objective, (4) abilities and experience of individual participants, (5) structure of the program (e.g., individual, group, makeup of group), (6) attitude of the participants (e.g., forced participation versus free selection, self-efficacy), and (7) learning styles of participants (e.g., multiple intelligences, cultural influences).

Consider a meaningful analogy to a task many college students may find difficult: cooking. The objective is to teach someone to successfully follow directions and bake a six-layer cake. For some people, following baking directions is simple. Others have problems when attempting to bake. The presenter needs to decide what method or methods should be used to teach cake baking. Reexamination of the variables listed previously can help the presenter determine how these might affect the methods chosen. So, if the students really wanted to bake a cake, would any of these variables affect their effort? If, for example, the presenter only had 30 minutes to teach baking to students, would it have an impact on the end result? Does the fact that there are six layers to this cake influence the task? If the participant never so much as cooked an egg, would it influence the methods chosen? If there were 30 people in the class, should the educator conduct the class differently? If the individual was forced to participate in the class, what might the educator do differently in the presentation?

These questions can also be asked by a health educator when determining what variables may affect a health education presentation and thus the methods chosen for the presentation. Consider the plight of a health educator trying to teach a person newly diagnosed with asthma to adjust to asthma, both to prevent complications and to enjoy quality of life. What variables or factors would affect the selection of objectives and subsequent presentation methods? Looking at the baking example, issues of time, patient attitude, class size, and complexity of the asthma are some variables that must be taken into account.

Identify and Select Appropriate Presentation Methods

It is important to recognize the link between the objectives, content, and methods. The objectives represent the tasks to achieve. The content reflects the information to impart to participants in order to accomplish the objectives. Methods become the critical strategies for delivering the content and, subsequently, helping participants achieve the objectives. A presentation outline or **plan** encapsulates these concepts and provides direction for the presentation. Figure 7-1 provides a sample presentation outline for the initial session of a ten-week stress management program.

Presentation methods offer the educator great flexibility in designing programs. It is important to recognize that there are many ways to address the targeted content and achieve objectives. Sometimes educators are presented with learners or audiences who are not responding to one or more of the chosen presentation methods. By being flexible and having alternative methods readily available that match the learning objective, the educator will be able to quickly replace the original method with an alternative. Table 7-1 lists various presentation methods available to health educators.

In addition to changing the type of methods used, one can also alter the sequencing (order) of the methods. Health educators should select methods

Target Audience: In-Service Teachers
Topic: Stress Management
Objectives
1. Participants will identify four common stress problems experienced by teachers and students. (knowledge)
2. Participants will discuss how stress has affected their roles as teachers and affirm their motivation for the program by discussing two reasons they want to participate in this program. (attitude)
3. Participants will develop a stress management plan. (skill)

Key Content
1. Definitions of stress
   Types of stressors
   Effects of stress
   Coping strategies
   Preventing stress

2. Possible motivations
   Have more energy
   Improve body image
   Improve self-esteem
   Reduce health risks
   Improve life expectancy
   Ease pain

3. Elements of coping skills
   Different types of techniques
   Massage therapy
   Music and relaxation exercises
   Exercise
   Diaphragmatic breathing
   Meditation skills
   Journaling

Methods

Method	Content Focus	Instructional Aids	Time
Lecture/Discussion	Defining stress Effects of stress	Handout	30
Brainstorm/ Lecture	How stress affects teacher and student performance Motivation for reducing stress	Overhead	15
PowerPoint/ Music	Overload stress	Computer/ Overhead	10
Break			10
Small group work	Stress management strategies Stress management planning	Butcher paper	25
Group discussion	Strategies Potential obstacles to implementing		15
Closure	Key concepts learned		15

Figure 7-1 Presentation Outline

Table 7-1	Potential Presentation Methods	
Method	Focus	Characteristics and Comments
Appraisals or inventories	Assessment of needs, attitudes, behavior, interests, skills	Provides quick overview and on-the-spot assessment; be wary of reliability and validity issues
Audiovisuals	Cassettes, slides, overheads, posters, displays, books	Works for multiple intelligences (MI)
Brainstorming	Group participation; quick generation of ideas	Avoid discussion; seek total involvement
Case studies	Review and critique true event	Aids analytical thinking
Computer-based	CD-ROM, software programs, Internet-based assignments, chat rooms	Hits MI; can be dynamic; need to validate accuracy; may require training
Critical incidents	Similar to case study, but without ending; can be made up	Provides critical thinking and problem-solving skills
Debates	Explore both sides of an issue (e.g., drug laws, abortion, teen rights, health care, advertising)	Works best with structure
Demonstrations	Provide visual performance of a skill (e.g., first aid, self-care, computer skills, cooking)	Helps visual learners; aids skill development
Dramatizations or skits	Can be scripted or improved	Works best with active participants and practice
Experiments	Can be done in session or on own	Ethical concerns; ranges from simple to complex
Fishbowls	Small inner circle discusses topic; outer circle can critique or partner up	Variation of debate
Games	Model TV games or be creative	Helpful review of material; fun
Large group discussion	Follow-up or part of lecture; can be structured or unstructured	Allows for questions; opportunity to check for learning

Table 7-1	Potential Presentation Methods (Continued)	
Method	Focus	Characteristics and Comments
Lecture	Knowledge; attitudes	One-dimensional; verbal learners
Problem solving	Focus on dilemmas such as peer pressure, conflicts, stress	Helps to use problem-solving models
Role playing	Participants act out scenarios; can be totally, partially, or not structured	Remind them it is a role; voluntary; needs processing
Sentence completion	Participants complete sentences with health implications	Follow-up discussion needed to process
Skill practice	Follow-up to demonstrations; pairing of learners helpful	Provide feedback; sequence properly
Small group discussion	Participants address issue prior to or as a follow-up to lecture or large group discussion	Have clear directions; move around groups to assist; keep focused
Values clarification	Participants choose sides or rank priorities	Helps clarify priorities for different dilemmas; often situational

that add variety to programs. It is wise to avoid the overuse of one method (e.g., lecture, video, group work) in order to maintain the attention of the audience. Methods that focus on skills should occur after the participants have adequate tools (e.g., knowledge, observations) to address skill-based activities. This is not to say, however, that an educator could not first try a skills-based activity, using it almost as a pretest. One example of this could occur when teaching about healthy eating. First the presenter could teach about what is desired in a healthy meal. The presenter could follow up with skills for reading labels and selecting healthy foods from the grocery store or when dining out. An activity could include a meal being planned or selected and then analyzed for its nutritional content to see how well the audience did in its selections. Additionally a pretest could be administered to assess present eating practices, to be compared with the new choices made after being educated. In this case the presenter would have used inventories, lecture, group work to analyze labels, individual or paired meal planning, and other methods to carry out these plans.

Although there are logical sequencing guidelines, it is beneficial for an educator to be prepared with a variety of presentation methods, to adjust to the dynamics of the group, and to not be afraid to experiment with sequencing of the methods. By following these guidelines, presenters will increase the likelihood of reaching their objectives and engaging the learner or audience.

Methods can effectively serve a variety of purposes. While the primary purpose is to support the attainment of objectives, methods can also be selected to address skills, influence the climate of the room, affect relationships, target learning styles, and address emotions. It is helpful for educators, new or seasoned, to be reminded of methods that address these specific presentation issues. Table 7-2 provides examples that can be used in special situations.

Many presentation methods exist other than those listed in Tables 7-1 and 7-2. The types of methods used are restricted only by a lack of presenter creativity. Being creative as a presenter is less about innate talent and more about hard work. The presenter must think of different ways to present the

Table 7-2   Presentation Methods for Special Situations
Methods to Liven up Audience
Audiovisuals, computer-based, debates, demonstrations, fishbowl, games, role playing, skits
Methods to Confront Conflict or Attitudes
Case studies, critical incidents, debates, fishbowl, role playing, skits, values clarification
Methods to Support Problem Solving
Brainstorming, case studies, computer-based, critical incidents, demonstrations, experiments, problem solving, sentence completion, small group work
Methods to Reach Emotions
Audiovisuals, case studies, critical incidents, fishbowl, role playing
Methods to Develop Skills
Computer-based, demonstrations, experiments, games, problem solving, role playing, skill practice
Methods to Enhance Cognitive Thinking
Brainstorming, critical incidents, debates, experiments, games, large group discussion, lecture, problem solving, small group discussion
Methods Suitable to Multiple Intelligences
Audiovisuals, computer-based, demonstrations, role playing, skill practice, skits
Methods to Build Interpersonal Skills
Debates, games, group experiments, role playing, skits, small group discussion

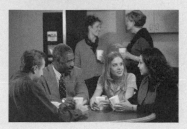

Community
connections 3

To aid in the preparation for her in-service presentation on stress for teachers, Natalie decided she must not only access the Internet, but also talk with teachers and school administrators. She would also look to other resources in her community, such as the county health department, health agencies, and other colleagues.

material and get the audience involved, and must try different methods to see what works best. He or she should also utilize the insights gained from needs assessments, as well as the results of both formal and informal evaluations of the program. It is not always the method that is "good" or "bad," but the dynamic makeup of an audience and how a presenter relates to the members. Factors such as age, gender, motivation for attendance, ethnicity, and time of day, among others, have the potential to affect the success of methods.

Gather Resources to Aid Program Implementation of Methods

The successful development and implementation of methods requires access to needed resources. These resources can provide the inspiration for ideas, be the method itself (e.g., CDs, audiovisual material), act as supplements to the method (e.g., handouts, pamphlets, data), and aid in ensuring that content delivered is accurate and up-to-date. Many resources are available at the local, regional, state, and national levels. Health education texts usually provide appendices that list resources.

Health educators should check that resources are accurate, up-to-date, and appropriate for the audience. While it is sometimes difficult to determine the accuracy of resource materials, their value can be determined through author credentials, evidence of peer review, and consistency with similar resources.

The proliferation of material on the Internet, along with its vast use, presents great opportunity as well as potential problems. The fact that anyone can create a Web site and call it the "Office on Scientific Health Research" warrants caution. Thus, the information found on the Web should be evaluated for accuracy and appropriateness by utilizing the same criteria as previously mentioned for any resource. Table 7-3 lists URLs that provide links to many meaningful Web sites that contain resources for presentation methods.

Table 7-3	Web Sites Containing Helpful Presentation Resources

Center for Research on Learning and Teaching
http://www.crlt.umich.edu/tstrategies/teachings.html

PBS Teacher Source
http://www.pbs.org/teachersource/health_fitness/high-nutrition.html

Center for Application of Prevention Technologies
http://modelprograms.samhsa.gov/template_cf.cfm?page=model_list

Health Finder
http://www.healthfinder.gov

Health Teacher
http://www.healthteacher.com/

Guidelines for Health Education and Risk Reduction
http://aepo-xdv-www.epo.cdc.gov/wonder/prevguid/p0000389/p0000389.htm

Association for Supervision and Curriculum Development
http://www.ascd.org/

Wired for Health
http://www.wiredforhealth.gov.uk/

Evaluate the Effectiveness of Methods

The importance of utilizing input from participants about presentation methods cannot be overstated. Participant feedback is particularly valuable in gathering information about how to improve programmatic efforts. Information related to the appropriateness of objectives, content, and methods should be collected. It is also critical, though not discussed here, to collect evaluation data on impact objectives. When collecting data, it is desirable to avoid yes-or-no responses and helpful to allow for subjective comments about the methods used in the presentation. This process evaluation typically occurs in the form of objective and subjective responses. Figure 7-2 provides sample items for a process evaluation of presentation methods.

Properly conducted, evaluation can provide further insights into the needs of participants, as well as their perspectives on the value of various methods employed in the session. Educators must be careful in their interpretation of evaluation results, since they often can be quite confusing. For example, an instructor could read 25 objective evaluations and find that 5 participants indicated the methods were fantastic, 5 stated they were horrible, and 15 were neutral as to the usefulness of the presentation methods. In cases such as these, the subjective comments become increasingly important because they could provide specific details regarding what was liked or disliked or what could be done to improve

Specific Statements Related to the Objective Evaluation of Methods

Please rate the following items according to the following scale:

5	Strongly agree
4	Agree
3	Neutral
2	Disagree
1	Strongly disagree

____   Methods utilized helped me to better understand the material.
____   Methods utilized helped me to improve skills in _____.
____   Methods utilized were appropriate for my desired learning style.
____   Methods utilized were helpful in staying focused on the presentation.
____   Methods utilized made it easy to become involved in the learning process.
____   Methods utilized allowed me to ask questions and seek additional information.
____   The session was presented at a level appropriate for my needs.
____   Resources and materials provided during the session were important to my understanding of the material.
____   The instructor provided clear directions for completing program tasks.
____   Methods utilized were significant in helping me to complete the program's objectives.
____   Methods utilized demonstrated an understanding of the needs of the audience.

Specific Statements Related to the Subjective Evaluation of Methods

Please provide feedback on the following items:

Describe what learning experiences were most valuable to you in this program and why.

Describe what learning experiences were least valuable to you in this program and why.

What suggestions do you have for improving the methods used in this program?

Figure 7-2 Sample Process Evaluation Items for Presentation Methods

Community connections 4

Even in the first in-service, Natalie was proud of her evaluation efforts. By conducting a process evaluation at the end of the in-service, she was able to glean some valuable insight on how to improve her presentation. As deflated as she felt after reading the evalu- ations, a week later she was able to value the honest comments and suggestions, and she took the opportunity to seek the advice of her mentors and peers in the field. The evaluation process was very important in directing her next presentation.

the session. It is equally important for presenters to critique themselves and to make use of peer evaluation. In being open to such honest reviews, it is likely a health educator will find ways to enhance presentation efforts.

Evaluation can also make for more effective presentations through emulation. There is nothing wrong with scanning the literature for presentation-based programs that work as long as they are based on audiences similar to the one targeted in the presenter's program, or they can be effectively modified to work with the needs of the target population. Public health literature is full of tried and tested programs. Health educators should learn from history and continue to improve upon existing methods.

Tips and Techniques for Selecting Presentation Methods

While experience is often the best teacher for presenters, a number of strategies can help increase the probability of conducting a successful presentation. This section discusses four techniques that will aid presenters in developing lessons and learning experiences that are likely to achieve desired outcomes and to be valued by participants.

Match Methods to Content, Presenter Expertise, and Audience Needs

Matching methods to content comes from having a clear idea of what information should be delivered, how in-depth the presentation will be, and what developmental stage the audience represents. Health content varies so greatly (from impersonal to very personal) that educators need to be aware of what methods will best blend with the audience and materials. For example, sexuality educators teach material that touches on values, beliefs, and attitudes regarding personal information. The methods used in these programs need to gradually progress from less threatening to more in-depth activities. The educator needs to do this without running the risk of offending the audience by using methods deemed as inappropriate.

Community connections 5

Natalie realized she made mistakes in her first presentation by using only lecture-style presentation methods in a dark auditorium, which did not allow for interaction, facilitation of discussion, or small group activities. The teachers had come to the presentation wanting to be engaged and to learn something valuable for use in the classroom. For her next presentation, Natalie felt that matching her methods and content with audience needs would almost guarantee a better response from the teachers.

Certain methods may be acceptable to one culture or group while being completely unacceptable to others. Health information is closely tied to one's values, beliefs, cultural nuances, geographical issues, and other personal attributes. Thus, it is the educator's responsibility before using a method to ensure that it is respectful and in accordance with the majority of the participants. Thus, planning ahead and conducting a needs assessment are vital to a well-prepared program. Cultural issues include much more than an individual's racial or ethnic background. Culture also includes one's religious beliefs, gender, age, familial background, disability, sexual orientation, language skills, geographical location, and political beliefs. The more a health educator can find out about the target population, the less likely the presentation will falter.

In general, objectives directed toward increasing knowledge can be met through more traditional methods, such as lecture and audiovisual (e.g., video, computer-generated presentations, overhead transparencies). Objectives that are directed to improving or developing skills, changing attitudes, and ultimately adapting new behaviors, however, need to include experiential activities that involve the audience in the learning process. By relying too much on traditional lecture methods, health educators limit many of the learning opportunities available to participants.

Health educators should also use methods that work well for their particular personality and expertise. In addition, health educators need to know the role they are serving in the educational setting. Is the role as facilitator, teacher, workshop leader, or a combination

Did You Know

When considering which presentation methods to incorporate in the classroom or community settings, the participants' learning styles may guide the methods to choose.

Auditory Learners
Like to be read to
Like to read out loud
Like to use mnemonics to help learn material
Like to talk with others about their ideas

Visual Learners
Like to learn from reading, taking notes, and using worksheets
Like to use highlighters to outline important facts
Like to see a visual representation of the information
Like to use multimedia materials such as computers and transparencies

Kinesthetic Learners
Like to move around to learn new information
Like to take frequent breaks
Like to use rhythms or music to learn
Like to learn in different settings

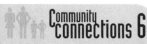
Community connections 6

Natalie realized after her initial presentation that she was not as comfortable delivering information in a speech or lecture format. She was much more comfortable the second time, when she conducted the teacher training in a more informal, workshop-style format. Understanding and experiencing her weakness as a lecturer in front of 150 teachers was a negative experience. As a result, though, she was able to build a better method or technique for herself when having to speak in front of large crowds. Future presentations would utilize computer programs, overhead transparencies, and note cards to guide her more comfortably in a traditional lecture format.

of these? Based on the role served, they can then modify a lesson or presentation to suit the types of information being disseminated.

The health educator should also determine the audience demographics and needs. Why are the individuals in the class or program? What are their needs? What are their expectations? Because information about audience needs is not always readily available to the educator, he or she must be flexible and prepared with alternative methods, such as knowing when a group activity would work best in small groups as opposed to a large group discussion. A presentation should be designed with two or more methods in mind, one that the educator is confident and competent in using and one that is possibly new or innovative based on the content or audience. An educator can begin to become competent in using new methods by preparing them in advance and being ready to implement them in new settings. When first implementing new methods, a health educator might want to combine them with proven methods, as there will be less pressure on the new method to carry the presentation. Starting with what one knows well and building upon those skills and abilities is the best way to improve one's method repertoire.

Involve Participants in Method Selection

People who feel they are a part of the learning process in terms of *how* they learn may be more inclined to participate. Increased participation improves the chance for increased knowledge, attitudinal changes, and subsequent behavioral changes. Traditional classrooms or presentation settings resemble an authoritative-style leader who dictates what will be learned, or, in many cases, not learned. Health education is a process that goes beyond the dissemination of facts. Thus, the need to include participants in the process is greater.

Organize Resources

Having organized resources can make or break a presentation. The following three suggestions can aid in organizing resources. First, develop strong networks within and outside the profession. A health educator may never know when a resource or idea will serve program needs. A network of resources and professionals can easily be created by obtaining national, state, regional, and local organization directories; maintaining an address book on email; or accessing a phone book. Second, create an organized, updated, and manageable file system of printed materials, lesson plans, and other reference material. How many times has a health educator found a resource that he or she really needed *last* week? The more resources one builds up, the less likely they are to be organized, and the more likely it is that they will not be quickly accessible. Third, to stay organized, utilize a system for prioritizing resources. For example, when material arrives via mail, email, or fax, deliberately file it, set it into a small pile for review in a few days, discard it, or pass it on to a colleague.

Sequence Methods for a Safe Environment

Health educators should ensure that the methods used are sequential. Properly sequencing methods means that one should not introduce a method that requires a lot of participant self-disclosure if the participants do not yet know each other. The beginning of the class or group should utilize methods and activities that help participants get to know each other. Other methods can then be added as a safe environment is established. For example, a role-playing activity is likely to fall apart if it is introduced to a group that has just met or whose members do not know each other. In a setting where the health topic is more personal or controversial, individuals in general will respond in a hesitant manner. The educator must lay the foundation for a safe environment that fosters respect, trust, and participant involvement. Once the foundation has been laid, the educator can progress toward using more involved activities, such as debates, role plays, and question and answer sessions. Audiences will be more inclined to participate in the methods if they feel psychologically and physically safe to engage in the activity.

A key activity that can ensure that the participants will progress sequentially is the use of ground rules or class guidelines. This activity is one that can be done early in the class or program, and sets the norms by which participants will be held accountable by the educator as well as by the other participants. Ground rules help in creating a safe environment, as well as set parameters in which the program or class can operate. An example of a ground rule is that there should be no put-downs or rejections of individual feelings or opinions.

Overcoming Challenges to Selecting and Utilizing Presentation Methods

When presenters are given an opportunity to reflect upon a presentation that did not go well, they often identify several barriers that created problems. Issues such as a lack of trust and problems with time can frustrate both the presenter and audience. This section identifies ways in which these barriers can be overcome.

Build Trust

Trust is an important factor for individuals to buy into messages. Health educators need to ensure that a lack of trust does not become an issue associated with a presentation. Building ground rules into the presentation is one of the first ways an educator can develop a trusting relationship with participants. Ground rules lay the foundation for a psychologically safe environment. In addition, there are numerous "get to know you" activities, icebreakers, and warm-ups that can be included in one's presentation to help build a trusting environment between the participants and the educator, and among the participants themselves. The proper selection of presenters, along with relevant training, can also help build trust.

Use Time Wisely

An issue that can cause stress is an over- or underestimate of the amount of time a method or activity will take. Many times an educator will allot 15 to 20 minutes for an activity on paper, but discover that in real time it only takes 10 minutes or lasts as long as 30 to 40 minutes. Being flexible is probably the best way to overcome time issues. A five-minute cushion can be added to each method or activity to help with time. Having extra activities ready to implement if time runs under, and having a backup outline if an activity runs over, can also help. Knowing when to move on or to let an activity continue is an important skill that will develop with time and practice. Newly practicing health educators should rely on a watch or timer to aid in timing. Using a timeline or a matrix to help outline the presentation from start to finish can greatly reduce these kinds of problems. Figure 7-3 is an example of a presentation timeline.

Time	Content	Method/Activity	Resources Needed	Backup
9:00– 9:25 A.M.	Welcome, introductions	Four-squares activity	Butcher paper, markers, tape	Interviews
9:25– 9:45 A.M.	Stress overview	Computer-generated presentation	Computer handouts	Transparencies
9:45– 10:10 A.M.	Coping skills information	Demonstration with art therapy, relaxation techniques, music	Drawing materials, CD player, CD	Chalk board

Figure 7-3 Sample Presentation Timeline

Expected Outcomes

Although the ultimate judgment of the success of a presentation should rest on attaining program goals and objectives, other presentation successes are measurable. The following points provide insight into four possible presentation outcomes that are realistic and desirable.

Achievement of Goals and Objectives

The primary mission of presentations should be to accomplish goals and objectives. Objectives should be realistic, with short-term impact objectives focused on knowledge gains, affective changes, or skill development; and long-term outcome objectives and goals focused on behavior changes and improved health status. One of the more difficult tasks for beginning professionals is to decide the degree of change necessary for participants. For example, what percentage of the target audience needs to successfully grasp the knowledge for a presentation to be considered successful? Be cautious of setting objectives that are unrealistic, such as lowering sexually transmitted infection rates after a three-day knowledge-based program.

Improved Health Status

Health educators conduct many short-term programs even though they are trying to initiate long-term change in program participants. Using sound theory to back such programs, such as the Transtheoretical (Stages of Change) Model,[8] can help ensure that short programs will be beneficial in leading to long-term change. For many individuals, the move toward the action stage may take years. Short-term programs, however, may play an important part in getting participants to contemplate or prepare for action. For

Did You Know

When planning the methods and strategies used to disseminate health information, it is crucial to respond to the needs of culturally diverse populations. The following are assumptions of multicultural education:

- Health educators can improve learning and achievement of students from diverse cultures if the learning environment is more consistent with their culture.

- Students or participants in programs will become more culturally competent if taught in an environment that is free of bias, prejudice, and stereotype.

- Students or participants can improve their self-concept when multicultural approaches are applied to learning and to the methods used in the classroom or community.

- Health educators who use culturally sensitive strategies, methods, and programs increase the likelihood that health messages will be internalized and will result in an overall improved health status of the students or participants.

Source: Association for the Advancement of Health Education. (1994). *Cultural awareness and sensitivity: Guidelines for health educators.* Reston, VA: Author, p. 2.

example, a smoker learns very early about the dangers of smoking. With each year that passes, the more antismoking messages he or she hears and the more information he or she learns about quitting, the greater the likelihood that he or she will move toward action. If, as the model suggests, change is a process, then there is room for programs that continue to keep people involved with methods that educate and work on attitudinal changes. Programs can also target skills for dealing with peer pressure to smoke, smoking cessation, and helping others to quit.

In many instances, improved health status among participants may never be known. There may be one person, however, who improved an aspect of his or her health because a health educator was part of a process that led toward that change. It is realistic to expect an outcome of at least an improved health consciousness from a presentation.

Increased Buy-In for the Program

Perhaps the most important early outcome to be accomplished from a presentation is participant buy-in to a larger program. For example, a few years ago, nurses at a local hospital implemented a weight-loss program. The program was 16 weeks long, and on the opening night they had television coverage and a turnout of over 100 participants. Unfortunately, by week 16, only four people were in attendance. The nurses had planned the program with absolutely no input from participants; consequently, there was no buy-in. It is critical that early presentation efforts look to accomplish buy-in as an outcome. No matter how pertinent the objectives and methods, if no one attends, it was not energy well spent.

Increased Self-Confidence as a Presenter

One of the outcomes of a presentation that is extremely important to health educators is the opportunity to grow as professionals. There are very few substitutes for real-world practice. As a result, new professionals will find growth opportunities from early-career presentations. Focusing on what went well and what can be improved should lead to an expectation of self-confidence that can come out of every presentation. As with most areas in life, the more practice and effort that go into the presentation, the more satisfaction is likely to result. Students often dislike participating in and delivering in-class presentations in their undergraduate preparation; however, many health educators report back to the faculty months or years later how beneficial the practice and feedback was for them. Improving one's presentation skills requires practice, and there is no better place than with one's peers in-class and with trusted faculty or instructors. Additionally, through proper planning and meaningful evaluation, presenters can gain confidence in their ability to both accomplish objectives and deliver effective presentations utilizing appropriate methods.

Conclusion

Natalie demonstrated how easy it is to ignore or overlook some essential steps in preparing for a presentation. Natalie's example should make it clear that it is vital for health educators, whether working in schools or communities, to spend quality time determining how they will disseminate or relay information. Natalie learned early on some valuable lessons about what not to do when giving a presentation and what to do when adversity arises.

Most individuals who present on a regular basis are likely to have stories to share and experiences they would rather forget. A commonality that many of them have regarding those "not too memorable" presentations is that they did not plan or prepare themselves for the topic, audience, or learning styles encountered. Seasoned educators will also report that the best way to improve one's presentation style is to practice; welcome opportunities to speak in front of different or diverse populations from oneself; ask others to evaluate the presentations for content, flow, and effectiveness; and continually improve and adapt the presentation methods as needed. This chapter has examined strategies for developing and implementing effective presentation methods so that health educators can position themselves for handling the diverse populations and presentation challenges that will confront them now and in the future.

KEY TERMS

method: A systematic approach, procedure, or strategy that is specifically carried out or conducted by teachers, presenters, and speakers to disseminate information, objectives, and lesson materials.

objective: A specific step or procedure used to reach an overall goal that indicates what learners will be accomplishing in one lesson, presentation, or specified time period.

plan: A specific outline that includes the topic to be taught, learning objectives, content to be disseminated, and methods or presentation activities to be used.

REFERENCES

1. Morris, W. (Ed.). (1981). *The American heritage dictionary of the English language.* Boston: Houghton Mifflin.

2. Gilbert, G. G., & Sawyer, R. G. (2000). *Health education: Creating strategies for school and community health* (2nd ed.). Sudbury, MA: Jones and Bartlett.

3. Anspaugh, D. J., Dignan, M. D., & Anspaugh, S. L. (2000). *Developing health promotion programs.* Boston: McGraw-Hill.

4. Green, L. W., & Kreuter, M. W. (1999). *Health promotion planning: An educational and ecological approach* (3rd ed.). Mountain View, CA: Mayfield.

5. McKenzie, J. F., & Smeltzer, J. L. (2001). *Planning, implementing, and evaluating health promotion programs* (3rd ed.). Boston: Allyn and Bacon.

6. Gilmore, G. D., & Campbell, M. D. (2005). *Needs and capacity assessment strategies for health promotion and health education* (3rd ed.). Sudbury, MA: Jones and Bartlett.

7. Armstrong, T. (1994). *Multiple intelligences*. Alexandria, VA: Association for Supervision and Curriculum Development.

8. Prochaska, J. O., Redding, C. A., & Evers, K. E. (1997). The transtheoretical model and stages of change. In K. Glanz, F. M. Lewis, & B. K. Rimer (Eds.), *Health behavior and health education: Theory, research, and practice* (2nd ed.). San Francisco: Jossey-Bass.

ADDITIONAL RESOURCES

Print

Forbes-Greene, S. (1993). *The encyclopedia of icebreakers: Structured activities that warm-up, motivate, challenge, acquaint and energize.* San Diego, CA: Pfeiffer & Company.

Hedgepeth, E., & Helmich, J. (1996). *Principles and methods for effective teaching: Teaching about sexuality and HIV.* New York: New York University Press.

Pfeiffer, J. W. (Ed.). (1989). *The encyclopedia of group activities: 150 practical designs for successful facilitating.* San Diego, CA: Pfeiffer & Company.

Tackman, D. L. *Hands-on health: Creative teaching strategies.* New York: Glencoe McGraw-Hill.

West, E. (1997). *201 icebreakers, group mixers, warm-ups, energizers, and playful activities.* New York: McGraw-Hill.

8

Developing Effective Presentations

Heather M. Wagenschutz, M.A.
Jason Rivas, M.P.A.

Author Comments

Heather: Understandably, public speaking is often ranked as a significant fear for many. Although this fear may never fully subside (to this day, I experience butterflies when speaking before a large crowd), awareness, preparation, and practice can give the speaker confidence, which allows for a much more enjoyable experience. What I hope the following chapter will provide is a foundation from which professionals can enhance their speaking skills. Simply put, we are all a work in progress, so please do not let the process of learning to become a better public speaker get you discouraged. Polished speakers can be powerful and persuasive and can help establish positive change in the fields of public health and health education.

Introduction

First impressions are generally lasting impressions. For many health educators, the first opportunity to make an impression comes during a formal presentation. So, proficient presentation skills are indispensable to the health educator. Public speaking provides an opportunity to impress, persuade, and sell others on concepts and ideas that directly affect individual and community health status. Public speaking is challenging, but it can be enjoyable and provide tremendous intrinsic and extrinsic rewards when properly planned. Because a great deal of health education involves presenting information to target populations, it is essential for the health educator to possess effective presentation skills. These skills not only decrease anxiety associated with making a presentation, but also increase the likelihood the appropriate message will be received by the audience. Effective public speaking is dependent on a number of factors, including the effort that goes into the preparation of a presentation and the presenter's speaking skills. Preparing for a presentation can be time-consuming. Effective preparation and delivery skills, however, can make the experience positive for the presenter and the audience. Through careful planning and preparation, a health educator can be effective in most speaking situations.

Steps for Conducting Effective Presentations

Few people are able to speak extemporaneously on a variety of health-related topics. Even those who possess the natural ability to speak well in public require the occasional skill builder. So, whether one is just starting, has a few years of experience, or is already a seasoned professional, solid preparation is required. This involves knowing the audience and the type of presentation to be given.

Prepare for the Presentation

Knowing the general audience, topic, and expectations are the first steps before planning a presentation. An audience could consist of young people in school, individuals attending a personal behavior change seminar, professionals attending a workshop, members of a community coalition committee, or community volunteers working as an advocacy group. Each group has unique needs and expectations. Information about the listeners, such as ages, occupations, religions, attitudes, beliefs, moods, and feelings, is needed to elicit a desired response.[1]

Presentation expectations are influenced by the setting in which the program takes place, such as a boardroom, auditorium, classroom, or community center. Prior to the presentation, the health educator should find out who will be attending, what needs to be covered, and the time frame allotted for the presentation.

Good speakers must be able to adapt their presentation to the surroundings. For example, the approach a health educator uses in a presentation about blood-borne pathogens in a factory setting may be quite different from that used for presenting the same information to public health nurses at a health department. Speakers are able to adapt better when they consider audience composition, knowledge levels, and attitudes.[2] Speakers who prepare by gathering information prior to a presentation make better connections and impressions with their audiences and are more likely to adapt to meet the needs of the audience than those who do not.

Understand Different Presentation Settings

There are three types of presentation settings: formal, semiformal, and informal. Each type shares commonalities, yet differences are evident.

Community connections 1

Rachel, a health educator of the Brazos County Public Health Unit, was asked by the local superintendent of prisons to give a two-hour program on women's health issues to 20 women at a local correctional facility. As Rachel prepared for the meeting, she gathered handouts and overheads she had used effectively many times with university women, failing to consider the unique characteristics of the target population she had been asked to present to. Upon arriving at the facility for the presentation, the health educator discovered that two of the women could not read and several of the women spoke Spanish only. The information she had used previously with university women was too complex, and the handout materials prepared for a young university audience were not appropriate for an older incarcerated audience. If Rachel had taken time to inquire about and consider the characteristics of her audience, she would have been spared a difficult situation and would have been more effective in her presentation.

Formal

Formal presentations center around organized functions, such as speaking to a board of health on future health promotion endeavors, or presenting at a legislative luncheon. The style of dress should be conservative and neat, taking care not to distract from the presentation.

The physical setup of a formal presentation usually includes a podium, with the speaker slightly elevated on a platform or stage. Audiences tend to be large, ranging from 50 to 100 or more individuals. Often, much is at stake because of the number of influential people in attendance. Solid impressions made in formal presentations can garner support and help further the cause.

Semiformal

Examples of semiformal settings include conducting employee in-services, facilitating an educational or behavior change workshop, speaking at a school, or conducting a community focus group. The environment of a semiformal presentation is generally more relaxed than that of a formal presentation. For example, chairs may be arranged in a circular fashion or in a U-shape to promote group cohesiveness. Group size usually does not exceed 40 or 50 people. Health education jargon (e.g., "epidemiological incidence and prevalence," "assessment and assurance," "cardiovascular disease risk reduction strategies") should be used sparingly so that participants are not confused, intimidated, or bored. Given that the setting is less strict than the formal environment, tasteful humor may be used.

It is easy for professionals to underestimate the importance of a semiformal speech or presentation and approach it with less rigorous standards. The same amount of time and energy given to preparing a formal presentation should be expended for a semiformal engagement. Semiformal, therefore, does not mean less effort and energy; it means a great opportunity to do more.

Informal

Informal presentations tend to offer the greatest amount of pleasure and the least amount of stress because they involve a much more relaxed atmosphere. Typical informal scenarios include sharing monthly accomplishments with coworkers at a department meeting or conducting focus group discussions with seventh and eighth graders. The room can be arranged in any of the previously mentioned ways, and can be changed upon arrival if needed. Group size usually consists of less than 25 individuals. For most informal presentations, speakers should make minimal use of complex vocabulary terms, jargon, or acronyms. Normally a conversational approach to speaking works best, with humor and activities to help the process. Informal presentations can provide an opportunity for speakers to get to know the audience. Do not, however, let the informal atmosphere be deceiving. Because informal presentations are less rigid, the speaker has tremendous latitude in presentation style; however, informal presentations need adequate preparation time to be effective.

Whether the presentation is formal, semiformal, or informal, the qualities of effective speakers are universal. Speakers who are considerate, genuine, trustworthy, enthusiastic, and proficient are more likely to capture and maintain an audience's attention than those who appear egocentric, uncaring, dishonest, and misinformed (see Table 8-1 for characteristics of effective speakers).

Table 8-1   Characteristics of an Effective Speaker

- *Considerate*. Listening to and validating the concerns, opinions, and reactions of participants shows that the speaker values the audience's input as much as his or her own.
- *Genuine*. Making up information, giving false compliments, or using overdramatic wording can lead the audience to believe that the speaker is only there to be liked.
- *Trustworthy*. Good speakers create trust by being honest and sincere and using credible sources of information. If the data seem out-of-date or debatable, the audience may ignore what is being said.
- *Enthusiastic*. The excitement that surrounds a speaker who genuinely appears excited about the information being presented is catchy. Enthusiastic presenters maintain audience attention because they convince the audience that the information they are presenting is exciting, interesting, and important.
- *Humorous*. Appropriate humor personalizes the topic and allows the speaker to make light of subjects that can be complex or intense.
- *Proficient in subject*. Being prepared and well versed in the topic being presented shows dedication and commitment. Having a degree of proficiency in the topic increases credibility and trustworthiness from the audience's perspective.

Set the Stage: The Presentation Opening

Prior to starting a presentation, the speaker must first greet participants. The type of approach will depend on the type of presentation. For example, the speaker may greet participants as they enter the room. In contrast, greeting the audience as a keynote speaker at a professional conference may simply involve thanking them for the opportunity to present.

The introduction of the presentation provides opportunity to garner the interest of the audience, sets the tone for the rest of the presentation, and makes a first impression. The introduction is a good time to acknowledge the person who made the arrangements for the presentation. Being invited to present is an honor, and the introduction time could be used to thank the organizers of the presentation. In addition, the introduction can serve as a time to acknowledge special interests of the audience and arouse interest in the topic of the presentation.[3]

The saying "You never get a second chance to make a first impression" is directly relevant to how a speaker should begin a presentation. The audience will draw conclusions about the presenter and the topic within the first minutes of the presentation. Therefore, speakers must carefully plan the opening of the presentation. Several techniques, such as humor, relevant stories, and audience questions, can be used.

Humor

Most audiences, regardless of the setting, enjoy humor, especially as an icebreaker. Humor, in fact, may be one of the greatest assets of a polished speaker. People like to laugh, and speakers like the audience approval associated with laughter. For humor to be effective, it must be tasteful, applicable, and nondegrading. A joke on the unpredictable nature of teenagers may not receive an encouraging response from a group of teens. A joke about parent quirks, however, may show a common thread of understanding. Humor does not always imply the use of jokes. Clever anecdotes or cartoons may be equally effective. In fact, showing an applicable cartoon prior to the time a program begins can help the audience understand what will be discussed, while eliciting an initial humorous reaction.

On the downside, humor may be politically incorrect, make the audience feel obligated to laugh, or create general discomfort. Because building rapport between speakers and their audiences is a process, creative and safe humor may be most valuable in the midpoint or end of an engagement, after the speaker has already established credibility.

Relevant Stories

Storytelling can help a speaker and the audience connect. Many speakers begin presentations with relevant news events or a short personal story. Before engaging in a program on nutrition, for example, a speaker may recall the difficulty an older person faces when making food choices on a restricted income. Stories express familiarity with the subject from a professional and personal perspective. When participants find it easy to relate to a speaker, a story, or a current event, they tend to make a stronger connection with the topic.

Posing Questions to the Audience

Posing a question is an effective way to get attention. For example, asking a question like "What household accident currently takes the lives of over 8,000 children every year?" helps the audience focus on a topic because it requires a specific response. In general, when posing questions, allow time for a response. Some questions are meant to be rhetorical and do not require a response. "How do we stop household accidents from occurring?" may not require a response but rather asks the audience to ponder the issue. These methods focus attention in the direction of the topic and assist the mental participation of the audience.

Deliver the Presentation: Use Effective Skills to Make a Presentation

Effective presentations involve the use of skills that may be practiced and learned. Effective speakers understand these skills and use them to their advantage. Effective use of **body language** (nonverbal cues) can help a speaker connect with the audience and ensure that the content is conveyed.

Know the Purpose and Material

The presenter should be mindful of the central purposes of the presentation,[3] which are to persuade, instruct, or inspire. Each theme anticipates a different outcome and may require varied approaches. One way to ensure this happens is by asking the question "So what?" while developing the presentation. For example, a speaker may say, "The number of Americans suffering from type 2 diabetes will increase rapidly over the next ten years." So what? What does this mean to a health educator? What does this mean to a group of high school students or to employees within a worksite? An effective speaker will show how this connects to his or her audiences in order to create direction. An example of the same opening statement, but with first considering the question "So what?" is: "In the next decade, type 2 diabetes will increase at a rapid pace. What this means for health care workers is that we need to work closer with county and city wellness groups to try to alleviate the soaring costs associated with mismanaged patients."

In addition to understanding the presentation purpose, it is important to become familiar with the material and content that will be presented. This is particularly true for health educators, who must be able to talk about a wide range of health issues and concerns. Presenters should take time prior to the presentation to become updated on the content of the material to be presented. Audience members may have questions, and their specific concerns should be addressed. Speakers should never answer a question with potentially false information, but rather let listeners know they will find the correct answer and get back to them as soon as possible. The advent of email allows this process to occur both swiftly and easily.

Understanding Body Language

Effective presenters are aware of the messages that the body (nonverbal) and voice (verbal) convey to the target audience. For example, part of understanding the words "Be careful!" comes from a person's movement, tone, and facial expressions. While saying "Be careful!" and trying to create the impression of a warning, the body moves with a quick jerk, the tone is high and shrieking, and the eyes are wide open. The picture is complete for the audience. These components of communication offer more than just uttering sounds. The presenter connects feeling to the sounds, and the feelings help make a presentation dynamic.

Only 7% of what an audience understands comes from spoken words; the other 93% comes from voice tone and pitch, facial expressions, and mannerisms.[4,5] In essence, the "meaning starts in your mind, flows to your body, then through symbols of gesture, tone and expression flows to your audience."[5] How a message is communicated may be just as important as what is said.

Community Connections 2

Rachel recently attended a statewide conference sponsored by the state public health agency. As she listened to the keynote speaker, she noticed that the speaker made little eye contact with the audience and often stared at a point in space. The speaker stood in one place and slumped over his notes. The speaker went over his allotted time and failed to entertain questions from the audience.

Without even hearing what was said, what impressions do you get? Regardless of how valuable the information might have been, Rachel was distracted by the negative nonverbal cues. Was the speaker nervous, uninterested in the topic, or simply unconscious of the real messages being sent? Lack of attention to nonverbal cues ruined what could have been a valuable presentation.

Nonverbal Cues

Nonverbal cues are those impressions given to a person, group, or audience with facial expressions, body movements, and other gestures. Nonverbal cues aid the speaker in a smooth presentation delivery by reconfirming the meaning behind a spoken word. Usually the first impression that audiences pick up from speakers is the way they *appear*, such as standing tall, staring at the ground, or fidgeting with objects. Delivery is crucial to presentation content.[2]

Important nonverbal cues in presentation delivery include posture, eye contact, body movement, and facial expressions.

Posture.   Good **posture** conveys confidence and expertise. Proper posture necessitates standing tall, with the chest slightly out and the head back. Presenters who stand with feet shoulder-width apart, hands at the waist, and weight concentrated on the balls of the feet appear attentive. Speakers who sit in a chair or hide behind tables or podiums may appear awkward if they do start to move around the platform. Standing center stage without any of the previously described crutches makes for a strong first impression.

Equally important is the ability to adapt posture to the type of presentation. The erect, stoic posture associated with a formal presentation may be intimidating or awkward for an informal setting. Similarly, resting on a table, which may be appropriate in an informal situation (e.g., facilitating a support group), would be inappropriate in a formal setting.

Eye contact.   Lack of eye contact may show distrust, apprehension, nervousness, lack of confidence, trepidation, or boredom. In contrast, appropriate eye contact portrays confidence and connects the speaker with the audience at a personal level. Effective use of eye contact includes connecting briefly (one to two seconds) with different listeners throughout the presentation. The speaker should take care not to focus on a single individual for an extended period of time, but rather scan the audience and focus periodically on individuals randomly. Whether in a job interview, presenting to a small group of 10 to 12 individuals, or giving a large lecture, skillful eye contact can make the difference in a presentation. Each person in the audience wants to feel a part of the presentation. Effective use of eye contact can allow this connection to occur.

Body movement.   Body movement is a nonverbal cue that can create different degrees of intimacy, warmth, and friendliness. Speakers who move freely demonstrate a greater level of comfort with themselves and the topic and tend to maintain a higher level of audience interest. Arm and hand gestures are appropriate ways to express feelings. Waving arms and hands about during a comment like "What can we do?" has a greater impact than if arms were resting on the podium or at one's side. Gestures like pointing or giving the "okay" sign help to clarify or define a point. Body movement is not effective, however, unless the speaker has a purpose behind the movement. Highly scripted presenters who carefully choreograph each movement can appear unnatural.

Movement may become distracting rather than enhancing. Overuse of arm movement can convey hyperactivity or nervousness. Similarly, pacing may become irritating to listeners trying to hear a trailing voice. Effective speaking involves being able to remain in one spot until a natural break occurs in a thought process (e.g., the end of a concept), allowing the speaker to move without disrupting the flow of information. In general, a speaker should avoid changing positions until a thought has been finished. Similarly, a speaker should not start a new thought until all movement has stopped and the speaker is firmly positioned.

Facial expressions. Facial expressions can be used to pull the audience toward unspoken insinuations. For example, lifting the eyebrows at the end of a question may show a desire for a response. Grimacing while reading the latest inoculation rates for infants could be used to show the need for improvement. The sincerity of a presenter can be conveyed to the audience through facial expressions.

Some speakers consistently appear to be unhappy. Others have a tendency to appear bored. These speakers fail to use one of the most powerful facial expressions for public speaking—a smile. A genuine smile can display warmth, affection, sincerity, or sympathy. As long as the information is not too serious, a smile can go a long way to win an audience.

Verbal Cues

The manner in which the presenter speaks has a direct impact on the conclusions an audience makes about the speaker's opinions and beliefs. Because "the voice is a flexible and complicated instrument," the feelings behind words should be considered before they are spoken.[1] What a speaker says and *how* he or she says it have a great deal to do with what the speaker is thinking. Presenters should consider how accurate and clear their message sounds to others. Concise oral communication tends to be the strongest driving force behind the final decision of a person, group, or company.[5]

There are a number of principal verbal cues: word accentuation, pitch, tone, pace, volume, and use of words. Appropriate use of verbal cues helps the listener connect to the presenter on a deeper level. Characteristics of good presenters include the ability to use vocal variety, emphasize key concepts with inflection, and gain attention through volume.[5]

Word accentuation. **Word accentuation** is the process of emphasizing certain words to let the listener know that a word or phrase is particularly important. Effective speakers are able to slow their pace in midstream to highlight important words or phrases, without the audience being consciously aware of this tactic. A short pause following an accentuation generally helps drive in the importance of the point.

Pitch. **Pitch** is associated with voice octave and can fluctuate from low to high. Like word accentuation, variation in pitch can be used to emphasize points. For instance, raising and lowering the pitch can create doubtfulness or uncertainty (e.g., "I think so"). Placing a higher pitch at the end of a phrase demonstrates uncertainty or questioning (e.g., "They are?"). A lower pitch usually represents endorsement (e.g., "It can be done"). Variation in pitch is a useful technique in situations where the speaker wants to elicit emotional reaction or support.

Tone.   **Tone** consists of the patterns in which a pitch is placed. Using a chant-like tone or a monotone can have a numbing effect on participants. Listening to someone who speaks in a monotone detracts from maintaining interest levels, however fascinating the topic may be. When practicing speeches, it may be helpful for presenters to record their voice and listen to it for tone fluctuations.

Pace.   **Pace** is the acceleration or deceleration of the presentation. Sometimes a speaker will slow the pace of a speech to create a sense of intrigue or suspense. Speeding up momentarily could represent an increasing level of excitement. Too much speed, however, may confuse an audience because of lost words and pronunciations. Speakers should make sure the tempo is comfortable for the audience. If members of the audience appear confused or irritated, ask if the presenter could repeat what was said, or begin talking among themselves in order to find out what was missed, then the pace may be too fast. The presenter may wish to ask the audience if the pace is adequate if individuals appear confused or frustrated.

Volume.   None of the previously mentioned verbal cues will matter if the presenter is not loud enough. Voice **volume** should be raised and lowered according to where the presentation is taking place (e.g., a large or small room, outdoors or indoors). The speaker should always ask the audience if the volume is adequate. If not, the speaker should make adjustments rather than asking the audience to "just move closer." It is not the responsibility of the audience to make sure a speaker's volume is satisfactory. It is the speaker's role to monitor whether the audience can hear and to change volume to accommodate the listeners.

Knowing the makeup of the audience beforehand may aid in planning appropriate voice volume. Older populations may have diminished hearing of high-pitched and soft-spoken sounds. Appropriate voice volume also is dependent on the room setup and structure. For longer rooms, speakers should aim their voice toward the back of the room so that those sitting near the back have a chance of hearing. A room that is short in length, yet wide, requires less volume from the speaker, but more turning while speaking to ensure that individuals sitting at both sides of the room can hear. Participants become extremely frustrated and may feel left out if they cannot hear the speaker.

Use of words.   A final verbal cue that the presenter should consider is the use of words. This includes word choice and use of proper grammar. Poor grammar or inappropriate choice of words can leave a negative impression of the speaker with the audience. Many times grammatical errors sprinkled through a speech can distract listeners and draw attention away from the content of the presentation. Likewise, use of regional colloquialisms or local jargon by a presenter may lead to misunderstandings by the audience.

Practice heightens awareness of verbal and nonverbal cues, thus ensuring a positive impression in a real presentation. Many courses in public speaking and in education require student presenters to practice in front of peers. In this way, the student presenters can receive feedback on their use of presentation skills. Others' impressions of the verbal and nonverbal messages can be discussed with the student presenter, and subsequent presentations may be enhanced by this awareness. Using a presentation evaluation form, similar to the one presented in Figure 8-1, may be helpful when practicing and evaluating presentation skills.

Did You Know

Listeners remember more of what they hear in a presentation that uses "picture" words. Presentations that use abstract words make it difficult for the average listener to recall content. Words that paint a picture when said, such as *alligator, umbrella, rose*, or *shark*, are more easily recalled than more abstract words such as *paradigm, configuration, generic*, or *prevention*.

Source: Business Communication Resources. Available: http://www.westwords.com/Guffey/did4.html.

Bring Closure: End the Presentation

The shortest part of the entire presentation is the closing. An effective closing is like placing the final ribbon on a wrapped gift. A poorly formed ending, however, can erase much of what preceded it. Effective presentation closings may include offering a challenge to the audience, summarizing major points that were presented, or calling on participants to improve the future by taking action.[6,7]

Audience Challenges

Challenges made to an audience are intended to promote a sense of commitment. They work particularly well in settings where change is desired. For example, a group can be challenged to donate at least ten hours a month to a volunteer organization, or to lower current rates of heart disease in a community by 15%. Challenges can be used to motivate action.

Reminders of Past Points

As previously mentioned, the presentation could open with a question or an anecdote. One way to help the audience remember key points is to finish with a summary of answers or a continuation of the anecdote. When properly planned, a concluding tie-in can be powerful. It has potential for creating many different moods.

	Excellent	Good	Fair	Poor
CONTENT				
Timely				
Accurate				
Research based				
Organization				
Comments:				
STRUCTURE				
Effective opening				
Smooth transitions				
Effective closing				
Effective question/answer period				
Comments:				
DELIVERY				
Nonverbal Skills:				
Eye contact				
Facial expression				
Gestures				
Voice:				
Volume				
Pitch				
Pace				
Word accentuation				
Tone				
English Use:				
Grammar				
Word choice				
Visual Use:				
Appearance				
Readability				
Coordination and use				
Relevance				
Comments:				

Figure 8-1 Presentation Evaluation Form
Source: Adapted from Stout, V. J., & Perkins, E. A. (1987). *Practical management communication.* Cincinnati: South-Western Publishing.

Community connections 3

Recently, Rachel was invited to attend a United Way banquet at which the guest speaker was the director of a local teenage pregnancy prevention center. The speaker began by telling a real-life story of a 14-year-old pregnant girl who was surrounded by violence and poverty. After this very effective attention-getting story, the body of the presentation focused on a new approach to working with at-risk teens in poor areas. At the end of the presentation, the speaker referred back to the story that was used to open the presentation. Rachel left the presentation with a sense of hope and motivation to help prevent teen pregnancy.

Call to Action

Effective presenters are able to grab the attention of the audience and guide them through various ideas and themes, resulting in audience agreement with how and why a conclusion has been made and why it is important to act. For example a call to action about seat belt safety could be "Buckle up! By remembering to buckle up, we could reduce the number of fatal accidents by over 30% each year. Life and health insurance rates would slowly decrease and severe injury rates would start to fall." The objective of this closing is to inspire individuals to become active participants in meeting the goals of the presentation.

Respond to the Audience: The Question and Answer Period

Following a presentation with a question and answer segment can be an effective means to convey concern for the audience and to gauge their understanding of what was presented. The presenter should stay relaxed and in control, while adequately and accurately responding to audience questions. In general, the presenter should make direct eye contact with the individual asking the question.

Did You Know

Although question and answer sessions are easier to implement in smaller groups, they also should be included in larger settings. The presenter should anticipate questions and prepare answers ahead of time, when possible. Sometimes it can be intimidating for members of an audience to question a presenter. It may be helpful to write some questions ahead of time and ask "friendly" members of the audience to ask them. Sometimes, this will open the way for more reluctant audience members to join. The way in which a presenter responds to questions from the audience will influence whether others will feel free to ask questions.

Listeners typically do not remember more than three points. The average listener has trouble recalling more than three compelling ideas and typically will recall the first and last points of a presentation most quickly. When possible, presenters should stick to three main points in making a presentation, and make the most important points first and last.

Source: Business Communication Resources. Available: http://www.westwords.com/Guffey/did4.html.

Tips and Techniques for Conducting Effective Presentations

In addition to effective presentation skills, speakers should be attentive to negative presentation characteristics that could potentially reduce the impact of the message being presented. This is not always easy to do, given that it is difficult to see one's own ingrained behaviors. A seasoned presenter, coworker, or supervisor can help improve the speaker's overall performance by offering constructive criticism.

Reduce Distracting Mannerisms

In addition to effective verbal and nonverbal cues, a speaker needs to be aware of distracting verbal and nonverbal **mannerisms**. For example, most speakers have a favorite nuisance word or phrase that tends to be inserted between thoughts and during lulls in the presentation. Words such as *um, okay, like,*

Distracting Mannerism	Number of Times Observed	
Nuisance word	_____	Word: _____
Fidgeting with personal item (e.g., hair, tie)	_____	Item: _____
Fidgeting with writing implement	_____	Item: _____
Adjusting clothing, jewelry	_____	
Fixating on ground/back of room	_____	
Pacing	_____	
Hands in pockets	_____	
Arms crossed	_____	
Poor posture	_____	
Low voice volume	_____	
Speed (too fast or slow)	_____	

Figure 8-2 Distracting Mannerisms Checklist

Table 8-2	Strategies for Overcoming Common Distracting Mannerisms
Mannerism	Strategy for Overcoming
Nuisance word	When ending a thought or sentence, be sure to close your mouth and avoid uttering sounds. Practice speaking short unrelated points while focusing on the transition between thoughts or sentences.
Fidgeting with personal item	Use arms and hands during explanations. If hands are part of the presentation, they are less likely to roam and distract the audience. Make a point of being able to see your hands out of the corner of your eyes throughout the presentation. Keep pockets empty to avoid the temptation of playing with keys and loose change. When finished writing with marking pens or chalk, place them on the table so that hands remain free to communicate. Style hair so it stays out of your face and eyes.
Fixating on a point in the back of the room or on the ground; no eye contact	Maintain eye contact with audience members, especially at the start of every new idea.
Pacing	Walk to a predesignated spot in the room and stay there until the point being made is complete. Be aware of the audience having difficulty in following your movement.

you know, and *ah* may be irritating and distracting to the audience. With overuse of these words, the audience begins to anticipate the next utterance of the nuisance word, drawing attention away from the information being presented. With practice, speakers can train themselves to connect thoughts without using nuisance words or phrases.

Another distracting mannerism is fidgeting with one's jewelry, hair, beard, or other item. Twisting a finger in a necklace, combing hands through hair, or constantly pushing hair behind an ear can distract from a presentation. While speakers usually are not aware of the distracting mannerisms, the audience becomes keenly aware and irritated with these actions. Practicing in front of a mirror or peers, or videotaping and critiquing the presentation, can aid in identifying these mannerisms and other distracting practices such as placing hands in pockets, jingling coins or keys in pockets, or "massaging" chalk or white board markers. A checklist, similar to that found in Figure 8-2, could be used by peers to identify unwanted mannerisms. Table 8-2 lists common distracting mannerisms and suggestions for overcoming them.

Be Attentive to Common Mistakes

In addition to distracting mannerisms, there are other ways a presentation can fail. Attentiveness to these common mistakes increases the likelihood of a successful presentation.

Some of the more common mistakes that speakers engage in include the following:[4]

- *Apologizing in advance for out-of-date, boring, or ill-prepared material.* Not all presentations engender the same level of interest because of the nature of the information. Starting a speech with "I know this stuff is really dull so I will try to be quick about it" is negative and suggests to the audience that the presentation will be boring and useless. Excuses for typographical errors, lack of current data, forgotten handouts, or laziness should not be made to the audience. If the visuals are ineffective, do not use them. It is better to present the information verbally than to use a distracting, hard-to-read overhead.

- *Not having a purpose.* The speaker should know the purpose for the presentation. Furthermore, the speaker must believe in what is being presented. Passion is persuasion, and persuasion means change.

- *Using the same presentation for different audiences.* Audiences have different needs, so use of the same presentation without updating or modifying materials will likely result in an ineffective presentation. For example, conducting a presentation on nutrition to high school seniors and then delivering the same presentation to a senior citizen group would have less impact.

- *Discussing too much information.* Presenters should adhere to the main objectives of the presentation. This is particularly true for data and presentation graphics.

- *Reading every word from every visual.* A copy of the visual should be placed in front of the presenter to avoid turning one's back to the audience to read the visual on the screen. Additionally, the visuals should be written at an appropriate reading level.

- *Delivering the presentation without rehearsing.* Improvisational presentations rarely impress an audience. Practice makes perfect.

- *Failing to start and end on time.* It can be frustrating to an audience when a speaker is late or runs over the time allotted for the presentation. Be aware of the time during the presentation. If needed, assign a colleague (or room monitor) to serve as a timekeeper to signal when time is up.

- *Heaving long, heavy sighs.* Expressions such as these show listeners that the speaker is not thrilled to be there. Why should the audience feel any different?

Focus on Presentation Design

It is quite difficult to offer a prescription for great presentation design when there are so many factors involved that affect design decisions, from type of audience to type of content being delivered. It is enough to cause almost all health professionals to squirm in their seats as they madly plug away at creating their presentations. As for the software available to create the presentation, many professionals approach it one of two ways. They either become overwhelmed with all the design and format options available to them and avoid having to figure it out by sticking with the less-than-exciting default settings or they get so excited at all the design possibilities and everything they can do with the software that they suddenly become the Picasso of presentations, adding outrageous sound effects, wild slide transitions, and odd, out-of-place clip art that requires a certain level of interpretation to follow along.

The unfortunate truth is that the majority of today's presentations have reached a point at which everyone in the audience knows what to expect, and the visuals that were intended to complement the presenter's spoken word more often than not just get in the way. But armed with a few basic design rules, health professionals have the power to avoid creating the mundane and predictable presentations that haunt audience members long after they exit the room. The design process should be viewed as an opportunity to separate yourself, your organization, or your cause from all the others out there. It is a time to show the audience passion for the topic being presented so they might experience it as well. A presenter has a captive audience that is often hoping for the best, but in reality expecting far less. By following a few basic rules, the presenter can exceed the audience's expectations and leave them wanting more.

Rule 1: Less Is More

Numerous PowerPoint presentations at various conferences or internal staff meetings typically involve a whirlwind of bulleted, small text crammed onto each slide and a presenter who reads each slide line by line. As the audience members catch on and realize the presenter is reading to them, they will often read ahead, creating a situation in which the presenter and audience are out of sync. This disconnect can lead to audience members only listening to a portion of what is being said and drawing their own conclusions.

Slides that contain a lot of small text usually mean the presenter is either an ineffective presenter or does not know the information as well as he or she should and is using the text-filled slides as a kind of support mechanism while speaking. Large amounts of small text are also used because many believe more text is more convincing, though the opposite is true. By using a larger font size (e.g., 30 point), the presenter forces himself or herself to list only those points carrying the most weight and to have a better understanding of the material being presented. With fewer bulleted prompts to lean on, it becomes the presenter's task to elaborate each point rather than read to the audience, making for a presentation that keeps the attention of all those listening. In the end it comes down to a single question: If the audience can understand the presentation simply by reading a copy of the slides, why is the presenter even there? The slides are not meant to do the presenter's job, which is to convey the overall message. They are merely there to emphasize crucial points and visually complement the presenter's voice. Without some kind of explanation from the presenter, what is written on the slides should mean very little to the audience.

Rule 2: Image Is Everything

Avoid using cheap-looking clip art images. This includes the majority of images that are bundled with whatever presentation software is being used. Good presentation design stands out from the crowd, something extremely difficult to achieve with clip art that practically everyone in the audience has already seen or used at one time or another. The truth about clip art is that the majority of images used lack the professional look most presenters want to exhibit, and most give the impression that the presenter simply did not put a great deal of thought into his or her presentation. Images used should be unique, high quality, and convey a sense of power. One way to deal with this issue is to look for sites on the Internet that sell royalty-free images. These images typically sell for $1 to $5 each and can be saved and used again in the future. Consider the money spent an investment, because a well-designed presentation can help the audience achieve the presentation objectives.

When selecting images to include on the presentation slides, focus on keeping them consistent. Include all photos or stick with illustrations that all have a similar look and feel. Inconsistent imagery translates into design chaos. Also, do not become overzealous with the style or number of fonts used within the presentation. Curly, flamboyant, carnival-type fonts have their place in design, and that place is not within the realm of PowerPoint presentations. Fonts used should be distinct and easy to read for audience members in the front and back of the room. The key is to have the audience focusing on the presenter, not the pretty words on the screen. Also consider the colors used within the presentation. Too much or too little contrast between the text and background colors can result in audience irritation and, eventually, disinterest.

The audience is not looking for a circus act. Words that tumble, dance, or swing into view only serve as a distraction; although it may seem boring, it is usually best to stick with the default text animation. The same holds true for slide transitions. A presentation is not the time to demonstrate crafty video transition skills. Stick to the default transition or another variety that is quite simple.

Rule 3: Be Original

When talking about the layout of design elements (e.g., header, subheaders, body text, images) within a presentation, there is often the mindset that one must follow the templates that come with the software. Those templates force the presenter to follow a rigid layout: There must be a title on every page. There must be bulleted text. Images must be placed directly to the right or left of bulleted text, and so on.

The fact that a large number of professionals follow these preprogrammed layouts does not mean it is the best choice to make. Keep in mind that as a presenter, your task is to make a statement, and doing so involves taking the time to create a unique visual complement to your verbal presentation. A decent level of originality can be achieved simply by following what photographers and artists refer to as the "rule of thirds." When applied to presentation slides, the rule works as follows: Imagine dividing the slide into thirds both vertically and horizontally (see Figure 8-3). All important design elements within the slide are placed where the lines intersect, called *power points*. The logic behind this rule is that placing design elements near these power points rather than directly in the center or scattered elsewhere creates more interesting and powerful visuals. The elements can also be placed so they align vertically or horizontally along one of the power points.

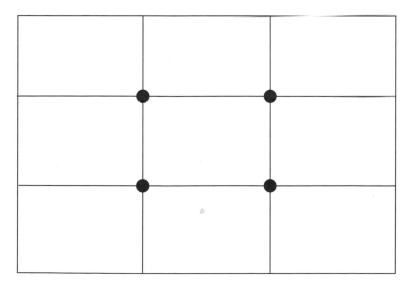

Figure 8-3 Rule of Thirds

Within PowerPoint, the guides can be set to create an outline for the rule of thirds. The example in Figure 8-4 shows a slide with the text positioned horizontally along the upper horizontal line while the woman running is aligned with the right vertical line. Audience members will first notice the woman, and their eyes will naturally follow the direction of her implied movement until they reach the text, thereby making a connection between text and image.

Following these three rules will separate health professionals from the majority of their peers and put them in a valuable class of presenters that are extremely hard to come by.

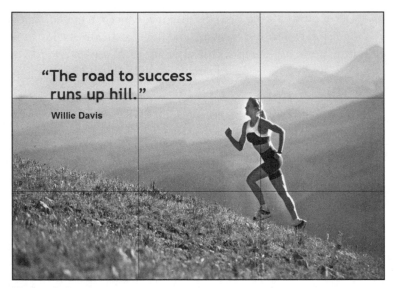

Figure 8-4 Rule of Thirds Applied

Prepare a Discussion Guide

A discussion guide can be a helpful tool to enhance a presentation.[8] The guide may consist of a brief outline and talking points or discussion questions related to the presentation. The guide can highlight major themes and messages, provide background information such as scientific facts when appropriate, suggest related activities, and list resources for more information. It provides the audience with an outline for the presentation, a convenient tool for note taking, and a way to take the information from the presentation home. A discussion guide also may include information about how to reach the speaker (e.g., address, phone, email), should members of the audience have further questions after the presentation.

Overcoming Challenges That Hinder Effective Presentations

Preparation and some forethought can help overcome barriers that may hinder effective presentations. Practicing techniques that help ease anxiety and anticipating problems that may arise during the presentation can ameliorate many of these problems.

Reduce Presentation Anxiety

Speaking in public is a common fear. Many presenters will experience anxiety before and during a presentation. The key to overcoming anxiety is to use it to help prepare and build a better presentation. Stage fright, or the butterflies, is commonly manifested by sweaty palms, trembling, and a dry mouth. A presenter can use various techniques to decrease the anxiety caused by public speaking:[9]

- *Organize.* Organization will provide confidence in the material and allow focus during the presentation.
- *Visualize.* Visualize delivering the presentation with enthusiasm and confidence, mentally rehearsing the sequencing of the presentation.
- *Practice.* Nothing can take the place of practicing the presentation. Sometimes it is helpful to have colleagues critique the practice sessions.
- *Breathe.* Deep breaths can help alleviate tension and resulting muscle tightness.
- *Focus on relaxing.* Focus on being relaxed rather than thinking about the tension of presenting. Clear the mind of tension-filled thoughts and insecurities about the presentation by consciously altering thoughts to a more relaxing theme.
- *Release tension.* Release tension prior to the presentation by consciously tightening muscles throughout the body and then releasing them; practice deep breathing during this activity.
- *Move.* Gesturing or moving about may be a way to release some of the built-up tension. Speakers who find themselves clenching the podium or standing stiff and erect due to tension may find movement a welcome relief.
- *Eye contact.* Eye contact helps reduce the feeling of being removed from the audience. It also helps speakers feel as if they were talking to a person one-on-one and lessens their focus on the vastness of the audience. Connecting with an individual in the audience builds confidence that the presentation is being understood.

Do Not Fret Over Technology Malfunctions

The use of technology is a way to make presentations come alive. Presentation software (e.g., PowerPoint), sound bites, and music add dimension. There are occasions, however, when audiovisual elements can malfunction: The graphics do not display correctly, the music does not play on cue, the microphone cuts out, or the computer locks up. In these instances it is best to adapt, adjust, and move on. Move around the room and speak louder if the microphone cuts out. Computers sometimes seem as if they have an agenda of their own, so carry handouts of the main ideas and key points. If the computer does not successfully reboot, hand out the copies and carry on from there. Do not dwell on the problem or overapologize, because this only magnifies the mistake and takes away from the presentation.

Anticipate Difficult Audience Members

Some audiences may include a select few who consciously or unconsciously seek to negatively influence the presentation. This is especially true with controversial presentations such as sex education or environmental issues. These participants demand extra attention for a variety of reasons. The initial response may be to give up authority for fear of confrontation. This may affect the audience's perception of the speaker's competence. The following subsections describe several types of audience distracters that presenters may face.

Community connections 4

During a program that Rachel gave at the local university on nutrition, a gentleman was in the audience who was studying to be a dietitian. Throughout the program, he interrupted Rachel and added comments to what she was saying. Several times he raised his hand for a question and instead would describe personal experiences with nutritional research. Rachel could sense that she was losing control of the situation. Soon audience participation in the presentation decreased as people gave up trying to compete with this "expert." By the end of the session, audience members were so irritated that one actually asked him to be quiet.

The Debater

One type of presentation distraction involves the *debater*. Debaters attempt to prove to the audience that the speakers are less competent or knowledgeable than themselves. The debater may sit silently until it is time for questions and answers, or rudely interrupt from the very beginning. Generally, the debater should be allowed to speak. Taking time to understand this person's perspective, however, does not mean an alteration of the presenter's personal viewpoints and convictions. Instead, it is meant to increase tolerance and participation by all audience members. A debater who sees that the speaker has no intention of engaging in a heated debate may feel calmed and validated. Validating the debater can occur by using phrases like "I have never thought of it that way; thanks for sharing your opinions with us," or "That is an interesting point." Most of the time, debaters simply want to know they are being heard.

The Expert

Experts are persons, or groups, who feel that their level of expertise exceeds that of the speaker. They may preface comments by announcing their credentials and years of experience to validate what is about to be said. Normally, experts mean well. They are excited about the topic presented because of their personal aptitude and tend to be a bit overzealous. Many experts have an abundance of useful information that can work to a speaker's advantage. When experts are given the freedom to interrupt and dominate the presentation, however, the speaker quickly loses credibility. Experts need to be gently persuaded that a need exists for others to participate. Possible responses include the following: "You sure do know a lot of information. I have found it very helpful. Could you *silently* critique my information and then we can discuss anything you would like to add or correct when I am finished?" or "Because you are up-to-date on this, I would like to focus my energies on those who are not. I am sure you understand." Make sure the expert knows this is not a personal attack, but a compliment. The presentation needs to be geared toward the needs of the entire audience, most of whom are not experts.

The Poor Listener

Sometimes individuals who are disruptive are so because they fail to listen to the information. This can be annoying for a speaker. Poor listeners miss a lot of the presentation's generalizations and interpretations. Because the poor listener is easily distracted, the presenter should intersperse the presentation with relevant quotes, video segments, or eye-catching visuals when possible. The better a presentation is organized, the greater the chances of reaching a higher percentage of audience members, including poor listeners. Poor organization can be especially difficult for poor listeners, because jumping from thought to thought can confuse them. Having a structured outline (either as a handout or overhead transparency) or a discussion guide to follow during the presentation helps keep everyone on track.

Did You Know

Even some "politically correct" labels may offend certain audiences. A survey sponsored by the Labor Department found that about 44% of black households want to be called *black*, while 28% prefer the term *African American* and 12% opt for *Afro-American*. The survey also found that while nearly half of all *American Indians* prefer that term, 37% prefer the term *Native American*.

Source: Business Communication Resources. Available: http://www.westwords.com/Guffey/did4.html.

Expected Outcomes

So how does the "perfect" presentation feel? Would the speaker even know if the established goals were accomplished? Although near perfection is possible with practice and solid organizational skills, there really is no such thing as the perfect presentation. Speaking is an ever-growing process of improvement. There are some ways, however, to tell if a presentation was on target.

When an audience both enjoys and learns a lot from a presentation, they will show it with some distinct behaviors. More often than not, people will stay in their seats during the presentation, have less side conversations, and make exceptional eye contact when they have connected to a speaker. It is almost as if they were hypnotized. Think about an instructor in college or high school who kept the class interested. The urge to use the bathroom or get a drink of water suddenly was not important or even formulated. As discussed throughout this chapter, a proficient speaker comes prepared, knowing the audience's needs and how to effectively meet them. Having a presentation be smooth and professional is simply a matter of research, organization, and practice.

A rule of thumb is to offer an anonymous questionnaire to participants at the end of a program. This simple evaluation offers the speaker a tangible source of audience perceptions. A Likert scale survey could be used to gauge people's opinions and thoughts. It should consist of no more than ten questions that address the main areas covered throughout this chapter, such as speaker preparation, knowledge, professionalism, interest, organization, and the quality of the program information presented. Postpresentation surveys take the guesswork out of "outcome" and offer valuable insights for future endeavors.

Conclusion

Learning the art of exceptional presentation preparation and public speaking is essential for health educators. Public speaking does not always mean a crowd of people and a podium; it involves a variety of opportunities for sharing health education messages. Regardless of setting, the more proficient the speaker, the more likely it is that the audience will absorb information that will assist them in maintaining their health.

Effective public speaking is a skill that can be learned. In fact, it is a skill that all health educators, regardless of current speaking skills, can and should improve. It takes a great deal of practice and experience, but the benefits outweigh the costs.

KEY TERMS

body language: Use of limbs and body parts in such a way as to convey a message, whether intentional or not, during a presentation.

mannerisms: Habits or characteristic ways of continually doing something during a presentation that can be annoying to audiences.

pace: The acceleration or deceleration of a presentation.

pitch: The height and depth of voice tones that a speaker uses during a presentation.

posture: The position of the body during a presentation.

tone: The quality of the sound of the presenter's voice.

volume: The fullness or quantity of the sound of the presenter's voice.

word accentuation: The process of emphasizing certain words during a presentation.

REFERENCES

1. Reid, L. (1972). *Speaking well* (2nd ed.). New York: McGraw-Hill.

2. Whitman, R. J., & Foster, T. J. (1987). *Speaking in public*. New York: McMillan.

3. National Press Publications. (1993). *Powerful presentation skills: A quick and handy guide for any manager or business owner.* Hawthorne, NJ: Career Press.

4. Peoples, D. A. (1988). *Presentations plus: David Peoples' proven techniques.* New York: John Wiley & Sons.

5. Whalen, D. J. (1996). *I see what you mean.* Thousand Oaks, CA: Sage Publications.

6. Miller, N. E. (1946). Speech introductions and conclusions. *Quarterly Journal of Speech, 32,* 181–183.

7. Bradley, B. E. (1981). *Fundamentals of speech communication: The credibility of ideas* (3rd ed.). Dubuque, IA: William C. Brown.

8. Center for Substance Abuse Prevention. (1994). *A discussion guide can enhance your presentation.* Washington, DC: National Clearinghouse for Alcohol and Drug Information.

9. Mandel, S. (1987). *Effective presentation skills.* Los Altos, CA: Crisp Publications.

ADDITIONAL RESOURCES

Print

Dale, P. (2000). *Speech communication made simple: A multicultural perspective.* White Plains, NY: Addison Wesley Longman.

D'Arcy, J. (1998). *Technically speaking: A guide for communicating complex information.* Columbus, OH: Battelle Press.

Holcombe, M. W. (1990). *Presentations for decision makers.* New York: Van Nostrand Reinhold.

Peoples, D. A. (1992). *Presentations plus: David Peoples' proven techniques* (2nd ed.). New York: John Wiley & Sons.

Rae, L. (1997). *Using presentations: In training and development.* London: Kogan Page.

Wilder, C. (1990). *The presentations kit: 10 steps for selling your ideas.* New York: John Wiley & Sons.

Internet

Creating Online Presentations. Available: http://www.microsoft.com/education/tutorial/online/pptHome.asp.

Making Presentations. Available: http://careerplanning.miningco.com/cs/presentations/.

Presentations Online. Available: http://www.presentationsonline.com.

Presentations.com. Available: http://www.presentations.com.

Toastmasters International. Available: http://www.toastmasters.org.

Virtual Presentation Assistant. Available: http://www.ukans.edu/cwis/units/coms2/vpa/vpa.htm.

9

Developing and Selecting Print Materials

Katherine Delavan Plomer, M.P.H.
Robert J. Bensley, Ph.D.

Author Comments

Kathy: I have been a health educator for the last ten years, working most recently in the area of literacy and health. Health information can be confusing and overwhelming for many people. In the current information age, health educators have the important job of clarifying and communicating the vast amount of available health information to wide and varied audiences. There is a growing divide between those who have access to information and those who do not. It is critical that no one miss out on needed health information, and print materials can be an excellent way to provide information to those who need it. Health educators can provide an important service by creating easy-to-read, audience-centered print materials that allow everyone, regardless of reading ability, language status, or other barriers, to get the health information they need to take care of themselves and improve their lives.

Introduction

Print materials play a vital role in health education and encompass a broad spectrum of media, from flyers to brochures, posters, newsletters, calendars, bookmarks, and books. They are useful tools that allow health professionals to provide needed information on diseases and self-care, convey important preventive health messages, and motivate people to take action to improve their health.

Even given the current use of technology, where information is readily available on the Web, print materials have an important place in health education. Print materials provide tangible take-home messages, and are effective at reinforcing oral communication or standing alone to convey information.

The written word can be posted, passed on, read many times, or unfortunately, thrown away.

People are bombarded every day with messages through television, radio, the Internet, billboards, and other media. With all of these stimuli, how can health educators develop print health materials that engage the people who need to be reached? How can materials be designed so they are effective, functional, and motivating?

Throughout this chapter, several themes vital to making print materials relevant and useful to people recur. The cardinal rule is to write health education materials simply and clearly so that key messages and action steps stand out. Another important rule is to pretest materials with the intended audience. They are the only ones who can accurately say what works and what does not. Pretesting and involving the intended audience in the production of materials can mean the difference between materials being used or thrown away.

Types of Print Materials

Print is a very diverse medium. Intended audience, purpose of the material, needs of a program, and length may all be factors in determining the type of material a health educator selects. The most common types of print materials are pamphlets, flyers, posters, and newsletters. Each type has a purpose, and a combination of materials can be used to reach an audience.

Pamphlets

Pamphlets are one of the most basic and common methods for disseminating health education information. Pamphlets may supplement presented material, supply information at health fairs, be mailed to a group of people with a common health problem or interest, or act as resource materials in clinics, schools, community centers, and other community facilities. Pamphlets are good educational tools because they can be easily distributed, tailored to meet the needs of a specific audience, and can reach people who would not be reached through other programming channels. Pamphlets allow readers to pick up information on sensitive topics they may be embarrassed to ask about in person. They also allow an educational message to be saved, read more than once, and passed on to others.

Flyers

Flyers are one-page documents, usually used to promote one-time events, activities, or services. In order to attract attention, they rely heavily on graphics and clearly visible headlines to differentiate them from other flyers in circulation and to motivate the reader to take a closer look. Flyers may be posted or distributed by hand to individuals. They are relatively inexpensive to develop and are an easy way of getting "who, what, where, how, and when" information out to the public to generate participation in an event.

Posters

Posters are also one-page documents but are intended to last longer than flyers. They are generally more expensive due to their larger size and use of color. Posters are good for raising awareness and communicating limited amounts of health information. They are popular for display in community centers, clinics, health departments, worksites, and schools. Posters often combine pictures or graphics with a strong written message and can be very effective at delivering straightforward messages designed to promote action. Personalized posters are getting easier to create and print. For example, schools can create posters about physical activity with pictures of their own students exercising.

Newsletters

Newsletters are different from other types of print materials in that they are used to communicate with specific groups of people on a regular basis. Newsletters are typically used for (1) communicating content information to a particular group (e.g., updating diabetes patients on the latest disease-related news, or informing members of a safety coalition about worksite safety issues), (2) raising awareness (e.g., about HIV/AIDS issues in the community), (3) promoting services and programs (e.g., health department services and events), and (4) raising money (e.g., charitable organizations sending updates to past contributors). Newsletters are useful educational tools because they have a defined audience and are sent to individuals who have a particular interest in the information being shared. Newsletters provide the opportunity for targeted communication and can incorporate audience participation. For example, readers can be invited to contribute articles, letters, or ideas for topics to be covered.

Nontraditional Materials

There are many creative ways of using print; fotonovelas and calendars are two such materials. For instance, a fotonovela tells a story using photographs and dialogue, much like a comic book.[1] This is an entertaining way of sharing health messages. Fotonovelas are designed to portray real-life situations and emotional or sensitive subjects.

Calendars combine the information people want to know regarding dates and holidays with useful information on health. The message is posted for an entire month and can be reinforced another month later in the year. For example, a state breast and cervical cancer screening program took pictures of coalition members statewide for the monthly calendar photos, developed motivational messages, and added facts and quotes regarding the importance of cancer screening to create an attractive, long-lasting, and very popular health education tool.

The sky is the limit for using print materials—some possibilities are bookmarks, place mats, bumper stickers, grocery bags, refrigerator magnets, car magnets, and comic books. Be creative!

Steps for Developing Print Materials

Before Writing Begins

A lot of discussion and planning needs to take place before the first word is written for an educational piece of material. Developing an educational piece is an investment of personnel time and project resources. Ensuring that print materials are a needed element of a program and that time, staff, and resources can be committed to the task before writing begins will increase the likelihood that the end product serves its purpose.

Questions to ask prior to creating written materials include the following.

- *Why is this material needed?* The need for developing the product may arise from any number of causes, such as requests for unavailable materials, the results of a needs assessment, available materials being out-of-date or inappropriate for a particular audience, available materials being too expensive to purchase, or the emergence of a new public health issue (e.g., avian flu).

- *Is print the best way to reach the target population?* Methods that use video, CD-ROM, the Internet, radio, or television are other ways to communicate health information. The decision to use print should be made after other methods have also been discussed.

- *How will this material fit with the program's existing goals and services?* Will the material be used to promote the program's services, supplement presented information, or be distributed as an educational tool in and of itself? For example, a nutrition program may use a poster to advertise its services and at the same time provide basic tips on healthy eating.

- *Are there existing materials that could fill the need or do new materials need to be developed?* This question can be answered by looking at existing materials both within and outside an organization. For example, many generic pamphlets about heart disease are available from nonprofit organizations, such as the American Heart Association; from governmental organizations, such as the National Heart, Lung, and Blood Institute; and from for-profit companies.

Once it is decided that new materials are needed or existing materials need to be revised, an internal assessment of resources should be conducted to ensure that there are adequate finances, sufficient time, and available staff or outside resources to complete the task.

Develop the Material

People generally read health information to fulfill a need—whether it is knowledge on how to manage an illness, information on where to go for services, concern over a health issue, or personal interest in a topic. Materials are effective if they take into account the intended audience and their information needs, are attractive so that the reader will be motivated to read the information, and are clearly designed so that key messages stand out.

The following seven steps will help to organize and plan materials development:[2,3]

1. Define the intended audience.

2. Gather information about the intended audience.

3. Develop goals and objectives for the product.

4. Develop content and visuals.

5. Internally review and evaluate material.

6. Pretest and revise as necessary.

7. Disseminate the material.

The following subsections discuss each step in more detail.

Step 1: Define the Intended Audience

Before writing begins, one must have a clear understanding of the needs, interests, and culture of the **intended audience**. Many factors will determine the intended audience; for example, a program may have a defined audience to serve, or an individual or group of individuals may request information be developed (e.g., breast cancer survivors may request information be printed on diet and exercise strategies to maintain their health). Other factors to consider are who is most at risk for a given health problem (e.g., injection drug users are a high-risk group for HIV/AIDS) and who might have missed previously developed messages (e.g., Vietnamese women may not be informed about cervical cancer screening due to a lack of culturally and linguistically appropriate materials). The creator of the materials needs to decide who most needs to receive this material.

Community connections 1

Heather works at a county health department in an area where West Nile virus is an emerging health problem. She has been given the task of developing a brochure to go along with a larger local public health information campaign. Her audience will be the community at large, but the population most at risk of viral complications includes people over age 50.

Step 2: Gather Information about the Intended Audience

Gather as much detailed information as possible about the intended audience. Finding out about audience demographics, needs, interests, concerns, knowledge, values, attitudes, beliefs, barriers to behavior change, motivators, cultural habits, and language preferences allows one to develop audience-centered messages and appealing materials. Information gathered is critical in helping to decide upon the goals and objectives for the print material, as well as how the document will be laid out and how messages will be presented.[2,4]

Community demographic variables such as age, gender, and education level can be derived from census data, government documents, reports, and statistics collected by the state or local health department or other agencies. A literature search of medical and public health sources will provide information on epidemiological data and health interventions. General information about knowledge, attitudes, and behaviors of the intended audience can be found by conducting a review of the behavioral and social science literature. Information published in a local newspaper or newsletters can also be helpful in background research on the intended audience.[1]

Local data can further be acquired through focus groups, in-depth interviews with community members, or surveys. Gathering this data is important to truly understand the specific needs and characteristics of the intended community audience. This local data collection will help to tailor materials so that they are relevant and responsive to audience needs.

Community connections 2

Because West Nile is a relatively new health issue in the United States, Heather needed to know what has happened in other communities related to this issue. What do people know and not know about the issue? What are the barriers to taking action? What messages have been effective? She conducted a literature search to learn about campaigns in other communities and an information search on the virus itself to learn more about modes of transmission and to see what information was already available. To learn more about knowledge and behaviors in the senior community, she conducted two focus groups at the local senior center.

Table 9-1	Sample Goals and Objectives for a West Nile Virus Brochure

Goal: Community members will learn about how the West Nile virus is transmitted and how to lower their risk of infection.

Knowledge objective: Readers can identify two ways of lowering their risk for mosquito bites.

Knowledge objective: Readers can identify at least one way to keep the community mosquito population under control.

Behavioral objective: Readers will apply mosquito repellent when engaging in outdoor evening activities.

Step 3: Develop Goals and Objectives for the Product

Setting goals and objectives focuses the direction of the written material and helps separate what the audience "needs to know" from what is "nice to know." The process for setting goals and objectives should be driven by what is learned from researching the intended audience: What are effective motivators for the intended audience? Do knowledge gaps exist? What are their barriers to change? Failing to set goals and objectives can result in creating material that is unfocused and too broad to meet the population's needs. Objectives should be limited in number and should focus on the change desired from the reader rather than on facts or principles (see Table 9-1). The tendency is to want to provide a lot of information in case people "want" to know it or it "may be useful." Focusing on the "need to know" information makes messages clearer and materials better focused on behavior change messages. For example, a message on how and why to reduce cholesterol may be lost in a brochure that puts too much emphasis on explaining the differences between HDL and LDL cholesterol. Including members of the intended audience in this phase will help ensure that the goals and objectives are appropriate and achievable.

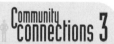 Community Connections 3

Heather formed an advisory group to help her as she developed the brochure. A lot of information was available about West Nile, but knowing she had limited space, she had to prioritize the information and set goals and objectives for the brochure. She and her advisory group decided it was most important to explain what West Nile is and how residents can protect themselves and the community. They would include Web links to direct people to more detailed information.

Step 4: Develop Content and Visuals

Content can be developed once goals and objectives have been determined. Again, participation by the intended audience in this phase is key and can greatly enhance the product and save time in making revisions later. This stage involves deciding how to best present the message: What motivates the intended audience to engage in the behavior? What are the barriers? It is essential at this stage to incorporate behavior change theory and models and to decide how to formulate messages based on theory principles. The development phase also requires decisions regarding layout and presentation of the material.

Improving readability, or "writing in plain language," is more than just good practice—it is now a requirement for the federal government. On June 1, 1998, President Clinton issued an order that by 2001 all federal regulations and written materials must be in "plain language." Listed in the president's memorandum were guidelines such as: use common, everyday words, use *you* and other pronouns, write in the active voice, and use short sentences. A guide to writing in plain language and a copy of the president's memorandum can be found at http://www. plainlanguage.gov.

Most public health materials should be developed for readers with limited literacy. The National Adult Literacy Survey published in 2003 confirmed earlier data that nearly 50% of the American population has limited literacy.[5] **Health literacy** is a person's ability to read, understand, and use health information to make informed health-related decisions. The 2003 study published by the National Center for Education Statistics indicates that over 75 million adults have either basic or below basic health literacy.[5] Education level is the measure most often used to estimate reading ability, but people generally read at a level below their last completed grade. It is estimated that the average person reads at an eighth-grade reading level, with one in five individuals reading at or below a fifth-grade level.[3] Thus, when developing materials for the general public, it is best to aim for a fourth- to sixth-grade reading level, with seventh to eighth grade being the highest level for the general public.[6-9]

Community Connections 4

Heather, in consultation with her community advisors, began to develop content and visuals for the brochure. The intended audience was the general community, with a specific focus on older adults, so a wide variety of images were needed. She discovered through her focus groups that the senior community did not feel they were at risk because the semi-arid climate in which they lived meant there were relatively few mosquitoes, and applying insect repellent was inconvenient and hard to remember. Heather used her knowledge of the Health Belief Model to make sure her audience members knew that it does not matter whether there is 1 mosquito or 1,000, everyone is at risk for contracting West Nile if an infected mosquito is present (perceived susceptibility); that applying insect repellent, although inconvenient, is effective at preventing a serious infection (perceived benefits); and that they can do something by using insect repellent and wearing long sleeves and pants (self-efficacy).

A higher level can be used if writing for a specific audience, but even an "educated" reader can appreciate a simple, direct, and well-written message.

A common misconception is that writing materials at a fourth-grade reading level is the same as writing materials suitable for a fourth-grader, which can imply a tone of writing designed for a child. Writing at a reduced reading level really means simplifying materials by reducing sentence length, explaining unfamiliar terms, and adjusting word selection to use simpler and more familiar words.

A number of **readability** tests are available that determine reading level. Many word processing programs have built-in readability tests. Also, online formulas to test the readability of a document are easy to access. Most **readability formulas** (e.g., SMOG, FOG, and FRY) are based on a system that compares the number of sentences to the number of polysyllabic words within a passage. Materials that contain several short sentences consisting of short words will score at a lower reading level.

Readability formulas provide a gauge of how easy or difficult a printed piece is to read. Formulas do not, however, provide a complete picture. Readability formulas should be one measure, but not the only way an educational piece is evaluated. Readability formulas do not take into account context, accuracy of language used, clarity of style, design, or the reader's experience.[3] Combining a readability formula with other evaluation methods such as pretesting and tools such as the Suitability Assessment of Materials (SAM) will provide the most accurate picture of how easy or difficult a document is to read. SAM provides a systematic way to review and rate print material in six categories: content, literacy demand, graphics, layout and typography, learning stimulation and motivation, and cultural appropriateness. The tool provides specific criteria for rating material as superior, adequate, or not suitable in each of the six categories.[3]

Because space is limited in written materials, newly developed materials should contain information on where the reader can seek more information on the Web. It is important to first check out Web sites you intend to cite to make sure the information is easy to understand and easy to navigate. Also, Web sites come and go or change addresses, so it is important to keep checking links if pieces are revised or reprinted.

Step 5: Internally Review and Evaluate Material

Before print material is submitted for pretesting, it should be extensively reviewed internally. The material should be proofread to identify spelling and punctuation errors. Coworkers, other health educators, and graphic designers should review the piece for accuracy, spelling, grammar, and design. A content expert should review the information for currency and accuracy, if needed. For example, it would be appropriate for an oncologist or representative from the American Cancer Society to review a pamphlet that focuses on breast cancer.

A checklist can be a helpful tool to assist in the evaluation of print materials. Checklists summarize and remind reviewers of the important points that should be considered when reviewing a document. Individualized checklists can be created for specific materials, or standardized checklists can be used.

Community connections 5

Heather planned early to line up places to pretest the brochure. She went back to the senior center with the brochure and a predesigned set of questions to make sure the brochure's content was understandable and the graphics were appropriate (see Table 9-2). She also took her brochure and assessment tool with her to community health fairs that were set up by a local news agency. She ran the brochure through the SMOG readability formula and went to a local adult literacy class and asked them to read through it for understandability. She provided a $10 grocery certificate to all her document reviewers.

Step 6: Pretest and Revise as Necessary

Developing print materials is time-consuming. One step that is frequently omitted because of time constraints is **pretesting** the material with the intended audience. However, this is one of the most important aspects of materials development and should *not* be overlooked, as it helps ensure that materials are well understood, responsive to audience needs, and culturally sensitive.[2] The pretest needs to take into account a variety of important factors, including how the material looks, whether the reader understands the key messages, whether the reader feels capable of following recommendations, and whether the material is offensive in any way. The creator of the material cannot accurately assess if the material is acceptable—only the intended audience can.

The following elements should be assessed when pretesting materials:[3]

- *Attractiveness.* Is this something readers would want to pick up? Are the colors, images, and layout appealing? If the material does not attract the reader's attention and invite him or her to read further, it will sit on the shelf or be thrown away.

- *Comprehension.* Is the content understandable? If key messages are not clear or are misunderstood, the material will not be useful. Make sure to use common language and define any words that may be misunderstood.

- *Self-efficacy.* Do readers feel they can do what is being asked? Many health messages are ineffective because they are seen as unrealistic. For example, a smoker who has tried to quit several times may feel overwhelmed by materials that focus only on the hazards of smoking. Materials that neither address the true challenges of quitting nor provide realistic strategies to help in the process may not be effective.

- *Cultural acceptability.* Is the message in any way offensive? Does it seem relevant? Images or messages that are acceptable to one culture may have an entirely different connotation in another. Similarly, recommendations that make sense to one group may not seem relevant to another. For example, a low-fat cookbook for a white audience may be viewed as out of touch for a Latino audience if it does not include alternative recipes for traditional foods such as refried beans or tamales. The developer may be surprised at what may be seen as offensive. The only way to be sure not to offend is to have the material reviewed by members of the target audience.

- *Persuasion.* Do readers feel compelled to act? Do readers feel the message is relevant to them? Was the message in the material convincing enough that the readers would now, for example, wear seat belts while driving?

Individual interviews, focus groups, and written feedback forms can be used to pretest materials. If written feedback forms are used, the form itself should be pretested to make sure the questions are clear and provide the needed feedback. It should also be made clear that questions on the form are not intended to be a quiz but rather to elicit feedback on the material. All questions should be worded in a neutral language to avoid biasing the reviewer. Ideally, 25 to 50 members of the intended audience should review materials. If this is not realistic, pretesting with at least 5 to 10 people is better than not pretesting the material at all.[2] When pretesting a document, ask open-ended questions whenever possible. Open-ended questions help determine if the reader understood the message as it was intended, and provide the greatest opportunity for eliciting all differing points of view (see Table 9-2). Close-ended questions can also be useful, especially if the question incorporates response categories to provide specific feedback to the reviewer (see Table 9-3).

If major changes are suggested as a result of the pretesting, have material reviewed again by members of the intended audience before the revised version is distributed.

Table 9-2   Sample Open-Ended Pretest Questions

1. How would you use this pamphlet if it were given to you?
2. Can you do what the pamphlet says to do? Why or why not?
3. What do you think of the colors used in the pamphlet?
4. What three words best describe this pamphlet?
5. Would your family or friends use this pamphlet?
6. What do you think of the pictures?
7. What else would you do to the pamphlet to make it better?

Table 9-3   Sample Close-Ended Question

In your opinion, was the poster designed to reach: (circle one response)

All people

All people, but especially teenagers

Just teenagers

Other (please specify what other groups)

Source: National Cancer Institute. (1989). *Making health communication work: A planner's guide* (NIH Publication No. 89-1493). Bethesda, MD: National Institutes of Health.

Step 7: Disseminate the Material

Consider the best method of disseminating materials. For example, is the printed material a brochure that will be displayed in a pamphlet rack in a health clinic? Will it be mailed to members of the intended audience? Will it be handed out during a presentation or program? Is it a poster or flyer that will be posted in locations with high visibility? Will it be distributed in mass quantities at a health

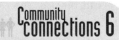

Community connections 6

Once she made changes to the brochure based on feedback, Heather showed it to colleagues at the health department and corrected grammar and punctuation errors. She gave them a checklist to give her feedback on layout, writing style, and content. She changed some technical information. Because she could not provide all the information she wished in the brochure, she reviewed several Web sites and provided the addresses so those seeking more information would be able to go to the best sites to do so.

fair or cultural event? Will it be available to download from an organization's Web site? If so, make sure it is easy to download and that there are options that allow those with older software and slower Internet connections to print it easily. Development plans should include how best to distribute materials so that they are accessible and seen by the intended audience.

Tips and Techniques for Developing Effective Print Materials

Most public health print materials are developed for broad constituencies. The key to effective print materials is to design them so that they are easy to read and clearly communicate the intended message. All the elements in presentation— content, layout, print and font choices, graphics, and readability—influence whether a document is appealing and readable. Many times health educators do a lot of learning on the job when it comes to designing and formatting materials. Each project is unique, but there are some general principles that can be followed to make a printed piece attractive, clear, and appropriate for the intended audience.

Determine Appropriate Content

Deciding on and prioritizing the information to include in a written piece is the cornerstone to disseminating the health message. There is more information on a topic than there is room for sharing it, and often (especially if a team does a written piece) there are different views on what content is important. The following guidelines help to ensure that a piece does not try to cover too much material and that what is covered is reinforced for the reader.

- *Limit goals and objectives.* During the planning phase, goals and objectives should be prioritized and limited to one or two main points. Trying to fit too much information in any one piece will make it difficult for the reader to retain *any* of the information.[2,3,10]

- *Present important information first.* Mention main points up front, and reinforce messages throughout a document. Organize information logically, in the order in which the reader will use the information.[3,11,12]

- *Summarize important points.* Key points should be summarized at the end of a document, particularly if a lot of information has been communicated. Summaries serve to reinforce action steps and refocus the reader on the key points of the material.[2-4]

Focus on Layout

Layout is the combination of text and graphics on a page. A balance between the two is important. A well-designed layout is one that works for the audience, organizes information in a way the reader will use it, and attracts attention.[11] The following guidelines aid in the development of an effective layout.

- *Create a cover that grabs the reader's attention.* Most people will take only a few seconds to determine whether they want to read a printed piece. If the cover does not appeal to the reader or provide enough basic information on the content, most people will never pick it up and read any further.

- *Always leave ample white space.* If materials are too crowded, it is difficult for readers to sort through information. Text should be balanced with graphics, graphical elements (boxes, lines, tables), and white space. White space may increase the length of the material, and a common mistake is to cut out white space to preserve content. Before doing this, review the content and decide if unnecessary information can be eliminated or any language tightened. If the content is acceptable, consider increasing the length of the document (e.g., going from a trifold brochure on letter-size paper to a trifold brochure using legal paper).[2,3,13]

- *Use headings to separate text.* Organize related information under an appropriate heading. This guides readers through the text. It also helps in directing readers back to sections of information that may be more relevant to their needs.[2,3,10,12]

- *Use bullets and numbering to highlight key points.* Using bulleted or numbered lists makes it easy for readers to identify main ideas without sorting through unnecessary information. Each list should have a simple, instructional heading. Limit lists to five or six items; if more room is needed, use subheadings. Lists also aid in the presentation of sequential information.[2-4,10]

- *Use a jagged right edge.* Readers have an easier time reading text with a jagged right edge (left justified). Right or full justification makes it difficult for a reader's eyes to follow text down the page.[3,4,10]

- *Use generous line spacing.* As a rule of thumb, multiple spacing should be used to separate paragraphs.[3]

- *Use horizontal print, rather than vertical.* People are accustomed to reading from left to right across a page. Vertical print can challenge even strong readers.[11]

- *Avoid orphan lines.* Orphan lines are those that do not fit on the same page or in the same column as the rest of the text. The layout should be rearranged so that a minimum of two lines are set off by themselves. It is better to move a whole paragraph or section to the next page than to leave a line stranded.

- *Plan materials so that important ideas follow a "Z" pattern.* Most readers are right-eye dominant, meaning they first look at the upper left corner and then crisscross diagonally across the page (in a "Z" pattern) toward the bottom right corner. Therefore, the most important idea should be in the upper left, with less important ones flowing to the bottom right corner.

Follow Print and Font Guidelines

Poorly chosen **fonts**, type styles, or type size can greatly impair a piece's readability. An abundance of literature is available that describes the intricacies of print and font choices. A few basic guidelines for printed educational materials include the following.

- *Use at least a 12-point type size.* In general, it is best to use either a 12-point or 14-point type size. Larger sizes may be used to highlight main ideas, themes, headings, or titles (see Figure 9-1). Anything smaller is difficult to read.[2-4,12]

- *Use only one or two different fonts within a single piece.* Although it may seem creative or fun to use more than two fonts, it can make the material appear cluttered and be more difficult to read. When using two fonts together, it works best to combine a serif font (letters have extensions or "feet" on the ends) with a sans serif font (letters do not have extensions on the ends) (see Figure 9-2).

- *Use serif rather than sans serif type.* Typically, serif type is easier to read than sans serif type (although sans serif is good for most headings). Sans serif is appropriate when trying to convey a sense of formality or professionalism. In contrast, serif is less formal and conveys a "softer" feeling (see Figure 9-2).[3,10,11]

- *Stick to simple fonts.* Fancy or script fonts are difficult for most readers and should be used sparingly. Script fonts are appropriate when trying to convey softness, sensitivity, or elegance. Be sure to use a large enough type when using script.[3,12]

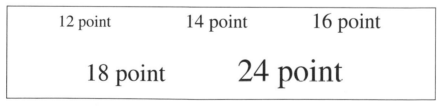

| 12 point | 14 point | 16 point |
| 18 point | 24 point | |

Figure 9-1 Typical Type Point Sizes

SERIF (with feet)   SANS SERIF (without feet)

Figure 9-2 Serif and Sans Serif Type

■ *Use dark-colored print.* There are many options for print color. Black is by far the clearest. Stick with dark colors like navy blue, dark green, or burgundy if choosing a color other than black for print. The print chosen should contrast with the paper or background color. Choose a white or light background for the best clarity.[11–13]

■ *Use capitals, boldface, or italics only to emphasize a word or main idea.* These tools are meant to enhance a point. If they are used for more than a few words at a time, it becomes difficult to read the text and to distinguish important ideas. Do not capitalize complete sentences or paragraphs. Full capitalization is hard to read and conveys a message of "shouting" (see Figure 9-3).[2–4,12]

■ *Do not use underlining or Courier font.* Both are holdovers from typewriters. Underlining was a practice used before modern word processors, to indicate to the printing house that the text should be italicized. Courier type font was the standard on typewriters and appears out-of-date when used on print materials.

■ *Use visual cues such as arrows, circles, or boxes to call attention to important points.* Set important information aside in a text box, or circle an important word or phrase to provide emphasis. Arrows can be helpful in pointing the reader to a specific spot on an illustration.[2–4]

Select Appropriate Graphics

Appropriate **graphics** can greatly enhance the effectiveness of health education materials. Clear graphics can make a complex idea or procedure more easily understood, improve recall of information, and increase readers' interest in a written piece. Graphics and illustrations can, however, confuse the reader if they are not linked to the educational purpose.[12]

THIS IS AN EXAMPLE OF USING ALL UPPERCASE LETTERS. WHICH DO YOU THINK IS EASIER TO READ, THIS PARAGRAPH OR THE ONE IMMEDIATELY FOLLOWING?

This is an example of using a mixture of upper- and lowercase letters. Which do you think is easier to read, this paragraph or the one immediately preceding it?

Figure 9-3 Inappropriate Use of Capitalization

Graphics relieve the monotony of large volumes of text and can reduce text by illustrating important points. Applying the following concepts to the use of graphics will ensure that they aid the reader and do not detract from the educational message.

- *Use graphics that aid in communicating the message.* Graphics should help the reader comprehend and follow the message. Individuals who have a difficult time comprehending text tend to use graphics as a guide. Therefore, a graphic should be placed near the text that illustrates the idea. Do not include an inappropriate graphic just for the sake of having one. For example, do not use pictures that are outdated (e.g., an individual wearing a leisure suit). The reader may believe that the information is just as outdated as the graphic.[2,4,11,12,14,15]

- *Use simple line drawings as opposed to complex graphics.* Simple line drawings do not contain large amounts of detail and are easily recognizable. Complex graphics generally contain shading and intricate detail. As such, complex graphics may not be understood by the reader or may lose their clarity during reproduction.[3,4,12,15]

- *Use captions to explain graphics.* Include a caption below a graphic to explain what is depicted (see Figure 9-4).[2,3,14,15]

- *Use graphics that are appropriate for the intended audience.* If the material is intended for the general public, graphics should depict positive health behaviors. Ideally, a person should be shown acting out the positive health behavior being described.

- *Use culturally appropriate graphics.* Graphics should depict a culture in a realistic and positive way. It is important, however, to avoid stereotyping or making assumptions about people or behaviors (e.g., not every family is made up of two parents, a boy, a girl, and a family dog, with

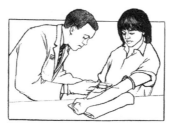

The doctor will take some blood to
check for hepatitis B

Figure 9-4 Example of a Captioned Illustration

Source: National Institute of Diabetes and Digestive and Kidney Diseases. (1997). *What do I need to know about hepatitis B?* (NIH Publication 97-4229). Bethesda, MD: National Institutes of Health.

Table 9-4	Graphics and Illustrations Checklist

__ *Necessity.* Was the graphic itself necessary to convey the educational goals of the material? Did it add to the patient's ability to understand the text?

__ *Suitability to convey content.* Did the graphic contain too much information to be helpful? Was it the correct type of graphic to convey the content?

__ *Familiarity to clients.* Would clients be able to recognize the graphic?

__ *Overall layout.* Were the size, print, empty space, and color appropriate for the concept being conveyed?

__ *Single concept.* Did the graphic convey a single concept or idea?

__ *Size.* Was the graphic itself sized appropriately for the type of material, type of text, and the concept itself?

__ *Labeling.* Was the graphic labeled? Was the size of print large enough relative to the graphic?

__ *Distracting elements.* Were ideas not relevant to the educational purpose eliminated?

__ *Cultural appropriateness.* Did the graphics present the culture in an accurate and positive way?

Source: Adapted from Rohret, L., & Ferguson, K. J. (1990). Effective use of patient education illustrations. *Patient Education & Counseling, 15,* 73–75.

the mother as the primary caretaker). Pretest graphics with the intended audience to be sure the graphics are not perceived as stereotypical, offensive, or irrelevant. Table 9-4 is a checklist that can be used to evaluate the appropriateness of graphics for written materials.[2,3,10,12]

- *Use recognizable graphics.* Graphics should be recognizable to the intended audience. For example, some may not recognize a drawing of the lungs unless it is put in the context of where the lungs are in the body.[2,3,12]

- *Leave ample white space around graphics.* As with type, use white space around graphics. This will help the graphics draw the eye into the type rather than vice versa. Also, avoid wrapping text around graphics, because this is often hard to read.

- *Use varying sizes of graphical elements.* Graphics that are all the same size are not very interesting. Instead, varying element sizes adds interest and shows what is most important. Size should depict the relative importance of each image.[12]

- *Anchor graphics to the edge of the page.* Graphics should not be floating in the middle of the page. Instead, try to anchor them to the edge of the page to help balance the graphics with the text.

- *Use shading with caution.* Gray shading adds contrast when it is not possible to print in color. Shading, however, should never exceed 20% gray unless printing in reverse (using white text on an all-black background). This method should be used sparingly, and only to highlight an idea.

Determine Readability

In addition to making sure information is written at an appropriate reading level, a number of other points will make a document easier to read.

- *Use common words.* Substituting words (for example, using *shot* for *injection* or using the word *flu* rather than *influenza*) makes materials much more understandable to people. Stick to common words whenever possible to create the easiest materials to read (see Table 9-5).[2,3,10] As a general rule, use words with fewer syllables whenever possible.

- *Use concrete language.* The more exact and concrete the language, the clearer the message. Spell out the exact recommendation whenever possible. For example, "Call the doctor if your child has a fever over 101°" is a clearer message than "Call the doctor if your child has a high fever."[2,3,10]

Did You Know

People take only about seven seconds to decide whether or not to read a pamphlet.

- *Use a conversational tone.* Writing in the third person is often the norm in writing. Using the second-person *you*, however, can be effective in personalizing information and focusing the message directly on the reader. For example, "Stop exercising if you feel short of breath."[2,3,10,11]

- *Explain technical terms.* Technical words, especially medical terms, are often unfamiliar to people and can be difficult to understand. Technical terms do not necessarily need to be avoided but should always be defined or explained. For instance, *mammogram* is an important term to understand in relation to breast cancer screening. A mammogram might be described as an "x-ray of the breast."[2–4,12,14]

- *Write in an active voice.* Use active rather than passive phrases (see Table 9-6). Vivid and active phrases make it clear to readers exactly what is expected of them and what action to take.[2–4]

Table 9-5	Substituting Common Language to Increase Ease of Reading
Word	Substitute
carcinogens	cause cancer
hypertension	high blood pressure
bacteria	germs
injection	shot
physician	doctor

Table 9-6	Active versus Passive Voice

Active: Eat five servings of fruits and vegetables a day.
Passive: Five servings of fruits and vegetables should be eaten every day.

Active: Exercise three times a week for good health.
Passive: Get regular exercise in order to have good health.

- *Use short sentences.* Keep sentences short when possible. Sentences that are too long and cover too many points can be confusing.[2–4]
- *Use slang words with caution.* Slang should be used with caution because it is not always appropriate and may offend some people. On the other hand, it is useful to use terms with which the target audience is familiar and to which they can relate.
- *Add interaction.* The more readers interact with the material, the more likely they are to remember and incorporate the information. Add interaction to materials by leaving blank spaces for readers to write goals, adding checkboxes, or posing questions for readers to answer (see Figure 9-5).[2,3,10]

Consider Special Issues

Older Audiences

Elderly people may have greater difficulty with vision, memory, and chronic illnesses, all of which can get in the way of comprehending printed material.[16] Font size is particularly important when writing for older audiences. A general

---

Am I at Risk for Breast Cancer?

You may be at risk for developing breast cancer if you can answer "yes" to any of the following*:

- I have a family history (mother, grandmother, sister) of breast cancer.
- I have a personal history of breast or ovarian cancer.
- I began my period before age 12.
- I began menopause after age 55.
- I have been exposed to great amounts of radiation (x-rays, treatments).
- I have the "breast cancer" gene.

*Even without one or more of these risk factors, you could still be at risk for breast cancer.

Figure 9-5 Adding Interaction

rule of thumb is to start with 12-point type and add a point for every decade after age 40. For instance, if a printed piece were to be targeted toward postretirement individuals, the appropriate type size would be 14 to 16 points (ages 50–79). As an individual's eyesight diminishes, it is easier to read larger type.

Colors should be chosen carefully. Seniors have a hard time reading light type on a dark background. Choose colors with a strong contrast between the text and the paper, preferably dark type on a light background.[17] Avoid using abbreviations, clichés, slang, and figurative language. Cues such as arrows, underlines, circles, and colors are useful in helping the eye focus on the most relevant information. A variety of graphics should be used to reflect the diversity of age, culture, and health status represented in the broad category of "older adults."[16]

Diversity

Making print materials culturally appropriate is essential for reaching members of different ethnic groups. For example, certain ethnic populations may perceive print materials that appeal to white audiences as unattractive, incomprehensible, or contrary to their cultural beliefs. Within different racial and ethnic distinctions, there are great variations in populations. Learning about the local population is important to developing relevant, appropriate materials. Many health messages are lost on members of minority populations because of poor translations, lack of attention to culturally specific motivators, and lack of involvement of the intended audience in the development and review of materials.[18]

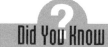

The English language itself can get in the way of writing clearly. Consider the following examples:

- The bandage was wound around the wound.
- After a number of injections my jaw got number.
- I had to subject the subject to a number of tests.

It is no wonder English is one of the hardest languages to learn!

Translation of materials into other languages is a challenge. Messages should be developed, whenever possible, in the language of the intended audience versus being developed in English and then translated. Literal word-for-word translations from English often result in the loss of meaning of the material. When translation is required, a bilingual team who represent the different ethnic groups or dialects of the intended audience should review the material. Three strategies that health educators can use to create accurate educational materials, no matter what the language, include (1) back translation—translate the printed materials in one language and then independently translate them back into the first language, (2) decentering—simultaneously translate printed materials into both languages, adjusting both until they have equivalent meaning, and (3) extensive pretesting.[18]

Internet-Based Material

The vast array of health-related information available on the Internet has led it to become a valuable resource for health educators searching for educational materials to use within their given professional setting, be that a community, school, or worksite. The beauty of the Internet is that practically anything found can be printed, copied, and distributed almost instantly. In doing so, however, there are several important things to consider:

- *Copyright violations.* Search for and read the site's copyright statement to ensure that using content from the Web site for educational purposes does not violate any copyright restrictions. If no such statement exists, then email the site's contact person and ask for permission to use its material for noncommercial purposes.

- *Advertisements.* Many Web sites are plagued with pop-ups, banner advertisements, and even the more subtle text ads. It is important to avoid using materials that contain any variation of these advertisements. Not only do the ads distract from the content, but they also can make it look as though the organization you work for advocates the product or service listed in the ad.

- *Scrolling.* A page from the Internet that has vertical or horizontal scroll bars visible within the browser window will not print out in the most ideal way. Words at the top or bottom of the page may be cut off, or paragraphs may be broken at less than ideal places. Always select "Print Preview" to determine whether what is to be printed actually corresponds with what is desired.

- *PDF files.* A PDF file is optimal for printing; in fact, that is its main purpose—to provide individuals with a way to effectively print online documents without having to be concerned with layout or formatting issues.

Overcoming Challenges in Developing Print Materials

There can be numerous challenges in developing print materials. Some common challenges include time and cost. Other challenges that might not be as readily apparent include finding people to help pretest materials and locating appropriate graphics. The following strategies can be used to reduce these challenges.

Manage Time

There is no such thing as developing a "quick pamphlet" or a "fast newsletter." Often the most clear and well-written materials—the ones that look like they must have been easy to develop—actually took the most time. Be realistic up front and allow adequate time to develop and pretest written materials. The following factors should be considered when creating a development timeline for print materials:

- The more target audience members included in the development process and the larger the team for developing materials, the longer it will take.

- Know the approval process for materials. Internal procedures and requirements and the proper approval channels can add significant time to development.

- The pretesting process takes time. Developing pretest questions, finding people to help review materials, and incorporating feedback adds time to the project, especially if the pretesting reveals that major changes need to be made to the piece.

- If new to using desktop publishing software, add time to the timeline. A simple brochure can take from several weeks to months to be conceptualized, researched, developed, pretested, printed, and distributed.

The development process almost always takes longer than anticipated. An important strategy for managing time is to have a clear action plan: What are the steps in creating the material? What is the timeline? Keep setting deadlines for the steps that need to be taken and stick to them. Knowing who is doing what is also important in managing time: Who is developing the content? Who is doing the layout? If multiple people are working on the piece, be sure to coordinate schedules and keep in constant communication. If key individuals in the organization need to approve the material, make sure they keep abreast of the process and the timeline of the project. Begin to develop pretest questions and make contacts to find pretesters early in the project instead of waiting until everything is finished.

Did You Know

At least 329 languages are spoken in the United States. In some U.S. cities, less than 60% of the people speak English.

Source: Smith, S., & Gonzales, V. (2000). All health plans need CLAMS: Culturally and linguistically appropriate materials. *Healthplan*, *41*(5), 15–18.

Keep Costs Reasonable

Even though cost can be a major limiting factor when designing printed health education materials, a product can still look professional and credible without costing a fortune. One strategy is to stick to one or two colors. The cost of printing increases considerably as more colors are added. Basic black print on white paper is the least expensive option. Use good-quality paper to improve the look and durability of the product. If white is too plain, try black print on a light-colored paper. Preprinted papers that have attractive borders and designs can also be used.

Learning how to lay out materials is another cost-saver. Desktop publishing software is relatively easy to learn, but the learning process is time-consuming. If time is more important than cost, consider outsourcing the material.

Find Pretesters

Finding members of the intended audience to help pretest materials can be challenging. Depending on the nature of the material being developed, individuals with certain characteristics are needed for the most accurate review. For example, African Americans should review a fact sheet on diabetes written for African Americans. A local health clinic that serves primarily African American patients may have individuals willing to participate. Enlist the help of office staff to find people or put flyers up to recruit interested individuals.

Develop partnerships in the community with varying groups (e.g., senior centers, schools, adult education programs, health clinics), as these sites often have groups of individuals who would be willing to help pretest materials. If possible, provide an incentive for reviewing materials, whether it is money, grocery certificates, or a small gift of appreciation. Let pretesters know that their time and input are valuable. Also, be sure to explain to participants that they are not being "tested," but rather that their input is needed to create an effective and appropriate printed piece.

Community connections 7

Heather had the brochure printed for community distribution. There was not enough within the budget for a color brochure, so she chose a light-colored paper with black type.

The brochure was also posted on the health department's Web site in a PDF form so it was easily accessible for those with computers and easy to download and print.

Incorporate Appropriate Visuals or Graphics

Finding culturally appropriate, health-related graphics can be challenging and time-consuming. **Clip art** is available through many software packages or can be purchased for a reasonable cost.

Photographs, clip art, and other art can be downloaded from the Internet, some for free and others for a fee. If a specific graphic is required, consider getting in touch with a local college or art school to see if a student can design what is needed. Graphic artists or other professionals can also be hired if the budget permits.

Expected Outcomes

Print materials, if developed properly, can be effective in providing information, motivating behavior change, and directing audience members to needed services. The development process takes time and requires attention to many details, such as content, font, layout, readability, and cultural appropriateness. The step-by-step process and the tips and techniques provided in this chapter provide a solid framework to use in print materials development. What can health educators expect by following the steps in the development process?

Materials That Fit a Need

As was discussed early in the chapter, taking time to ask and answer key questions before beginning development work is important. Answering preplanning questions will ensure that other channels have been explored before print is selected to reach the intended audience, that the proposed document is clearly needed, and that the print material fits within a program's existing goals and services.

Clear and Understandable Materials

Each step in the development process provides important information to guide in the development of the material. Gathering information on the intended audience and developing goals and objectives for the product ensure that health educators understand the population they are trying to reach and that materials developed will have a clear purpose. Developing content and visuals in partnership with the intended audience and internally reviewing and externally pretesting a document will lead to materials that are accurate, clear, motivating, and audience centered.

Audience-Centered and Culturally Appropriate Materials

Involving members of the intended audience in developing and pretesting materials is extremely beneficial. The most important outcome is creation of materials that are culturally appropriate and centered on audience needs, preferences, and motivators. Materials that are pretested with audience members are more credible and give the community a sense of ownership of the end product. Including audience members also helps health educators to better know the community, build relationships, and create partnership opportunities for future projects.

Conclusion

Designing or choosing printed health education materials is an important job of health educators. Even with expanding technology, print is not obsolete. It is easy to forget that there are people without access to computers or the Internet. The process of materials development and review is continual, since printed health education materials can quickly become dated as research uncovers new information on health and health behavior. Technology is increasing access to information and is providing new tools for health educators to disseminate materials.

Developing print materials requires health educators to draw upon their knowledge and skills in many areas. Knowledge of behavior change theory and of social marketing and health communication principles can aid in content and message selection. Skills in conducting focus groups and facilitating meetings are important in gathering input from the intended audience and working with a team to develop materials. Creating written materials also requires skills in writing, design, and readability assessment. Developing written materials is one way that health educators can utilize their many skills to communicate vital health information to the public. Print materials development can be a fun and rewarding part of a health educator's job.

KEY TERMS

clip art: Ready-to-use graphics that are not copyright restricted.

font: Style of type.

graphics: Visual aids such as illustrations, line drawings, photos, boxes, arrows, and art, used in a document to enhance and accompany text.

health literacy: A person's ability to understand and process basic health information to make appropriate health decisions.

intended audience: The audience designated as the population to reach. Also referred to as the target audience.

layout: The arrangement of text and graphics on a page.

pretesting: The process of testing materials with the intended audience through individual interviews, focus groups, or written forms to be sure materials are understandable, attractive, and culturally appropriate.

readability: How easy it is to read a document is based on such factors as approximate grade level, clarity of writing style, layout, design, and vocabulary.

readability formula: A mathematical formula generally used to calculate the approximate reading level of a piece of material. The formula takes into account the number of sentences in relation to the number of polysyllabic words within a passage.

REFERENCES

1. AMC Cancer Research Center. (1994). *Beyond the brochure: Alternative approaches to effective health communication.* Atlanta: Centers for Disease Control and Prevention.

2. National Cancer Institute. (1994). *Clear and simple: Developing effective print materials for low-literate readers* (NIH Publication No. 95-3594). Bethesda, MD: National Institutes of Health.

3. Doak, C. C., Doak, L. G., & Root, J. H. (1996). *Teaching patients with low literacy skills* (2nd ed.). Philadelphia: J. B. Lipincott Company.

4. National Cancer Institute. (1989). *Making health communications work: A planner's guide* (NIH Publication No. 89-1493). Bethesda, MD: National Institutes of Health.

5. National Center for Education Statistics. Available: http://www.nces.ed.gov/NAAL.

6. Davis, T., Bocchini, J., Fredrickson, D., Arnold, C., Mayeaux, E. J., Murphy, P., Jackson, R., Hanna, N., & Paterson, M. (1996). Parent comprehension of polio vaccine information pamphlets. *Pediatrics, 97*, 804–810.

7. Estey, A., Musseau, A., & Keehn, L. (1994). Patient's understanding of health information: A multihospital comparison. *Patient Education and Counseling, 24*, 73–78.

8. Weiss, B. D., & Coyne, C. (1997). Communicating with patients who cannot read. *New England Journal of Medicine, 337*, 272–273.

9. Root, J., & Stableford, S. (1999). Easy-to-read consumer communications: A missing link in Medicaid managed care. *Journal of Health Politics, Policy and Law, 24*, 1–26.

10. Doak, L. G., Doak, C. C., & Meade, C. D. (1996). Strategies to improve cancer education materials. *Oncology Nursing Forum, 23*, 1305–1312.

11. Farrell-Miller, P., & Gentry, P. (1989). How effective are your patient education materials? Guidelines for developing and evaluating written educational materials. *The Diabetes Educator, 15*, 418–422.

12. Hussey, L. C. (1997). Strategies for effective patient education material design. *Journal of Cardiovascular Nursing, 11*, 37–46.

13. Siebert, L., & Ballard, L. (1992). *Making a good layout*. Cincinnati, OH: North Light Books.

14. Cory, J., Bottum, C., & Haddock, C. (1995). Evaluating print health education materials. *Cancer Practice, 3*, 54–56.

15. Rohret, L., & Ferguson, K. J. (1990). Effective use of patient education illustrations. *Patient Education and Counseling, 15*, 73–75.

16. Murphy, P., Davis, T., Jackson, R., Decker, B., & Long, S. (1993). Effects of literacy on health care of the aged: Implications for health professionals. *Educational Gerontology, 19*, 311–316.

17. Canadian Public Health Association and National Literacy and Health Program. (1998). *Creating plain language forms for seniors: A guide for the public, private and not-for profit sectors*. Ottawa, Ontario: Author.

18. Sabogal, F., Otero-Sabogal, R., Pasick, R., Jenkins, C., & Perez-Stable, E. (1996). Printed health education materials for diverse communities: Suggestions learned from the field. *Health Education Quarterly, 23*, 123–141.

ADDITIONAL RESOURCES

Print

AMC Cancer Research Center and Centers for Disease Control. (1994). *Beyond the brochure: Alternative approaches to effective health communication.* Atlanta: Centers for Disease Control and Prevention. A free copy is available at http://www.cdc.gov/nccdphp/dcpc/publica.htm#breast or by calling 770-488-4751.

Centers for Disease Control and Prevention, Office of Communication. (1999). *Simply put* (2nd ed.). Atlanta: Author.

Culture, health and literacy: A guide to health education materials for adults with limited English literacy skills. Guidebook available for free from World Education, 44 Farnsworth St., Boston, MA 02210-1211. Phone: 617-482-9485.

The health and literacy compendium: An annotated bibliography of print and Web-based health materials for use with limited literacy adults. Guidebook available for free from World Education, 44 Farnsworth St., Boston, MA 02210-1211. Phone: 617-482-9485.

National Cancer Institute. (1994). *Clear and simple: Developing effective print materials for low-literate readers* (NIH Publication No. 95-3594). Bethesda MD: National Institutes of Health. To order a free copy call 1-800-4-CANCER. Publication T936.

Internet

Federal government's guide to plain language writing. Available: http://www.plainlanguage.gov.

10

Working with the Media

Michael Young, Ph.D., FSSSS, FAAHB

Author Comments

For more than 30 years I have been a health education faculty member in higher education. Beginning as a graduate student coordinating a community education project, and now as a faculty member, I have had a number of opportunities to work with the media. This has included providing media outlets with press releases to publicize various projects and recruit participants for training workshops. I have also provided regular community education articles to local papers and have even written a sexual advice column. In addition, I have worked with radio station personnel to create public service announcements that were distributed on a statewide basis and have been a guest on a number of radio and television talk shows.

I have been interviewed on many occasions. Sometimes reporters wanted an interview because we had won an award or received some recognition that they wanted to publicize. On other occasions the reporter was looking to me as the expert to provide background information or commentary on a situation within my area of expertise. There have also been several times that the interviewer wanted to talk to me because I had played a role in a controversial situation. Additionally, I have written to editors to suggest a feature story or to encourage the investigation of a particular issue. Finally, on some issues, to get my point across, I have simply written a letter to the editor for publication on the paper's opinion page.

My task in this chapter is to provide you with tips for working with the media. I am not a press agent who works with the media every day, but over the years I have gained some experience and am pleased to have the opportunity to share what I have learned. I hope this chapter will be of benefit to you and your organization as you work with the media.

Introduction

Why would a community health educator want to work with the media? There are numerous reasons, such as educating the public about an important health issue, publicizing activities, and encouraging people to take some type of action related to a particular health problem or concern. Sometimes the information to be shared is mundane, such as announcing the place and time a public meeting will be held. At other times, media exposure may be the result of a controversial issue. Just because it is publicity does not necessarily mean that it is good publicity. It is important to learn to work with the media so that, insofar as is possible, the publicity received by the organization is good publicity. Remember, the media can be powerful allies for furthering a cause.

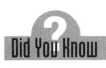

Did You Know

In addition to inventing the Franklin stove, bifocals, daylight savings time, and electroshock treatment, Ben Franklin also invented newspaper editorials.

Other chapters within this text deal with issues associated with social marketing, health communication, media advocacy, and legislative action. Many of the media methods and tools used are the same. This chapter focuses on developing technical skills used to apply these tools. In particular, this chapter addresses skills associated with public service announcements, news releases, letters to editors, fact sheets, interviewing, and press kits. Also included are tips for working with the different media outlets, with real examples of what has seemed to work well and what has not.

Steps for Utilizing Media Avenues

The father of the author of this chapter worked as an engine mechanic for one of the major airlines. At home, he spent much time working on the family car and truck. He often talked about the importance of having the right tool for the job. There were many tools in his toolbox, and he knew how to use them well. Good mechanics do not attempt to overhaul an automobile engine using only a hammer and a screwdriver, but rather make sure they have the right tools for the job. That which is good advice for the mechanic is also good advice for those working with the media: Have the right tools for the job and know how to use them. This section explores several of the tools that should be in a media toolbox and how they can best be used when working with media channels.

There are a number of channels for working with media—all of which should be used in a comprehensive health promotion effort. The steps for using each differ, just as the steps for using different types of mechanic's tools differ. Media channels that are typically more accessible to health educators include radio, television, and newspapers. Although all three are interested in what health educators have to share, the tools used to share that information vary.

Work with Print Media

Newspapers, radio, and television complement each other, yet differ relative to time and senses used. A newspaper is focused on sight and involves reading, which is a vastly different way of learning than auditory learning. That is not to say that the audience is necessarily different, but rather that the sense used in conveying information differs greatly. As such, a different set of tools is needed for sharing health information.

News Releases

News, or **press**, **releases** provide information about an organization and its activities. Radio, television, newspapers, and regional or local magazines consume news releases. For example, an organization could use this technique to announce new board or staff members, a grant award, or a special activity. News releases are often used by organizations to gain community recognition for the organization, its activities, and its members. They are often used to announce special events (see Figures 10-1 and 10-2). They may also be used to make position statements or to address controversy.

The news release is a one- or two-page double-spaced typed document. In addition to the source, contact person, Web page and email information, and release date and time, the release should include both a headline and a story.

- *Headline.* The headline provides the overall concept of the information and should be typed in capital letters. For maximum effectiveness, keep headlines one or two lines in length. There is no guarantee the media outlet will use the supplied headline. Not providing a headline, however, is an invitation for the media to write their own. This is fine when they use a headline that accurately reflects the story. If they make a mistake, however, their headline may actually be detrimental to your cause. Help them get it right: Provide an appropriate headline.

- *Story.* The story is the content of the news release and can be either a news story or a feature article. A news story provides information about an announcement or is an account of an activity that readers may find of interest. A feature is a story that is a main attraction or headline. For example, a news release pertaining to a breakthrough in cancer research or other research findings that affect human lives could be front-page news and the basis for a major feature story.

News stories follow the basics of journalism. In the first paragraph, they answer the questions who, what, when, and where. Stories should be written

DATE: April 14, 2008

FOR IMMEDIATE RELEASE

Re: The Society for the Scientific Study of Sexuality—Mid-continent Region Annual Meeting in Little Rock

This year's meeting of the Society for the Scientific Study of Sexuality (SSSS)—Mid-continent Region, will be at the Excelsior Hotel in Little Rock, May 19–21. The theme of the conference is "What is sex"? This will be a great opportunity for university faculty, students, public school teachers, counselors, therapists, and health professionals in Arkansas to attend a regional SSSS meeting. It will also be a great opportunity to hear, meet, and visit with some of the leaders in the field of sexology and sexuality education. Tim Turton, director of the Kinsey Institute, will be the speaker at the Saturday awards luncheon. Denise Albar and Carla Barnes, both of whom have served as president of the Society and are accomplished researchers, will also be convention speakers. A number of other nationally known sexologists will be on the convention program. Several speakers are from Arkansas, including John Wilson, Jim Anderson, and Jenna Condor, from the University of Arkansas; Lonnie Smith, from the Arkansas chapter of the American Civil Liberties Union; Rod Prahl, from the Arkansas Department of Health; and Amber Ptak, member of the Arkansas House of Representatives.

Enclosed please find a preliminary program that also includes registration information. Participants can save $25 by registering prior to May 1. Questions about the meeting and this release can be directed to co-program chair Michael Young, Ph.D., University of Arkansas 501-575-5639.

XXX

Figure 10-1 Sample Short News Release

through the eyes of a reporter, organizing material in the way that is appropriate for appearing in the newspaper. Place important elements early in the story, while saving those of lesser importance for later in the story (using an inverted triangle approach, where the most important information appears in the first paragraph and the least important near the end). If the release is used as written but is shortened to meet space constraints, the most important messages are still conveyed.

Feature stories contain more information in the body of the release than a news story. The writing should gain the attention of the editor and draw him or her into the story, because the editor is the person who will decide if the story is used at all. The objective is to get the entire story printed. This, however, does not always happen. Sometimes an editor may use only a portion of the material submitted. At times the objective might not be for the paper to publish a feature that was submitted, but rather to encourage them to write a feature themselves (see Figure 10-3).

FROM: American First Aid
        123 Eagle Drive
        Northport, MI 49670
        paxson@afe.org

CONTACT: Rebekah Paxson

PHONE: (312) 456-2367

FAX: (312) 764-2938

DATE: October 15, 2008

                                        FOR IMMEDIATE RELEASE

              FREE FIRST AID/CPR TRAINING AVAILABLE

The American First Aid Institute is offering free first aid/CPR training. A total of 10 training programs, each limited to 12 individuals, will be available. Trainings will be conducted over an 8-hour day, beginning Saturday, June 6, 2008. Enrollment is on a first come, first serve basis. For more information or to register for a class, call (312) 456-2367 or stop by the American First Aid at 123 Eagle Drive.

                            ###

Figure 10-2 Sample Short News Release

Many times reporters or editors receive a call from a person who tells them "Your paper/station should do a story about . . ." something that is of interest to them. Often the person calling is upset and wants the media to expose an injustice or wrongdoing. Just as often the calls may have plenty of emotion without having a lot of facts. How is it possible to get the paper to do a story about an issue?

Letters to the Editor

In many communities, the letters to the editor section is one of the most-read sections of the local newspaper. This section gives people an avenue for providing information, expressing an opinion, or saying "thank you" to an entire community (see Figure 10-4). Many times it will be appropriate to write a letter to the editor on behalf of an organization. The letters to the editor section also provides individuals with an opportunity to be heard as private citizens in situations in which the organizations that employ them may not want them representing the organizations on a particular issue. They offer the rare instance to tell a story without it being interpreted or given a different slant by a reporter.

Newspapers usually have specific limitations that guide the length of letters. Usually these guidelines are listed in the editorial section of the paper or can easily be obtained by contacting the paper's editorial department.

October 28, 2008

Matt Devoe
Record Eagle
Gardenton, Michigan

Dear Mr. Devoe:

The purpose of this letter is to request your paper do a feature news article regarding the use of materials, published by Abstinence Plus, in a countywide abstinence education project coordinated by Gardenton School District. As a trained health educator and coauthor of nationally known abstinence curricula that have demonstrated positive behavior (as per published evaluations in scholarly journals), a director of projects that have received numerous state and national acclaim, and a taxpayer living in Gardenton School District, I am deeply concerned about the use of these materials. My concerns are summarized below. In addition, please find a SIECUS Fact Sheet and an article from *Contraception Evaluation*—a journal that focuses on contraceptive effectiveness.

- Abstinence Plus materials are nationally known. They are known, however, for their medical inaccuracy, scare tactics, and lack of any evaluations published in scholarly/professional journals indicating their behavioral effectiveness.
- Abstinence Plus materials once were used in projects funded by the Office of Youth Pregnancy (OAYP). As part of a settlement of a court case that went all the way to the state Supreme Court, OAYP established a review process for materials proposed for use in their projects. Materials now must be medically accurate, neutral on religion, and neutral on abortion. Abstinence Plus materials are no longer approved for use in OAYP projects.
- Examples of inaccurate information: *Look At Me Grow*, an Abstinence Plus curriculum, includes a section about condoms that indicates there is "a 15 to 20% risk of transmission of HIV even with training and proper usage" and a statement that one author found, based on "a thorough review of condom effectiveness," that "condoms reduce the risk of heterosexual HIV infection by only 60%." In addition, the curriculum reports, "a large family planning clinic found that 80% of respondents had experienced condoms tearing or slipping off."

    Contraception Evaluation, which is the state Health Department's standard for medical accuracy, indicates that 2% of the couples who consistently and correctly use condoms to prevent pregnancy have a pregnancy at the end of a year of use. This is a failure rate due to failure of the method on an order of 0.02% of the times a condom is used. *Contraception Evaluation* also describes the failure rates of condoms in preventing the transmission of HIV between serodiscordant couples as extremely low, citing several studies, one in which the failure rate among couples who used condoms consistently and correctly was zero, and others that showed extremely low rates (see enclosures).
- From a public health perspective, the approach of these materials is inaccurate, irresponsible, and dangerous. Programs designed to prevent adolescent pregnancy and sexually transmitted diseases should emphasize abstinence.

(Continues)

Figure 10-3 Feature Story Letter

People need to understand that condoms are not 100% effective. They also need to understand that for them to work they must be used, not some of the time, but every time. To send the message, however, that condoms and other contraceptives do not work and are of no help is to discourage those who do engage in sexual intercourse and other risky sexual behavior from trying to protect themselves. After all, condoms are inconvenient to obtain and use, and if they do not work, then why bother?

Thus, based on evidence regarding medical inaccuracy and violation of required assurances, I respectfully request that your paper consider doing a feature article on this curriculum, with the intent of having it withdrawn from Gardenton Schools and the other school districts in Jackson County.

Sincerely,

John Berry, M.P.H.
1382 5th St.
Gardenton, MI 49203

Daytime phone: 712-289-3982
Evening phone: 712-892-0382
Email: jberry@jacksonco.mi.gov

Figure 10-3 (Continued)

Community connections 1

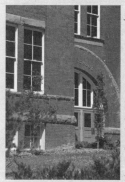

John was concerned about an abstinence education curriculum promoted by a local school district located within the intermediate school district's boundaries. He had expressed his concerns in writing to the project coordinator and the district superintendent (with copies to school board members), but to no avail. John had extensive experience with abstinence education, having coauthored an abstinence-based curriculum himself, and was considered by many to be an expert in the subject. The school district in question, though, had chosen to implement a different curriculum, one that was highly subjective and not based on accurate information.

Many people perceived John's protest as simply a case of being a "poor loser." John thought if he could enlist the support of the local paper to do a feature story on the issue, using, in part, factual information he could provide, it might bring some pressure on the district to remove this curriculum and install one that provided accurate information to students.

John called a friend, who also happened to be a newspaper reporter in a different state. He suggested John write a letter to the editor, not for the letters to the editor page, but rather one providing factual information about the situation. He also told John to make a phone call or send an email letting the editor know the letter was coming and to make a follow-up call to ensure the letter was received and see if a reporter would be assigned to cover the story. John wrote a stirring letter (see Figure 10-3), which a reporter then followed up for a feature story.

Guest Editorials

An additional avenue might be through a guest editorial. Many local newspapers provide opportunities to write an opinion editorial on a specific topic. An excellent example is a local slant on a national campaign (e.g., National Drunk/Drugged Driving—December). Typically, these allow for more print space. If guest editorials are available in the area, contact the editor first to confirm his or her interest. Obtain the guidelines and deadlines for submission. Make sure

---

May 28, 2008

Editor
Northwest Arkansas Times
Fayetteville, AR 72701

Dear Editor:

I could not believe it when I read the guest editorial in the *Times* concerning "Healthy Smoking." There is no such animal. Smoking is the number one cause of preventable disease and disability in this country. Smoking is responsible for 85% of all lung cancers and plays a role in the development of cancer of just about every other body part as well. At least 30% of all cancer deaths are the result of cigarette smoking. Smoking is the number one lifestyle risk factor in heart disease. It has also been found that nearly 82% of all deaths due to chronic obstructive pulmonary disease can be attributed to cigarette smoking.

Smoking is not only a health hazard for people who smoke; it is also a health hazard for those who are exposed to their smoking. People who live with someone who smokes are also exposed to increased health risks. For example, the rate of lung cancer in female nonsmokers married to smokers is up to 3.25 times the rate of lung cancer in female nonsmokers married to nonsmokers. Smoking during pregnancy is also linked to a number of health problems in babies. In addition, children of parents who smoke have an increased frequency of respiratory infections and show reduced lung function as they mature.

Let me repeat. There is *no* such thing as healthy smoking. It is a free country. People have a personal right to make the unwise and unhealthy decision to smoke. They should not attempt, however, to convince themselves and others that the choice they have made is a healthy one. Neither should they expose nonsmokers to the hazards associated with their unhealthy behavior.

Sincerely,

Michael Young, Ph.D.
Professor & Coordinator, Program in Health Science
Director, Health Education Projects Office

Figure 10-4 Sample Letter to the Editor

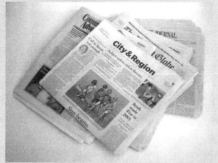

Community connections 2

John's letter to the newspaper resulted in a feature article that appeared on the front page of the newspaper's education section. Much to his delight, John found the newspaper had done an excellent job investigating the issues he shared and had reported them thoroughly in the paper. Within a week, the letters appearing in the letters to the editor section of the paper were primarily devoted to the curriculum selection issue. It appeared that many local citizens were just as concerned as John was with the use of the abstinence curriculum. The newspaper had its fair share of supporters for the curriculum, but each such letter seemed to focus on repeating the same argument over and over. Letters from opponents to the curriculum expressed numerous views as to why the abstinence-only curriculum should not be implemented.

to prepare the piece as directed. The newspaper may still cut portions based on available space. Use the same journalistic techniques previously described when preparing the information.

Work with Radio and Television

It is important to remember that the unit of exchange for both radio and television is time. In contrast to print media, which are not necessarily confined by time, radio and television are limited with respect to offering broad coverage of information with target audiences. Health educators most often interact with these media channels through public service announcements and interviews (which will be discussed as a separate media avenue).

Public Service Announcements

Public service announcements (PSAs) are short informational announcements typically used by charity, nonprofit, and community organizations. PSAs are used on the radio or television to educate the public, promote programs or services, and provide resources for behavior or community change. PSAs are one of the most common means of conveying messages to the public. Some PSAs are designed to evoke an emotional response in the listener or viewer. Other PSAs are more cognitively focused, informing listeners of dates and times of events, and are thus less dependent on emotional response.

Almost all agencies have, at one time or another, developed and used PSAs in their programming efforts. Because PSAs are relatively easy to produce and use, they have become a standard means for agencies to communicate messages to the public. Some PSAs are developed and aired nationally and are shown on local affiliate stations. Others are developed by national organizations and made available to community groups, who often add a tag line to identify their local organization and who work with local media sources to secure airtime in local markets. Increases in technical knowledge and skills have opened more options for creating PSAs at the local level.

There are basically two types of PSAs, those aired on the radio and those that appear on television. Of the two, radio announcements are usually easier to develop, cost less, and have a greater likelihood of receiving airtime. A radio PSA consists of a short message, which takes less than 60 seconds to read aloud, typed double-spaced on 8.5-by-11-inch paper (see Figure 10-5 for a sample PSA). The PSA should include the following:

- *Source*. Who is sending the announcement? Both the individual and the organization should be identified. The name of the organization, city, state, and zip code should be located at the top of the first page, as should a Web page or email address, if available.

- *Contact person*. Who is the contact person? This person may be different from the person actually sending the material (source). Include the contact person's name, title, phone number, email address, and fax.

- *Release date and time*. Is the information ready for immediate release, or is there a particular date when it should be used? For example, a PSA about Labor Day travel should be broadcast immediately prior to and throughout the Labor Day weekend. A time range should be included if a PSA is designed to be aired at a specific time of day. For instance, some PSAs may be more appropriate if aired during the late afternoon when adolescents are out of school or workers are commuting home. Be aware, however, that there is always competition for airtime. Airtime is what stations have to sell. The availability of some time slots (such as morning and afternoon drive times) is extremely limited. PSAs with fewer constraints for airing are more likely to be used.

Television PSAs are either components of broader state and national campaigns or are developed locally by the agency. A PSA that has already been developed is much easier and less costly to use than one that needs to be created from scratch. Usually PSAs obtained from a national campaign or agency (for example, the National Campaign for the Prevention of Teen Pregnancy, the Environmental Protection Agency, or the National Highway Traffic Safety Administration) can be tailored to include a message at the end identifying local contacts and action. In contrast, developing a PSA locally allows the issue to be customized for specific community needs, populations, and problems. Often local personalities will give their time to appear in television PSAs. Although personnel at local health agencies

FROM: Jack Holliday, Community Educator
       Community Safety Partners
       1224 Jefferson
       Kalamazoo, MI 49001

RELEASE DATE: February 18, 2008
TIME: 30 seconds

Zip, Zero, Zilch

JUST ONE DRINK BEFORE DRIVING CAN GET YOU BUSTED. YOUNG ADULTS
MAY THINK THEY KNOW EVERYTHING ABOUT DRINKING AND DRIVING, BUT DO
THEY KNOW THE "ZIP-ZERO-ZILCH" LAW? THIS LAW STATES THAT IF YOU'RE
STOPPED, YOU'LL BE TESTED FOR ALCOHOL LEVELS. IF YOU REFUSE THE
TEST YOUR LICENSE IS CUT UP ON THE SPOT AND GONE FOR SIX MONTHS.
IF THE TEST SHOWS YOU'VE BEEN DRINKING EVEN ONE BEER, YOU'LL LOSE
YOUR LICENSE FOR 30 TO 90 DAYS AND PAY UP TO $250 IN FINES.

IN MICHIGAN, THE ONLY WAY YOU CAN DRIVE SAFELY IS IF YOU HAVE HAD
"ZIP-ZERO-ZILCH" TO DRINK.

THIS MESSAGE IS BROUGHT TO YOU BY COMMUNITY SAFETY PARTNERS.

-END-

Figure 10-5 Sample Public Service Announcement

may like the idea of starring in their own PSA, they may be better served by using someone who is well known in the community or region.

Radio and television broadcast stations are interested in airing PSAs for a number of reasons. One major reason is that the Federal Communications Commission (FCC) reviews a station's public service when deciding whether to renew its broadcast license. Stations that provide an adequate amount of free airtime are more likely to receive a license renewal. In addition, most local stations are interested in airing information about events and issues that directly affect the local community. Many of their listeners reside within their broadcast range and have an interest in local activities and issues. For instance, many neighborhood members rely heavily on radio and television to inform them of free cholesterol screenings, immunizations, health fairs, and other health promotion activities. Stations in competition for listeners

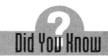

The number of daily morning newspapers in the United States has more than doubled over the past 40 years. During the same period, daily evening newspapers have decreased by 50%, while the number of Sunday papers has steadily increased.

have a vested interest in airing public service announcements that are both appealing and informative. Some stations are interested in health-related PSAs because they feel a responsibility to their listeners. PSAs that promote positive health and discourage negative health behaviors help stations meet this often unspoken responsibility to the public for providing messages that can improve the well-being of society. Finally, a station that airs PSAs that are designed to promote positive health behavior may generate community goodwill. The listener views the station as a good citizen of the community that provides a valuable service.

Conduct Interviews

The media may contact health educators to obtain further information about a topic, to answer questions about a controversial issue, or as a follow-up to information that was sent to them. The contact may be in the form of an interview, which can occur via telephone, radio, or television. The interview can be either formal or informal, conducted over the telephone, on-site at the radio or television station, at the interviewee's agency, or at some off-site location.

Maintaining a good relationship with the media requires being flexible and accommodating their schedule. In most cases they will be working on a tight deadline, so returning calls promptly and doing what is necessary to accommodate them will improve relations. Working cooperatively with the media may result in future interviews.

Telephone and Radio Interviews

A telephone interview is generally initiated by a reporter who calls requesting an interview or a statement related to a particular news item. Sometimes an initial call is made to arrange a time for an interview, which provides time to prepare. The reporter may be from a newspaper, magazine, or radio or television station gathering material for a story. The interview may be taped, so the reporter will have an accurate record of the interview, or, if it is for radio, to play on the air later. Finally, the telephone interview may be one that is conducted as part of a live on-the-air radio show, perhaps with call-in questions from listeners. During an interview, remember to promote the organization and provide a contact person name and phone number.

Television Interviews

The information, and actual audiotape, from telephone interviews can be used in radio or television stories. Like telephone interviews, television interviews are sometimes arranged in advance, such as being a guest on a local talk show devoted to community events (e.g., a *Talk About Town* type of show). Other times there is little notice. The interview may be a part of a story or series that has been developed over a period of time, or it may be an attempt to determine local response to a news story the station has just received from the wire service.

Community Connections 3

John was amazed at the amount of newspaper and television coverage of the abstinence-only curriculum issue. In fact, he had been called by three local radio stations and the local television station, all of whom wanted to interview him. Two of the three radio interviews were conducted over the telephone, and one actually took place at the radio station. In preparing for the telephone interviews, John double-checked all his facts and had copies of published research papers associated with the issue available. During the interview, John made certain to only express that which he knew to be true, and was careful not to express opinions that he could not back up. His answers were short and succinct. Each radio station appreciated his comments and aired exactly what he said. Although he was prepared, none of the interviews involved call-in questions from listeners.

It is important to remember that television, especially a news program, broadcasts video clips and sound bites that are measured in seconds. Often television reporters will tape an interview in the field, which will be aired later that day. Instead of showing the entire interview, the television producer will make the decision as to which segments to broadcast. The more time the person interviewed spent on camera, the more material the producer has from which to choose, and the less likely it is that the material that was thought to be important will actually be aired. It is best to keep the interview short to ensure that important information is presented. If the interview has to do with a controversial issue, it may be wise to speak from a short, prepared statement.

The most obvious difference between television interviews and other types of interviews is that there is a viewing audience. A telephone interview can be conducted in a bathrobe, but a television interview cannot. Many television interviews are requested at the spur of the moment. Professionals who are often called upon for interviews usually keep a change of clothes available for such occasions. Men can keep an extra pressed shirt and tie on a hanger at the office. Women can keep a blazer and nice blouse hanging in the corner. It is important to look good, even on short notice.

Last-Minute Interviews

Last-minute interviews often require an expert in a subject area to respond to questions. Time may not allow for background research. When contacted by the media for an interview on short notice, it is important to have a clear picture of the topic and the length of the interview. It is okay to decline the interview if the reporter is looking for factual information and expert opinion on a topic that is unfamiliar. Let the reporter know that the invitation is appreciated, indicate topics that may be more suitable based on level of expertise, and make a referral to someone who can better meet the reporter's needs.

Conduct a Press Conference

A press conference is often held in conjunction with a major announcement. It may be related to a new building, organization, or services provided in the area. Press conferences are also held to announce major projects, fund raising, or the latest statistics on health or safety issues. Media personnel from every media avenue (e.g., newspaper, television, radio) are typically invited to attend this forum.

A prepared statement is used and provided to the media, along with background or supporting material. The media usually ask for additional information that will help them build a good news story, so it is important to have a thorough base of knowledge pertaining to the issue. A press kit is usually distributed to the media, which includes background information about the issue. Even so, it is important to be able to respond intelligently and succinctly to their questions.

Tips and Techniques for Effectively Working with the Media

Become Familiar with Media Personnel

Using the media to benefit a cause involves becoming familiar with the personnel associated with the radio and television stations and newspapers that serve the community. For instance, it is good to know who writes and edits feature stories for the community morning newspaper. It would also be helpful to know something of the feature writer's personal interests and views on various topics. What if the feature writer is also president of the local chapter of the National Rifle Association? Would he or she be the best person to approach with an idea for a story to advocate local restrictions on purchase and possession of handguns? Knowledge is not a one-way street. It is good to know something about news personnel, but it is even better if news personnel know and view health educators as reliable sources of information—someone they can call when they need information. Establishing this rapport provides an avenue for contact with the news media. Cultivating such relationships can create a win-win situation for both parties.

Becoming a trusted resource for news personnel can also foster a strong working relationship. Media personnel need to be aware of a multitude of topics and issues. Trying to keep on top of all the changes that constantly occur can be overwhelming. In many cases, the media rely on their trusted sources for up-to-date information and late-breaking news. Emailing new findings or resource information reduces the need for a media contact to spend time searching for new and innovative information. Ensure that what you give to the media is correct and pertinent, because misleading or inaccurate information can be detrimental to fostering a strong working relationship.

Increase Chances of a PSA Being Aired

There are a number of ways to increase the likelihood that a PSA will be aired, including the following:

- Remember to keep PSAs short; most PSAs are less than 30 seconds long. Time is a precious commodity in broadcasting, where every second is tracked. Time blocks are typically available in 10-, 15-, 20-, 30-, 45-, and 60-second lengths. Thus, material to be included in the PSA will have to be carefully selected.

- Write the PSA in a concise manner, which may be difficult at first because this is not a skill often used in academic settings. Have colleagues and members of the target audience proofread the PSA. Read the copy aloud to determine approximate length. When doing so, it is important to read at the same pace as will be used on the media. Timing does not have to be exact, as the station may trim the copy to fit its time slot. The station usually will call if it needs more information.

- Call the stations being targeted and ask for the person who deals with PSAs. Let him or her know about the PSA, explain why it is important, and ask the best way to get a PSA on the air at that station. Follow the advice. When not able to visit directly with a person at the station, mail or fax the PSA to the station. Include a cover letter that explains the importance of the announcement and requests airtime. Stations receive many requests to air PSAs, so if there is a specific time period being targeted for the PSA (for example, a PSA pertaining to Halloween safety targeted during the week of Halloween), then submit it at least six weeks ahead of time.

- Sometimes stations (both radio and television) will work with organizations to help them produce taped PSAs. Spending funds to produce a quality product and to purchase particular airtime slots may be worthwhile. Paying for at least part of the process, instead of asking for it all to be donated, may result in more free airtime than would otherwise be received. For instance, a drug education program with the slogan *Be A Winner—Choose Not to Use* is implemented in Arkansas public schools at the fifth- or sixth-grade level by local law enforcement officers in partnership with school counselors and classroom teachers. Sometimes, grants have been acquired to support the training of officers and educators and for the purchase of materials, such as leader's manuals, student workbooks, and T-shirts. Most of the time, however, police officers raise money locally to purchase materials. To provide an antidrug message for young people

"This is Clint McDaniel of the National Champion University of Arkansas Razorback basketball team, encouraging you to be a winner on the court, in the classroom, and in life. Be a winner; choose not to use. This message brought to you by the University of Arkansas' Be A Winner drug education program, your local law enforcement agency, and this radio station."

"This is Jason Allen, quarterback for the University of Arkansas Razorback football team. Score a touchdown on the field, in the classroom, and in life. Be a winner; choose not to use. This message brought to you by the University of Arkansas' Be A Winner drug education program, your local law enforcement agency, and this radio station."

Figure 10-6 Be a Winner

around the state and to assist officers in their fund-raising efforts, the developers of this program worked with a local radio station and the University of Arkansas' athletic department to produce several short PSAs on a single tape. A small charge for production costs was paid, and the radio station made multiple copies of the tape. The tape was sent to *Be A Winner* officers around the state, who took it to their local radio stations. Rather than simply request free airtime for the PSAs, airtime was purchased from the station that had produced the tapes. In response, the station provided three times the amount of airtime for which it had been paid. Figure 10-6 contains two examples of the PSAs that were aired.

Increase Chances of a News Release Being Published

There are a number of ways to increase the likelihood that a news release will be published:

- Keep the news release short. Make each sentence concise and avoid using jargon. Imagine a reader who is trying to read words that are unfamiliar. At the same time, do not embarrass the reader by using words that may be misleading or have an underlying message that may be construed negatively.

- Write the news release so that it does not need a cover letter to explain the contents. It should be a complete story that stands on its own. This is not to say a cover letter is unimportant. Rather, the release should be able to be printed as is and still make sense.

- Make it easy for editors to read and follow. Use wide margins, and double space material. This white space provides editors with the room they need for editing the release. For submitted stories, triple space between the headline and the first paragraph of the story. Do not split paragraphs between pages. If a paragraph will not fit on a page in its entirety, move the paragraph to the next page. Each paragraph should stand alone, with or without the previous or following paragraphs. Be able to provide documentation for any assertions made. If stating, for example, that aspirin reduces the risk of heart attacks, then have copies of supporting research articles on hand. News releases designed to solicit a response need to include contact information in the last paragraph (e.g., "For more information, please contact Tom Broekema at 800-875-4422). With the advances in communication technology, including a statement to visit the agency's Web site or providing additional Internet links increases credibility. Typing "END," "###," or "XXX" at the end of the story text identifies the end of the release.

- Email news releases no sooner than one week before requested date of publication. Newspapers may receive hundreds of faxed news releases on any given day. An emailed copy ensures the news release is received by the party intended and provides a convenient method for the news reporter to contact you if more information is needed.

- Make a phone call to the media outlets in which the release is appropriate to appear. This helps in developing contacts so that the release can be sent to a person, rather than to a newspaper. A "newspaper" does not make the decision as to whether a release will be printed—a person working for the paper makes that decision.

Enhance Interviewing Skills

Ways to increase the likelihood of a successful interview include the following:

- Prepare for the interview. If called about doing an interview, be sure to know who is calling, the organization represented, and the purpose of the interview. Know if the agency you represent has a public relations policy that states that only specific individuals may talk to the press. Take a moment to gather background information. Offer to call back. The first few times doing an interview may be stressful. That is normal. Try to relax, and act normally. Remember that anything said may be heard on the air or printed in the paper.

- Provide the reporter with appropriate background information. Often reporters may have only a small amount of information on the topic, perhaps only that which has been included on a wire service fact sheet. Most reporters will appreciate assistance, especially if the information provided is relevant.

- Know in advance who will conduct the interview. If not familiar with the person, listen or watch the show (or read newspaper articles written by the interviewer) prior to the interview. Become familiar with and understand the format and interview style.

- Find out the target audience. Is the audience primarily teens? Elderly? High income? Audience information may be available from the marketing department of the media station or publication or from discussions with people who are familiar with the program or articles.

- Prepare to answer as many questions as possible. Some interviewers will provide samples of questions that will be asked. Other questions, however, may come up during the interview or from outside callers.

- Consider speaking from a prepared statement, and do not stray far from it. Stay focused on the topic that is of concern to you. Do not be led into answering loaded questions or talking about issues that would be better left alone. And do not be surprised if the question you are not prepared to answer is the one that is asked. It may be helpful to work out a few ground rules with the reporter before anything is recorded. If there is something that the reporter wants to ask but which you do not want to address, let the reporter know that ahead of time. If the reporter agrees to the conditions but asks the question on-camera anyway, politely indicate the interview is over. Realize that the question that was poorly answered or the statement that was made during the interview that you do not desire to be shown on television will often be what actually is aired.

- Make a list of major points to share during the interview. If the interviewer does not ask for the information, try to add it to the conversation.

- Have organized reference material available. The key term is *organized*— shuffling papers is not a positive image and sends a message of uncertainty. Being able to locate information quickly is a benefit.

Did You Know

The Federal Communications Commission (FCC) is an independent U.S. government agency, directly responsible to Congress. The FCC was established by the Communications Act of 1934 and is charged with regulating interstate and international communications by radio, television, wire, satellite, and cable. The FCC's jurisdiction covers the 50 states, the District of Columbia, and U.S. possessions.

- Do not be afraid to say, "That is a good question. I do not have the answer for that at this moment. I will have to do some additional research and get back to you." Admitting lack of knowledge is much better than providing inaccurate or incorrect information.

- Have a final statement prepared. Typically, the interviewer will ask if there is anything else to add. Take advantage of the opportunity to advertise the agency or make a significant statement about the topic.

- Do not be late to a scheduled interview. Remember, time is a precious commodity for media.

- For a television interview, dress for success. This means selecting apparel that is conservative, professional, and not likely to clash with other colors on the set. Avoid clothes that are white, light colored, or patterned. Accessories should be limited, because overaccessorizing may make noise or cause reflections from studio lights. Wear glasses if you usually wear them.

■ For a television interview, maintain good posture. Sit comfortably in the chair but do not slouch. Keep legs crossed or feet flat on the floor and lean slightly forward toward the interviewer. Do not gesture with hand movements, as this can be distracting on television.

■ Remain calm and professional. Nervous reactions are likely to be recognized over the telephone and on the radio.

Follow Up after an Interview

After the interview, check to see if what appeared in the newspaper, or on television or radio, accurately reflected statements made. Sometimes reporters take what they hear and put together a news story that clearly represents all aspects of a situation. Sometimes reporters simply mess up. The quote taken from the interview may not be close to individual or agency true positions on the issue. The reporter may not understand all that is involved and, working on a tight deadline, might make an honest mistake. In other cases, the portions of the article that are based on an interview, or the short segment of videotape or audiotape that is aired, may not be at all representative of the entire interview.

If reporters do a good job, let them know about it. If there are problems with the story, let them know about that too. It is important that views are correctly represented and the information provided to the public is factual. Reporters want to correctly represent their sources and have good stories. They may never know there was a problem unless they are informed.

Over the last few years my name has been in the paper and on radio and television in Arkansas on a number of occasions. Sometimes this has been in connection with something quite positive: announcement of a program award, scheduled upcoming training workshop, or receipt of a federal grant. Sometimes, however, the news is not entirely positive. The heading "State Lawmaker Threatens to 'Beat the Crap' Out of U of A Professor," for example, was the headline that appeared on the front page of Arkansas' largest newspaper. At a public meeting, a state representative sitting across the table interrupted discussion to yell (from about six feet away), "I'm about ready to come across this table and beat the crap out of you." He was quickly escorted from the room. The (now former) state representative evidently had forgotten, or perhaps was not aware, that a newspaper reporter—with tape recorder running—was present and had recorded every word he had said.

Community connections 4

After he listened to his radio interviews, John sent a thank-you note to each reporter, expressing his appreciation for being able to share information and for their willingness to accurately address the topic. He even received a call back from one of the reporters, who said, "I received your letter and just want to let you know that it is I who appreci-ated your candid responses. I hope you don't mind, John, if I keep you on my list for any future programs I develop that have to do with school-based sexuality issues." John felt honored to be acknowledged for his efforts and felt pleased to be able to serve as a future source for providing research-based guidance regarding sexuality issues.

Follow-up stories appeared in one or more papers nearly every day over the next two weeks. In addition, there were requests for television interviews. A lot was learned, in a short period of time, about how newspapers and television work and ways to deal with them. The author would try to provide newspaper reporters with as much information as possible so they would have a clear understanding of the issue. They would do a story, usually using a small portion of the information they had been given. Often, the stories missed the point. They included information, but not always the essential information. One of the television interviews generated over an hour of tape. About 15 seconds of it actually aired. It was not the 15 seconds that the author would have picked.

Use Media Fact Sheets

Media **fact sheets** are tools that can be used to support media bits and secure feature articles in a newspaper or magazine. Members of the media do not always investigate or seek out stories based on their own interests. Most articles are the result of some impetus provided from a reliable source. The fact sheet is sent to the media for encouragement and consideration for further investigation, perhaps to use in a feature story.

Often media sources will receive phone calls or letters encouraging reporters to do a story on a particular topic in which the caller has an interest. Many times the caller will make a case for a story, based on much emotion and little fact: "You've got to do a story about what's going on down at the school. It's criminal the stuff those teachers are trying to teach the kids." A fact sheet provides factual information about a situation.

A fact sheet is not a PSA or a news release. The fact sheet provides a structured format of information to the editor to assist in developing a story idea. It does not provide all of the details of the story, but does provide an idea and supporting information that can be expanded into a longer, more detailed article. The editor may make a decision whether to assign a reporter the task of developing the story idea based on the information provided in the fact sheet.

The fact sheet should be accompanied by a brief cover letter that provides a summary of the basic concept, gives a description of the problem, and identifies possible solutions. Both the cover letter and the fact sheet should identify the source of the fact sheet (both the organization and individual) and the contact person who is responsible for answering questions related to the fact sheet. Phone numbers, extensions, fax numbers, and email addresses should be included.

It is important to follow up the submitted fact sheet with a phone call to the news editor. "Last month I sent you information about the abstinence curriculum used at Fayetteville High School. I believe the program they are providing students is irresponsible and dangerous. What can I do to encourage you to do a story concerning the program?"

Use a Press Kit

A **press kit** is a packet of prepared information about a particular topic, story, or event that is provided to the media and other interested agencies. Press kits are typically prepared when a press conference is scheduled or special event is planned, such as a political rally or other public news event. A press kit could be developed for the opening of a new museum or library, or in conjunction with the release of the latest local statistics on AIDS or hepatitis by the local health department. A press kit ensures that the same information is disseminated to all interested persons

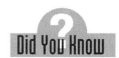

Over 5,000 newspapers can be accessed via the Internet.

and, to a large degree, eliminates the need for individual interviews or extra copying of materials. By providing the material to the media, the organization can also better maintain control over the information that is released.

There are no specific rules as to what can or cannot be included in a press kit. Usually included are fact sheets or other documents that provide answers to questions about the organization, the topic, and key personnel. A copy of a speaker's prepared remarks (if for a public address) provides reporters with the exact language presented. Include 5-by-7 (or larger) black-and-white photographs of speakers, products, or the event, if appropriate. If personnel from your organization have published journal articles on topics related to the press conference or event, then include reprints of such articles. Catalogs or other organizational materials can also be included, as long as the main focus is on that which is presented at the press conference or event. Having a press kit available can avoid the extra work of preparing responses and fulfilling numerous individual requests for information.

Press kits are usually presented in pocket folders and prepared in a visually appealing manner. Well-organized information that provides the answers to most of the questions reporters might have, contained in an attractive folder, conveys a positive image of the organization. Remember, however, that elaborate presentation style cannot substitute for quality content. Reporters are interested in the value of the information presented. Strive for quality, but not necessarily expensive, presentation.

Overcoming Challenges to Working with the Media

As with any of the other methods described in this text, there are many barriers, or problems, health educators routinely encounter in working with the media. Anticipating these problems and understanding how to overcome them are as important as mastering the techniques associated with media tools previously described in this chapter.

Ensure Media Coverage

What happens if PSAs are used rarely, if ever, or news releases never wind up as news stories? Unfortunately, this may be the case. The media are bombarded with many groups vying for airtime and print space, so at times there is great competition for media attention. Taking time to develop personal relationships with the people at the radio and television stations who make the decisions regarding airtime for PSAs and the people at the newspapers who decide which stories to print can increase the likelihood of success. Do not be afraid to engage in open and honest communication if the time or print space that should be allotted to an issue is not forthcoming. Find out what needs to be changed in developing materials in order to increase the likelihood of airtime or making it to print.

Limit Statements Taken Out of Context

Many times only a fraction of what an interviewee says is actually aired or printed. Unfortunately, statements used may then be out of context or include that which the interviewee hoped he or she would not have said. Media sources have limited time or print space in which to fit a whole host of competing stories. Providing interviewers with much more information than can possibly be used gives them the opportunity to choose what is important and what is not and, subsequently, what appears in the story and what does not. When a controversial issue is involved (and the interviewee or his or her organization is directly involved in that controversy), consider operating from a brief, prepared statement. Take few, if any, questions and when answering ques-

Did You Know

Modern-day radio broadcasting was pioneered by Frank Conrad in the backyard garage of his home in Wilkinsburg, Pennsylvania, in 1919 to 1920. Conrad was the first person to ever air an advertisement over a radio.

tions, stay close to the prepared statement. This strategy gives editors the bulk of what is intended to be shared, reducing the probability of misrepresentative statements being aired or printed.

Make Time for Fostering Media Contacts

Why spend precious time becoming involved with the media? After all, is that not the job of a reporter? As with other activities, it is hard to find the time needed to work with different media channels. Health educators are busy people. Working with the media, however, can be a great investment of time. This investment, if managed properly, has the potential to pay big dividends, as previously described in this chapter. The investment, if poorly managed, may bring little, if any, positive return. Building positive working relationships with the media early on is essential for making the most out of time spent. At the same time, be considerate of media personnel time. Contact them with new information, but be careful not to demand too much of their time. It is best to share information with them and let them know how best to contact you if they should have further questions.

Expected Outcomes

What outcomes can one expect from working with the media? It is reasonable to expect that attempts to publicize an event or to disseminate a message will receive some airtime or print space. It is probably unreasonable to expect that the station or newspaper will take on the cause as its cause and provide free daily publicity. Airtime and newsprint space are valuable commodities, and, as such, competition is high. The better the relationships built with news reporters, the greater the likelihood of being seen as a valuable source of information.

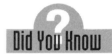

Did You Know

A newspaper is considered a "publication of record." As such, curious legal notices appear in the paper. In Michigan, newspapers are required to devote at least 25% of the paper to covering news-related issues.

It is also reasonable to expect that the media can be used as a means for providing health information to the public. But it is probably unreasonable to expect use of the media alone to substantially change individual health behaviors. As part of a more comprehensive approach, however, consistent use of the media and the development of positive working relationships with newspaper, radio, and television reporters increase the likelihood of creating positive change.

Finally, it is reasonable to expect that media coverage will increase community interest in the issue at hand, especially the more controversial the issue is. In contrast, it is unreasonable to expect media coverage to always be favorable to particular positions. Media are bound to provide a broad coverage of what they deem as being newsworthy to the community, while at the same time maintaining their right to hold diverse opinions. Thus, it is essential to ensure that any information shared with the media is both reliable and valid.

Conclusion

Working with the media provides individuals and organizations with opportunities to provide information to others on a broader scale than would otherwise be possible. The information provided may be directed toward an awareness of healthy and unhealthy behaviors, address controversial issues, or promote a particular organization, cause, or event. Each of the tools presented in this chapter may be used in any community health education agency, with some more applicable than others. The tools assist in making audiences aware of inappropriate social behavior that should be changed in order to ensure a safer and healthier life. Typically, attitudes are not changed as a result of media tools, because most attitudes are deeply rooted in social culture. An effective PSA or news release, however, may increase awareness and initiate a questioning process in individuals. Both legislators and the public can be influenced through the use of appropriate media tools. Consistent use of media tools and development of positive working relations with the press and media increase the likelihood of effecting change.

KEY TERMS

fact sheet: A tool that provides factual information about a topic or situation to the media in a structured format to assist in developing a story.

news (press) release: A one- or two-page document that provides information about an organization and its activities to the media. Also known as a press release.

press kit: A packet of prepared information about a particular topic, story, or event that is provided to the media and other interested agencies, usually in conjunction with a press conference or special event.

public service announcement (PSA): A short information announcement typically used by charity, nonprofit, and community organizations to educate the public, promote programs or services, and provide resources for behavior or community change.

ADDITIONAL RESOURCES

Print

Mallory, C. (1989). *Publicity power: A practical guide to effective promotion.* Los Altos, CA: Crisp Publications.

Goldman, K. D., et al. Tools of the trade. *News & Views* (multiple volumes and issues). Society for Public Health Education.

Goldman, K. D., & Schmalz, K. J. Tools of the trade. *Health Promotion Practice* (multiple volumes and issues). Society for Public Health Education.

Internet

Center for the Advancement of Health. *Communicating health behavior science in the media: Tips for researchers.* Available: http://www.cfah.org/pdfs/research_tips.pdf.

Dupree, C. *Tips for press release writing and effective media relations.* Available: http://www.internetnewsbureau.com/tips/.

Federal Communications Commission. Available: http://www.fcc.gov.

SECTION

III

Implementing Methods and Strategies at the Community or Policy Level

11

Facilitating Groups

Kathleen M. Roe, Dr.P.H., M.P.H.

Kevin Roe, M.P.H.

Frank V. Strona, M.P.H

Author Comments

Over the past 25 years, in different parts of the country, in different settings, and with diverse groups, each of us has had the pleasure of learning the art and skills of facilitating groups. This aspect of our health education practice is always interesting, sometimes challenging, and definitely rewarding. Whether facilitating or watching others, we have seen firsthand the transformative power of sensitive, culturally responsive group facilitation. We have witnessed facilitation that moved a group from frustration and conflict to communication and productivity. We have seen the way that a facilitator can assist people to find their voice in a large group, engage with others in new ways, and contribute to participatory democracy. Each of us has enjoyed discovering facilitation styles that draw upon the best of our own leadership qualities. We have found that, through facilitation, we can nurture the identity and commitment of often diverse groups of people brought together by chance, assignment, or common interests. In short, we have seen the way that facilitation strengthens and supports our common wealth. We hope this chapter encourages new health educators to stretch their facilitation wings and reflects the experiences of those of you who have been doing this for years.

Introduction

Facilitation is one of the basic tools in the health educator's toolbox. Across diverse practice settings, content areas, and populations, health educators are involved with all kinds of groups, including committees and subcommittees, ad hoc committees and task forces, planning groups, advisory councils, steering committees, commissions, boards, and coalitions. Most groups meet face to face, but technology now allows groups to meet by conference call and communicate over the Internet. Group settings, players, purposes, and politics vary, but the facilitation principles are the same.

Facilitation can be defined as actions that "promote, aid, simplify, or make a task easy."[1] Health educators' facilitation skills promote group communication and collaboration, aid participants in making individual contributions and working as a group, conceptualize and organize the tasks and group processes so that they are accessible and achievable, and help make the overall experience meaningful, rewarding, and productive. Effective group facilitation is both a skill and an art. It is refined with practice, requires discipline and focus, and draws upon the facilitator's intuitive insights. Health educators often make good facilitators because of their professional commitment to participation, inclusion, democracy, and diversity. Although health educators draw upon these commitments and make significant contributions both as leaders and members of groups, this chapter focuses on the art and skills of the specific leadership role of facilitating groups.

Did You Know

The National Association of Parliamentarians (NAP) was established in 1930 and is the largest professional nonprofit association of parliamentarians in the world. The group has a membership of over 4,000 parliamentarians from all over the world, including all 50 U.S. states. Their Web site, http://www.nap.org, offers information on **parliamentary procedure** and Robert's Rules of Order, a resource catalog, and a calendar of upcoming events.

Group facilitation is one of the ways in which health educators can become successful community change agents. Sometimes, health educators facilitate groups that they create or convene. Other times health educators are elected or persuaded to serve as facilitators of groups of which they are members. Health educators may be invited to serve as "outside" facilitators, bringing a calm, organized, and neutral voice to a forum or meeting. Regardless of the role or relationship, facilitating is very different from directing, advocating, or persuading. Effective facilitators focus more on process than content. In fact, facilitators often have to separate themselves from the issues under discussion in order to attend to the communication exchange and the progress of the group. This is not always easy. However, to an effective facilitator, *how* the group works together is often more important than the content of *what* they do or decide.

This chapter offers suggestions and guidelines that we have found helpful in facilitating many different kinds of groups. First, the types of groups that health educators frequently facilitate and the roles they might be expected to play are described. Next, attitudes and orientations to facilitation are suggested, followed by the nuts and bolts, including planning a meeting, developing the agenda, arranging for minutes, attending to other formalities, establishing a climate of inclusion, keeping discussions on track, evaluating the meeting, and appropriately managing facilitation challenges. Finally, the ways in which facilitation can stimulate, nurture, and celebrate community health and positive change are noted.

Community connections 1

Jade Smith has been a community health educator for nearly 20 years. One day, she received a call from her colleague Valerie, who had just been named project director of a large, multi-year community development project. This project required all kinds of group work—a planning committee, working groups, an advisory group, a community advisory board, and ongoing meetings of the staff who will support the work over the next three years.

"Jade, this has got to be a participatory process, and the timeline is tight. I need someone to help me with facilitation. We've been in so many meetings together and I've always admired the way you handle group dynamics. Any chance you'd like to take this on?"

At first, Jade was stunned. True, she's been in a lot of meetings and often served as an informal facilitator. But the extent of her formal training in facilitation was a group dynamics course in graduate school. But Valerie made the grant sound so interesting, and she was thinking of taking on one more project . . . so, taking a deep breath and wondering what she was getting herself into, she said, "Sure, Valerie. I'd love to help."

Types of Groups

Community health education practitioners facilitate many different types of groups. Sometimes, the health educator forms the group in order to accomplish specific program objectives or mobilize community involvement. Some groups are formed by funding mandate, others by community initiative, and still others by the priorities of an organizational or community leader. Groups can be large or small and can stay together for years or disband when a specific task is accomplished. Group members can be elected, appointed, or volunteers. Groups can have oversight responsibilities, advisory roles, specific tasks to accomplish by a designated deadline, or be formed merely to explore and share ideas and experiences. This diversity keeps group facilitation fresh and exciting, even for seasoned practitioners.

Communication and Decision-Making Groups

Groups established for communication and decision making are often the backbone of organizational units and community groups. The following subsections describe staff groups and various kinds of committees, as well as briefly introduce the roles of facilitation in each type of group.

Staff groups.   Staff groups typically exist to enhance communication and decision making among groups of people with long-term roles in an ongoing organization. Staff meetings, department meetings, faculty meetings, and their associated committee and subcommittee meetings all benefit from effective facilitation. A unique challenge of effective staff group facilitation lies in bringing the group together across office alliances, engaging participants despite differences in position and authority, and working within the constraints of the workplace to serve the organization's mission. Similarly, a unique contribution of effective staff group facilitation is the ability to stimulate and nurture vision, camaraderie, and shared commitment among people working together within an organization.

Standing committees.   Standing committees are those key subgroupings that are considered necessary to the overall work and productivity of the organization or effort. Resource Development, Outreach and Recruitment, and Evaluation are examples of standing committees an organization might establish. Standing committees vary between groups and may change over time, depending on the essential functions that the group or organization feels should be handled by its members. Standing committees should have a charge, specific objectives, and a scope of work. The facilitator then assists the committee by establishing and managing group processes that help the group meet that charge, while allowing adequate time and support for the work to be accomplished.

Subcommittees.   Subcommittees are smaller groups formed from members of an existing committee. For example, the standing Outreach and Recruitment Committee might have three different subcommittees to focus on youth recruitment, rural outreach, and publicity. Subcommittees take on a specific segment of the larger committee's charge. Effective facilitation helps the members stay focused and relate to the larger committee.

Committee-of-the-whole.   *Committee-of-the-whole* is a term often used for a discussion group that provides an opportunity for members of a larger group to address issues that may be beyond the scope of the usual meetings or that require additional time and broader input. This type of meeting may be held in conjunction with a regular staff or organizational meeting (e.g., the prevention staff of a local health department tuberculosis control program) or at a special meeting held for that specific purpose (e.g., discussing whether fees for family planning services should be increased). The committee-of-the-whole consists of interested members who would like to discuss certain topics without the formalities or protocol of the larger group. This type of meeting, sometimes not allowed under public government open-meeting laws, is not used for formal action or decision making, but simply to discuss issues pertaining to a pending decision or policy.

Task-Specific Groups

Ad hoc committees, task forces, commissions, and coalitions are groups that are formed for a specific period of time to explore a specific issue and take specific action. Once the task has been completed, the group may be disbanded.

Ad hoc committees.   Ad hoc committees typically have a charge and a specified timeframe. This type of committee is often formed to give issues a "quick study," explore options, and formulate recommendations for a larger body. For example, a health education unit of a college health service may decide to review its promotional materials to determine whether they should be merely updated or completely revised. An ad hoc group, composed of two staff members, the summer intern, a clinician, and two students, could be formed to look at the materials, research what other campuses are doing, solicit opinions from clients and marketing experts, and make a recommendation to the full staff within two months. An ad hoc committee's membership is usually open to anyone in the larger group who wants to participate. Its facilitator serves the committee by keeping it task-oriented and productive.

Task forces.   A task force is a formed for a slightly longer time to complete a specific task. Task force members often come from an existing group and may be supplemented by participation from others with complementary expertise, perspectives, resources, or energy. For example, a task force might be formed to assist with a health fair at an elementary school, arrange for volunteers for a blood drive, or develop proposals for a professionwide accreditation system. Task force members contribute the human power; they do the work. The facilitator provides strategic leadership, may actively help in member recruitment, and often arranges for the resources the group needs to accomplish its task. Once the defined objective is achieved, the task force is discontinued. The parent group, however, may convene a new task force—or reconvene the first one—should a similar need arise in the future. Facilitators of ad hoc committees and task forces are often able to ensure that the group's work becomes part of the historical memory of the larger group, thus facilitating action in the future and documenting the contributions and insights of participants at the time.

Coalitions.   A coalition is a large group formed from other groups, with the specific purpose of sharing information, raising awareness, producing an event, or advocating for an issue. Coalitions may disband once the focal campaign is over or last for years. The facilitator may be elected or drafted from participating organizations or provided by the convening agent (e.g., the funder, parent organization, or individual volunteer). A coalition facilitator's primary task is to keep the coalition energized, productive, and adequately supported to accomplish its goals.

The decision to create a committee, task force, or coalition is usually made when specific work needs to be done outside of the structures and expectations of

an existing group. The "work" can be exploration, thinking, discussion, delibera-
tion, or actual physical labor. The facilitator plays a key role in the group's success
by envisioning the entire process through to achieving the end product; making
sure that the charge, resources, and timeline are SMART (strategic, manageable,
achievable, realistic, and time-specific); creating and maintaining group focus and
productivity; celebrating the group's effort and accomplishment when the task
is completed; encouraging ongoing evaluation of the group's performance; and
making recommendations for future group structure and support.

Oversight and Advisory Groups

Community health efforts often rely on information and guidance from
experts. For example, the local health department may be charged to develop
an intervention strategy for an emerging health issue in an underserved part
of the county, or a community coalition may decide to tackle a content area
beyond its usual domain.

Oversight, partner, and advising groups.   Advisory groups enable health educators to obtain direction and guidance from people who understand the key
issues and dynamics of a community-based program or initiative. An advisory
committee might be created to discuss the implementation of a public act in
a local school district (e.g., removing soda machines from public schools), to
oversee a community-based research project (e.g., needs assessment of kinship
care families), or to advise on the community health education curriculum
of a local university. Individual members are selected for the expertise and
perspective they bring to the group, and typically include several members
of the focus population. For example, the advisory board for a clinic's new
Vietnamese breast and cervical cancer screening outreach program might include Vietnamese community leaders, Vietnamese clients from other clinic
services, screening providers, and cultural competency experts. Similarly, the
advisory committee for a health education training center might include local
employers, recent alumni, and experts in the program's content areas. While
advisory groups have a clearly defined role in the design and implementation
of the program of interest, they often operate in a less formal style than some
other kinds of groups. The facilitator's primary role is to create an environment
conducive to full participation and dialogue, and to help the group move their
ideas to recommendations.

Planning Councils

Planning councils are a specific kind of advisory group, created, often by
government, as a way of soliciting broad participation in program priorities
and resource allocation. For example, HIV prevention planning councils

bring together representatives of all those involved with and affected by HIV/AIDS: people living with HIV; caregivers and those who have lost loved ones to the disease; researchers; health educators; staff of community-based organizations; and professionals involved with the schools, justice system, funders, and other HIV prevention initiatives. Some planning councils have decision-making authority, whereas others are advisory to a key policymaker, such as a mayor or health department director. Planning councils have a specific charge, formal operating procedures, and clear objectives. The end result of their work is their decisions or recommendations. For example, the HIV prevention planning groups mandated by the Centers for Disease Control and Prevention (CDC) in all funded jurisdictions are responsible for developing five-year prevention plans that reflect the epidemic, risk factors, organizations, and cultures of their respective areas, and then ensuring that the cooperative agreement application submitted to the CDC by their health department reflects the plan's priorities. The CDC has specified inclusion, parity, and representation as core processes of the HIV prevention planning councils. Effective facilitation establishes and supports ground rules for parity and inclusion in council meetings while helping to ensure that the council achieves its objectives and meets its funding requirements.

Commissions

A commission is another type of formal body, usually appointed by an organizational or government leader, charged with making recommendations on a specific issue or problem. For example, the leader of a professional organization might want guidance on how the organization can increase the diversity of its membership. In that case, the leader could appoint a commission of experts—individuals within and outside the organization with complementary expertise and insight into the organization, diversity, and the professional field. Commissioners meet periodically over a designated time frame (usually one to two years), discuss the issues, explore alternatives, and develop recommendations. Resources for a commission are provided by the sponsoring organization. The designated head of the commission usually provides the meeting facilitation, often with staff support to organize the scope of the inquiry and manage communication between commission meetings. Some commissions are short term, whereas others, such as county health commissions, are part of ongoing resource allocation processes in communities or local governments. Facilitation of this type of group often involves artful management of competing interests, passionate advocacy, and deliberative decision making within a specified time frame.

Steering Committees

Steering committees oversee the implementation of programs or initiatives. Some are involved only in early stages (e.g., integrating peer volunteers into a clinical facility), whereas others become standing committees to oversee the operation of an ongoing program (e.g., a statewide asthma coalition). Steering committees may be made up of members of the larger group alone, or complemented by the addition of at-large members from the community. The roles of the facilitator of a steering committee are similar to those of the other kinds of oversight groups.

Members of effective advisory groups, planning councils, commissions, and steering committees serve specified terms, meet periodically, and commit to the specific and significant responsibilities of their positions prior to joining the group. They benefit from facilitation that establishes a climate of inclusion and active participation, maintains the group's focus, and reinforces the importance, and boundaries, of their advisory roles. The facilitator can also be the bridge between a group's recommendations and subsequent program design and implementation, policy decision, or resource allocation. Effective facilitation of advisory groups, planning councils, commissions, and steering committees is one of the most powerful ways a health educator can ensure that a community-based program reflects and serves community interests, needs, capacities, and possibilities.

Steps for Effective Group Facilitation

What skills are needed for effective group facilitation? Generally speaking, exemplary facilitators are able to plan effective meetings, develop productive agendas, arrange for minutes, attend to other meeting formalities, establish a climate of inclusion, keep group discussions on task, evaluate the meeting, and

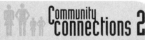

Community Connections 2

Over the next few weeks, Jade and Valerie met with various groups and individuals who would be involved in the project. It quickly became clear that Valerie's facilitation needs covered everything from a formal group of highly experienced advisors to informal groups of youths, community workers, and the general public. Jade felt fairly confident about her ability to facilitate many of the groups, but realized she did not have the experience or skills for others.

With Valerie's agreement, she invited her colleague Justin to join her. She had worked with Justin in the past and always enjoyed his sense of humor, ability to get along with almost anyone, professionalism, and integrity—important qualities in a facilitation partner. Justin agreed to come on board. Together, they felt they could help this process meet its goals and objectives, as well as contribute to community capacity and leadership.

appropriately manage facilitation challenges, whether the group is meeting in person or via conference call. The facilitator may also be involved in establishing group membership, outreach and recruitment, publicizing meetings, recording key decisions and collaborating on the minutes, and process evaluation. Numerous resources are available to assist facilitators with these tasks.[2-9] Regardless of the specific responsibilities, the facilitator's overarching goal is to nurture the group's confidence and capacity to work together effectively. Four steps of effective facilitation are discussed in this section, followed by recommendations for dealing with communications technology during meetings and conducting meetings in which one or more of the participants (or even all of them) are in different physical locations.

Plan the Meeting

The following questions can help the facilitator begin to plan a useful and productive meeting.

- What is the purpose of the meeting?
- Who should attend?
- Where should the meeting take place?
- What should we do if not everyone can attend?
- When should the meeting be held and how long should it last?
- Where does this meeting fit in the ongoing work of the group?

Each group is different in its preferred meeting times and location, appropriate meeting length, and optimal composition. Even within a group, each of its meetings may be slightly different, given the point of group development or progress on its charge. The facilitator's sensitivity to these dynamics helps create an appropriate structure and purpose for each meeting of the group.

There are times when a group meeting is not appropriate or possible, such as the following:

- The group may decide that the goal or mission is beyond their expertise and that the charge needs to be redefined before the group convenes again.
- There is a need for immediate action and time does not allow for a meeting.
- There is no reason to meet—no pending or urgent action, no necessary discussion.
- A meeting would be ineffective at this time—further recruitment, orientation, or conflict resolution needs to occur before the group can function effectively.

The facilitator's judgment is crucial in deciding whether a group should meet. In some cases, the facilitator makes the decision alone. Most often, however, the facilitator is working with a leadership group or support staff that will also be involved in the decision. If a meeting is to be held under difficult circumstances (e.g., dwindling membership, unsolved conflict), they will be key partners in planning its purpose, timing, location, structure, and agenda.

Develop an Agenda

The meeting **agenda** is one of the facilitator's most important tools. The agenda serves three basic purposes during the meeting: (1) It establishes the order of events, (2) it provides a road map for the facilitator while the meeting is in progress, and (3) it limits and focuses discussions so that the crucial **action items** are dealt with. The agenda also has implications beyond the few hours of the meeting. It serves as a benchmark of progress toward meeting the group's responsibilities. It focuses the group on its "need to do" versus "could do" actions and deliberations. It communicates the group's issues and productivity to a broader public. Even before the meeting, an interesting and relevant agenda generates interest and enthusiasm for participation.

The facilitator is ultimately responsible for the agenda. He or she should ensure, however, that overall agenda planning is developed with key group members (e.g., steering committee, subcommittee chairs, staff). Agenda planning should begin well before the scheduled meeting.

Most groups function best with a relatively formal agenda. Table 11-1 lists standard agenda elements. Additional agenda items might include public comment, small group exercises, training presentations, and meeting evaluation. Once the format for a group's agenda is determined, it is helpful to use the same broad outline for each subsequent meeting. This consistency serves three purposes: (1) Committee members and the public are assured that all meetings will follow a definite plan of order; (2) the facilitator has a predeter-

Table 11-1	**Key Agenda Elements**

Call to order
Welcome and introductions
Consideration and approval of minutes
Standing reports and announcements (written or oral)
Discussion and action items (each listed separately)
New business (for this meeting or for future consideration)
Closure
Meeting adjournment

mined outline to follow for each regular meeting; and (3) ongoing participants become familiar and comfortable with the flow, pace, and momentum of the meetings.

Less controversial, easy-to-handle, and informational items are often placed early in the agenda, in order of increasing difficulty. Once easier decisions have been made, participants may feel more confident and are ready to deal with more difficult issues. The business portion of the agenda (e.g., specific presentations, action items, unfinished business, new business) is often placed in the middle of the agenda. This provides time for latecomers to arrive before important issues are discussed. After difficult items have been resolved, the group can move on to lighter items for discussion, new business, input into future agendas, and meeting closure.

Specified time allotments can be an important addition to the printed agenda (see example in Table 11-2). Allocating time in advance allows the facilitator to be confident that the group's business can be conducted within the time set aside for the meeting. In order to reconcile all of the potential agenda items and the total available minutes, some items may need to be handled more quickly than others, some may be dropped from the agenda altogether, and others may need to be moved to a future meeting. Specified time allotments also let group members know what to expect. They help members make focused presentations, pace the discussion, and understand why the facilitator may move an item to closure or limit discussion.

The agenda should be distributed prior to the meeting (this is actually a requirement of open meeting laws in many governmental jurisdictions). Advanced distribution serves a number of purposes:

- Alerting participants to the issues to be covered, action items to be deliberated, and any guests or special presentations that will be part of the meeting
- Reminding presenters of the time limitations on their items and allowing them to see their role in the context of the entire meeting
- Ensuring that participants are aware of new issues to be covered so that they can conduct necessary research prior to the meeting

Table 11-2   Agenda with Time Allotments

Welcome and introductions	2:00
Agenda review	2:15
Review and approval of minutes	2:25
Budget review	2:35

- Building interest and enthusiasm for the meeting ahead
- Serving as a public or organizational notice of the meeting and its action or discussion topics

The agenda may be modified during the meeting, but this is unlikely to occur if it has been carefully prepared and is sensitive to pressing deadlines, group dynamics, and events in the broader organizational or community context. Members have a vested interest in items listed on the agenda because of the time spent prior to the meeting preparing to discuss them. Moreover, visitors or guests may have organized their own schedules to be at the meeting for only specific items. If the agenda is modified, particularly if items are deleted or the schedule is significantly altered, participants may lose confidence in the group's leadership and facilitation. A clear and reasonable agenda, created with stakeholder input and managed with discipline and good humor during the meeting, is one of the facilitator's most important assets.

Arrange for Minutes

The **minutes** of a meeting are the impartial, written record of what happened. Minutes must be accurate, as they will be used by participants and others to recall or understand what occurred at the meeting. Most groups are well served by even brief minutes that document that the meeting happened, the date and location, who attended, what was covered, any decisions, and who recorded the minutes. Accurate minutes require active and attentive listening during the meeting, making notes throughout, and careful attention to wording and detail when writing them up to ensure that the text and tone are brief, unbiased, and accurate.

Most facilitators find it too difficult to monitor group processes and take the minutes during the meeting. A formal group may have a secretary or historian with this specific responsibility. Some groups have support staff responsible for minutes. Less formal groups may decide to rotate responsibility for minutes among participants. The most important detail is to have someone designated as the recorder and to have **consensus** on the type of minutes to be produced. If the group wants detailed minutes, tape record the discussion so the person responsible for the minutes can check the notes against the tape before circulating the minutes to participants. If more concise minutes, or action-only minutes, are preferred, the recorder will most likely be able to get all the necessary information through notes taken during the meeting, by hand or on a laptop computer.

There are several styles of written minutes. A formal style is particularly useful for decision-making groups. If important organizational priorities or resource allocations are being decided, the group may need minutes that provide detailed summaries of the discussions and record the decision-making process.

Depending on the meeting procedures, the names of individuals who moved and seconded all motions, and the numbers voting for, against, and abstaining, may need to be recorded. Some groups may not require such detailed summaries of their discussions; others may need action-only minutes.

Selecting the appropriate minutes style is an important part of meeting planning. The **facilitator**, meeting staff, and/or chair (who may all be the same person) should think about the meeting's overall objectives, the interested parties and stakeholders who will want to know what transpired, and the nature of the record that group participants want or need to leave behind.

Once the meeting is over, the recorder should prepare the draft minutes and circulate them to the chair and facilitator for review. Reviewing the draft minutes is very important, because it ensures that what gets entered into the public record is both accurate and necessary. Minutes, particularly action minutes, should be circulated to all group members within a few days of the meeting if possible so that all participants can refer to the minutes as a reminder of actions they promised to take before the next meeting. Regardless of when the minutes are distributed, one of the first actions of the next meeting should be review and formal approval of the minutes of the previous meeting.

Attend to the Details

Once the meeting is planned, the agenda developed, and the minutes arranged, the effective facilitator can attend to other meeting details, including the setting formalities.

Setting

The setting of the meeting is important. An attractive, comfortable, and appropriate setting encourages attendance and invites participation. The room, lighting, and furniture can promote a positive atmosphere, one in which participants feel relaxed, focused, and inspired to be productive. Sometimes it is important to hold the meeting in a formal setting, such as city hall or the health department. Other times, it is important to hold the meeting where people work or in venues where the public can easily attend as observers. Working meetings need tables and appropriate work space. Presentation meetings require visibility and proximity to the speaker. Discussion meetings may be best held around a conference room table, or, if the discussion topic is more personal, a more casual setting may be most conducive to a successful meeting.

Participant Identification

Name tags, name plates, the wording on the roster . . . these details matter. How participants are identified may seem a minor detail but can have a major impact on the way group members interact. Everything printed on a name tag or name card should be specifically chosen. The facilitator can help staff or other stakeholders decide what should go on the name tags or other method of member identification. For example, will listing degrees on the name tags positively establish the credentials of group members or create imbalances of prestige and presumed authority? Will emphasizing first names in bold facilitate conversation between members or appear uncomfortably familiar and disrespectful? Will preprinted name plates communicate inclusion or spotlight and embarrass those who were not expected but are still welcome? Does the roster and its contact information establish parity within the group or identify status and resource differences that will affect members' comfort with each other? Do participant profiles allow all members to offer something that will be recognized as being valuable to the group? What kind of background information on group members will help them work together most effectively? There is no single right answer—the best decision is based on the culture, purpose, and experience of the group.

Meeting Tone

The beginning of the meeting sets the tone for the rest of it—formal, informal, warm, inviting, serious, urgent, focused, or brainstorming—which is communicated by the facilitator's behavior and opening words as the meeting gets under way. Arriving early, making sure everything is set and ready to go, being calm and focused, and perhaps greeting people as they arrive, all communicate important messages to participants about the focus and dynamics of the meeting ahead. When the facilitator is rushed, anxious, or distracted before the meeting, the group process starts awkwardly. Conversely, a calm and engaging facilitator is ready for participants and begins facilitating the group process when the very first participant arrives.

Whether to begin exactly at the appointed time is a matter of culture and meeting needs. Some groups have developed a punctual tradition, beginning and ending exactly on time. Other groups have a more relaxed attitude, either starting when the majority of expected participants are present, or at a commonly understood "real" start time (e.g., 15 minutes after the stipulated time). Whatever the group culture, it is important that the facilitator take these group norms into account in planning the agenda, assigning times to each item, and moving the group through the material in the time that is available.

Closure

The facilitator or designated timekeeper is responsible for watching the time and alerting the group throughout the meeting when they need to move along in order to meet their objectives during the time remaining. Ending a meeting on time is extremely important to most people. Running overtime may make individuals late for their next commitments or require them to leave before the meeting is over, and perhaps before agenda items they are very interested in are discussed. In addition to the *time* at which the meeting ends, the *way* in which it ends is important. The facilitator can bring closure to the meeting by summarizing what has been accomplished, reminding people of the next meeting time and location (if another meeting is scheduled), and thanking the group for their attendance and participation.

Other details that can enhance a meeting's tone and productivity include the following:

- Ensure the meeting site is accessible to all potential participants
- Set up and test audiovisual equipment in advance or during a break so that its setup does not disrupt the group process
- Use microphones if needed (standing or tabletop mikes) to enhance communication in a large group
- Provide meeting packets and handouts with information and guidance so that all participants can participate fully
- Provide refreshments appropriate for the time of day, group budget, and participant customs and dietary preferences
- Take planned breaks, particularly in long meetings
- Provide tables for additional materials and member exhibits
- Attend to ambiance details, such as lighting, noise, and temperature control

Attention to the power of these seemingly minor details to create the appropriate atmosphere is always a wise investment.

Consider Meeting by Conference Call or via the Internet

The last ten years has seen an increase in the ability of groups to meet together, in real time, without being in the same place. These are meetings in which one or more participants—sometimes all participants—call in through a phone line, mobile phone, or an Internet portal. This technology allows participants to hear and sometimes view presentations and participate in group discussions. Internet conferences and teleconferences increase access to meetings for many people, particularly professionals with office equipment and settings conducive to extended phone or computer use. These technologies also allow people to participate from far distances, decrease meeting costs, and enhance attendance and participation by eliminating travel time and expense. However, it should be noted that not everyone has access to the equipment or contexts that make Internet and teleconferences possible.

Facilitating groups meeting by conference call or the Internet follows many of the same guidelines of in-person facilitation. However, a few specific considerations apply:

- Organize introductions at the beginning of the meeting. Periodically check to see if anyone else has joined the call.

- Remind participants to speak clearly and slowly into the communication device.

- Ask that people listen with their phone on mute. People often multitask on teleconference calls, which can create a disturbance when everyone else can hear them typing, talking to coworkers, or washing dishes.

- Consider using programs such as Skype, Yahoo! Messenger, or Microsoft Messenger that allow participants to send a message via text message technology to the facilitator. Most of these programs are free or low cost and can be run on most technology platforms.

- Send materials, including the agenda, in advance to all participants. Be sure to include sign-in or call numbers and passwords.

Tips and Techniques for Effective Group Facilitation

Group facilitation can be extremely challenging. It requires the individual be relaxed yet alert, confident yet open to change, disciplined yet warm and inviting, consistent yet adaptable. Facilitators must keep their "eyes on the prize" while fiercely guarding group process. Most important, a facilitator must learn to be a productive leader with each new group, focused on nurturing the group's capacity to address its charge, learn from each other, and contribute to the broader effort of which they all are a part. The way a facilitator responds to the group, specific individuals, the tasks at hand, or unanticipated events directly affects the group's effectiveness. Artful facilitation thus requires the ability to think quickly, see the big picture, be sensitive to nuance, and act with confidence. Indeed, a confident, responsive facilitator sends a steady nonverbal message to the group and invites similarly calm and responsive participation.

Several basic health education orientations support this kind of effective, engaging, and rewarding facilitation. Key among these orientations are genuine belief in the power of groups, interest in others and an attitude of inquiry, an open and respectful interaction style, commitment to capacity development, and a sense of humor. Besides these orientations, paying particular attention to a few other basic issues greatly enhances facilitation success. Among the most important are establishing a climate of inclusion, keeping discussions on track, and evaluating the meeting.

Have a Genuine Belief in the Power of Groups

Facilitators are often leaders, but the strategies and techniques they use while in a facilitation role are very different. Effective facilitators, like leaders, often have a clear vision of the future, passion for the issues, personal commitment to a cause, and persuasive advocacy skills. They must carefully hold these in check, however, when facilitating. Facilitators place their faith in the power and wisdom of the group. That does not mean that they have no influence on the group's vision, strategies, decisions, or subsequent advocacy. But the facilitator must be willing to give more attention to the *process* of the group than the *outcome*. This is really only possible when the facilitating individual truly believes in what people can do when they work together and is willing to support that process over any specific outcome. Facilitators who wish to offer content to the discussion should state that they are "stepping out of the facilitator role" to make the comment, and then return to facilitation duties.[7] Stepping out in this way, however, should be reserved for extraordinary circumstances. A facilitator who does this too often will be seen as distorting the role and privilege of facilitation.

Have a Genuine Interest in Others and an Attitude of Inquiry

Effective facilitators know that good group decisions require active input and participation from all members. The facilitator needs to be genuinely interested in the attitudes and perspectives of all participants. This can be challenging, particularly when a group includes individuals or perspectives the facilitator has found troubling in previous contexts. As facilitators, however, health educators need to shift their frame of reference from past experiences to the potential for positive participation that always exists with new groups. One of the best ways to learn about the perspectives and potential contributions of both new and familiar participants is to ask questions. An attitude of inquiry on the part of the facilitator establishes a group tone of engagement, interest, and potential. By asking questions and listening to the responses, both facilitator and participants can visualize from new perspectives, work together in new ways, and imagine new strategies for community health.[10] Interest and inquiry also help avoid misunderstandings and a false feeling of agreement regarding decisions being made by the group. The facilitator's genuine interest in each participant's contribution, and consistent outreach to all participants and points of view, protects the integrity and potential of the group process.

Exhibit an Open and Respectful Interaction Style

Integrity and authenticity are two of the most important aspects of a facilitator's reputation. Health educators' professional commitment to honesty and informed participation provides a familiar foundation for this aspect of facilitation.[3] Even in the most trying circumstances, facilitators should not resort to deception or coercion to obtain involvement. Participants will quickly see through each. Insincerity is counterproductive because individuals will either anticipate it or be irritated by it.[11] Manipulation leads to a lack of confidence and low levels of trust between members of any group, which then results in an inability to function. Remaining neutral while facilitating a group, both during and outside of meetings, is also crucial to the facilitator's integrity. This means avoiding gossip, judgmental small talk, or other forms of divisive group noise. As any health educator knows, the greater the trust between group members, the higher the capacity for learning and, thus, the greater the level of group effectiveness.[12]

Maintain a Commitment to Capacity Development

Effective facilitators support and assist group members in accomplishing their tasks. When the tasks are relatively simple, interest is high, and adequate support is available, capacity development is easy. In this case, the facilitator can play a key role in capacity development by helping participants see that what felt easy was actually the result of very specific skills, responsibility, and group work. Not all group activities, however, are so simple. Facilitators perform their most important work when problems arise. This is not to say that the facilitating health educator "helps" the group by solving its problems. As in other helping relationships, facilitators have to be extremely careful in the way in which they offer assistance. Self-reliance (the ability to act on one's own initiative) is important to individual members,[13] and collective problem solving is central to group development and efficacy. Appropriate facilitator support includes helping a group learn from both its successes and its missteps. For example, if a news release was sent out too late to be effective, the facilitator can help the group move from blaming the individual who missed the deadline to understanding the process, analyzing the organizational or social context that failed to prevent the problem, and planning so that it does not happen again.

Have a Sense of Humor

Effective facilitators enjoy the process, the people, the challenges, and the rewards of groups, which is bolstered by a healthy sense of humor. Being able to see the humor in situations, laugh at oneself, heartily relish the unpredictable, and find the fun in even mundane situations prepares a health educator to facilitate almost any group under almost any condition. A facilitator who enjoys life, people, and groups is a flexible, grounded, and effective vanguard of group process and productivity.

Community connections 3

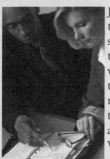

Jade and Justin spent time together, brainstorming and discussing the commitments they were about to make to this project, to the communities with which they would be working, and to their colleague, Valerie.

"I want to make sure that people aren't being used just because the funder specifies *community involvement*," said Justin.

"I agree. And I want to make sure that people get something out of each group meeting they attend," added Jade, "whether it be new contacts, new information, reassurance and encouragement, or a sense of what's really possible when people work together."

"I want to ensure full participation by everyone, not just the ones who are the loudest or the most assertive," said Justin. "And I want to make sure that everything we do, from the little details to the big decisions, strengthens community capacity."

"I'll need to make sure that I don't get frustrated by the pace of group process," noted Jade. "And I really want to experiment with a variety of styles and facilitation techniques."

Justin thought for a moment and then said, "Jade, I'm going to need you to help me with some of the politics of this project." Jade replied with a smile, "And I'm going to need you and your sense of humor to help me keep it all in perspective."

The facilitator's style and the behavior that it models will have a direct impact on group interaction and productivity. In his book *Groups That Work (And Those That Don't)*, Richard Hackman, a well-known scholar in the field of small group research, illustrated the importance of the modeling aspect of facilitation. Trying to resolve the problems that a committee experienced due to his own ineffective leadership, he concluded: "By finally modeling in my own behavior what I expected from others, I was able to rescue what many members were beginning to feel was a doomed project."[12]

Effective and artful facilitation requires an alert, honest, and adaptable facilitator. A genuine belief in the power of groups, interest in others and an attitude of inquiry, an open and respectful interaction style, commitment to capacity development, and a sense of humor all serve a facilitator well.

Establish a Climate of Inclusion

The facilitator is one of the most visible group participants, particularly during meetings. It is the facilitator's responsibility to set the tone that welcomes all members, invites participation, and honors contribution. This may be challenging in diverse and multicultural groups, groups with different vested interests, or groups with an unhappy history. Sometimes, the power is in the "little" things, such as learning people's names, pronouncing them appropriately, and remembering them from one meeting to the next. Inclusion is enhanced by the facilitator's attention to who has spoken and who has not, and then active solicitation (during the meeting or on break) of perspectives from people who have not yet been heard. The power of an inclusive embrace is transformative, particularly when backed by fair and understandable operating procedures and consistent facilitation. These are all dependent on the foresight, leadership, and skill of the facilitator. Health educators are particularly well suited to these challenges, as they are not unlike challenges faced in other aspects of their work. Health educators know how to make individuals comfortable, demystify procedures, stimulate interest, and nurture the stages of change. Inclusive facilitation is the same concept, but with groups instead of individuals.

Keep Discussions on Task

Every group needs operating procedures that explain, in advance, how discussions will be handled, how decisions will be made, how votes will be taken, and how actions move within and beyond the group. Most deliberative or decision-making groups find **Robert's Rules of Order**[14] to provide a smooth and understandable framework for discussion and decision making. Some groups modify the rules slightly ("**Bobby's Rules**") to better serve a less formal group culture. Some groups feel that both Robert's and Bobby's Rules are based on cultural assumptions that promote argument over consensus, individual expression over group dialogue, and forceful persuasion over understanding. The facilitator needs to be sensitive to these concerns, helping the group develop and then commit to operating procedures that encourage discussion, informed decision making, and respectful engagement.[15]

Once the procedures have been established, the facilitator needs to fully concentrate on the committee's discussions and deliberations, attending not so much to content as to process. More than anyone in the room, the facilitator is responsible for keeping the group focused on its task and moving toward the action that needs to be taken in order to fulfill its charge. The facilitator can help the group stay focused in a number of ways, particularly if the discussion starts to wander. For example, the facilitator can introduce each item by highlighting its relation to the group's charge and specifying the time allotted and the desired end result (e.g., discussion or decision). Once items are being discussed, the facilitator can periodically summarize what has been said, thus helping group members avoid repeating the same points, and gently moving the group toward closure. The facilitator who loses track of the group's direction or conversation should not try to cover up his or her confusion or become defensive. Instead, he or she can ask the group directly (e.g., "Where are we going with this?" or "Who can summarize where we've been?"). A short break is often useful, even if not on the agenda, so that the facilitator can consult a colleague or the committee's recorder. A summary of the discussion is then an effective way to refocus the group after the break and align it with the action or conversation that needs to happen next.

Evaluate the Meeting

The facilitator can learn a tremendous amount of useful information by taking a few minutes at the end of a meeting for evaluation. The most formal way to do this is to distribute a written evaluation form to each participant and allow a few minutes at the end of the meeting for its completion. Figure 11-1 provides an example of a short meeting evaluation form. This kind of simple survey can also be sent out electronically immediately following the meeting.

Less formal evaluation methods can bring warmth and closure to a meeting, while also providing the facilitator with invaluable process insight. For example, a facilitator who knows a meeting has gone particularly well might invite each person to share one word that describes his or her experiences. Sessions that involved a presentation might end with each person around the table mentioning one point he or she learned that will be particularly helpful in his or her work. Even a meeting that was difficult might benefit from this sort of one-minute evaluation, asking members to each say or write down details that worked well for them at the meeting, as well as those required to help them more fully participate next time. Asking for "three words to describe your experience of the meeting" is a wonderfully evocative evaluation question, providing both substance and context from each participant. Brief process evaluation techniques such as this provide the facilitator with important information about participants' experiences and are rich with suggestions to maintain or improve the quality of future meetings.

Today's meeting was. . . (1–5 scale, 5 = strongly agree, 1 = strongly disagree)				
Productive	5	4	3	2	1
Important	5	4	3	2	1
Organized well	5	4	3	2	1
Facilitated well	5	4	3	2	1
Useful information	5	4	3	2	1
Good discussions	5	4	3	2	1

Three words that describe your experience of today's meeting:

_____   _____   _____

Thank you for your feedback!

Figure 11-1 Meeting Evaluation Form

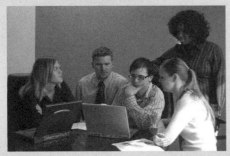

Community connections 4

Six months into the project, Justin and Jade found themselves loving the work. They were challenged, excited, and learning every day. They met regularly with Valerie and her staff leader, Tracey, to debrief past meetings and plan for those ahead. They dedicated considerable time to preparing for group meetings and always found that the investment paid off. Their agendas were workable, the groups were engaging, the tasks were clear, and people kept coming back. That is not to say, however, that the work was easy.

"I have the hardest time keeping the Clinic Directors group on task," exclaimed Jade one day. "They go off on so many tangents. I'm nothing but a timekeeper and a grouch in that group!"

"Have you considered listing the two or three primary objectives of the meeting at the top of the agenda?" asked Justin. "That might help them see what absolutely must be accomplished in the coming hour, no matter how excited and off-topic they get about other agenda items."

"That's a good idea," said Jade. "Another issue that is really distracting is the way some advisory group members constantly rustle through the handouts I pass out for each item. I think I'll ask our assistant Lei to help me make meeting binders containing all the necessary handouts for the next meeting. At the end, they can take home the handouts and leave the binders for the next meeting."

Brainstorming about a group that had trouble completing the agenda, Justin suggested, "You might consider asking one of them to be the timekeeper next time. If you're too focused on time management, they're not getting all they could get out of a good facilitator. Having someone else watch the time might allow you to watch and nurture other aspects of the group process—including helping those youngest members find their voices and start speaking up."

Overcoming Challenges to Group Facilitation

Group facilitation is both important and rewarding. But it can also be extremely challenging. Any group will face challenges as it learns to communicate and work together, meet its objectives, and reconcile internal differences. Even the most successful groups exist within broader contexts (e.g., personal, cultural, organizational, social, political) that place demands on members that will affect group dynamics and may present facilitation challenges. Among the most common facilitation challenges encountered are uneven participation, poor group attendance, disruptions caused by technology, conflict, and burnout. Each of these challenges is described in this section, followed by specific strategies we have found useful for overcoming the challenge and using the experience to benefit the group.

Encourage Participation

It is not uncommon for meeting participants to have different levels of comfort speaking in groups. Some members may feel intimidated by the expertise, position, age, or style of other members. Some participants may be more or less prepared than others. There may be different levels of risk or vulnerability among group members. There may be cultural differences in interpersonal communication, the use of silence, deference, and respect that are not understood by all. Some members may be eager to participate in the group process, while others might be there because they were told to attend. Add to that all of the ongoing "background" dynamics of participants' lives and jobs, and it is no wonder that group members participate in different ways at meetings.

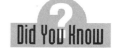

One of famous anthropologist Margaret Mead's most well-known statements is about the power of groups: "Never doubt that a small group of thoughtful, committed citizens can change the world. Indeed, it's the only thing that ever has."

The most important participation concerns for the facilitator are (1) establishing a process that honors differences and encourages communication, (2) monitoring the emerging dynamics to encourage all members to participate in the manner in which they are most comfortable, and (3) ensuring that the group process benefits from as much participation and group input as possible. Several specific strategies can help the flexible facilitator overcome uneven participation in a group meeting.

- Establish full participation as an explicit goal when opening the meeting.
- Include a round of introductions or a brief icebreaker at the beginning of the meeting, so each participant gets a chance to hear his or her own voice—and be heard by others—within the first 15 minutes of the meeting.
- List "full participation" as a criterion in the meeting evaluation, both as a way of reinforcing its importance and in order to gather information on participants' perspectives and needs related to full participation.
- Periodically remind the group of the importance of full participation, inviting members who have not yet spoken to comment or share their perspectives.
- Note the number of people who have spoken, and the number who have not, as the discussion progresses. Share observations with the group before calling on the next person. As facilitator, it is appropriate to say, "I'd like

to hear first from those who haven't offered their opinion yet. Then I'll call on those who have already spoken."

- Try small group discussions for five or ten minutes in the middle of a larger discussion, as some people will be more comfortable talking with two or three others than speaking before an entire group.

- Consider adding a co-facilitator who brings additional insights into the participation dynamics of this particular group and who might be able to bring out greater participation naturally.

- Check in with participants privately, both those who do not participate and those who may be dominating the discussions. The latter may not realize their own patterns or their effects on others. People who do not participate may feel honored and surprised at the facilitator's interest in their perspective and thus encouraged to join the group dialogue. In both cases, ask for recommendations on how to balance group participation.

- Offer to facilitate or coordinate training on multicultural communication, group dynamics, or decision making for the group, an orientation for those who are feeling behind, or a social event to allow participants to interact in a less formal way. Sometimes merely adding a working lunch to a regularly scheduled meeting or hosting a drop-in gathering with light snacks 30 minutes before the scheduled starting time changes the dynamics and lets participants warm up to each other outside of the roles and structures of the meeting.

- Report on the "full participation" evaluation results as a way of stimulating discussion of ways to make group discussions more inclusive. Seeing in print that the group gave "full participation" an average low rating of "2" on a scale of 1 to 5 can stimulate group discussion and suggestions for change.

    Each of these techniques will help the facilitator deal with uneven participation at individual meetings, while establishing and reinforcing a norm of full and respectful communication over the longer life of the group.

Maintain Attendance

Groups that meet on a regular basis often encounter attendance problems. Sometimes they are due to structural issues, such as where the meeting is held or the purpose of the group. Other times, poor attendance is purely personal, the result of busy people having too much going on and the meeting not being their primary or pressing priority. For example, health problems, family responsibilities, car trouble, or work crises can all interfere with a group member's intention to attend a meeting.

Facilitators should be prepared for uneven attendance from time to time, but also be alert to the meaning of persistent absences. The following are techniques for understanding, improving, and maintaining meeting attendance.

- Send reminder notices well in advance, even if the next meeting date and time have been well publicized.

- Make sure that the meeting time and location work for participants. Sometimes, a change in time or venue makes all the difference in a member's ability to attend regularly.

- Make personal calls or email contact to ensure everyone feels welcome prior to the meeting.

- Check in with people who have not been attending. Find out why and see if there is anything that can be done to make it easier for them to participate regularly.

- Conduct a survey to gather opinions and recommendations for enhancing meeting attendance and participation, and share the results with the group.

- Review meeting procedures and the meeting formalities to make sure that members encourage and honor participation.

- Make sure that all participants have meaningful roles. No one wants to go to a meeting in which they have no role or feel ignored. Similarly, people do not want to waste their time at meetings that do not really make a difference.

- Do not take it personally. Things happen, the office gets busy, child care falls apart, people get overwhelmed, traffic gets backed up—there are many reasons why people may miss a meeting here or there. It is best to just check in to see what happened, let them know they were missed, and welcome them back when they return.

Minimize Technology Disruptions

Skilled facilitators used to be able to create a meeting space with limited outside interruptions. The advent of mobile technology has changed all of that. Participants may now come to a meeting with pagers, cell phones, short messaging systems (SMS), electronic calendars, and Internet access. Time pressures, multitasking, and the desire to be always in touch have made these technologies a "must have" for many, and a unique facilitation challenge. The following are suggestions for dealing with the reality of communications technologies and meeting facilitation:

- Make sure the opening remarks include the instruction that cell phones and other devices be placed on vibrate or, better yet, switched off until the break or completion of the meeting, and that SMS/text messaging be kept to a minimum.

- Do not assume everyone shares the same rules of mobile phone courtesy. Some people consider it fine to answer the phone as they stand up from their seat or walk out of the room. The facilitator may need to include in the ground rules of the meeting that calls that must be taken should be answered outside of the meeting space so as to minimize the disturbance to the working group.

- Pay attention to whether SMS/text messaging is creating a disturbance to the group process. Many people use SMS/text messaging to communicate with others when talking by phone is not possible or appropriate, such as in a meeting. On most occasions, this is not a problem. However, in some circumstances and with some groups, use of text messaging can create the appearance of a silent "cross-talk" that can be chilling to group communication. Effective facilitators are familiar with the technologies used by group members and not afraid to request SMS/text messaging be kept to a minimum. Similar rules should apply with the use of laptops and email.

Resolve Conflict

Facilitators work with groups of individuals with different backgrounds, multiple perspectives and motivations, varying degrees of comfort and commitment to group process, and, sometimes, history together that predates the new committee or task force. This can be the source of stimulating exchange and invigorated group action. It can also be the source of both minor and profound conflict. It is the facilitator's responsibility to ensure that conflict enriches the group's explorations, decisions, and actions.

Avoiding *all* conflict is not an effective facilitator's goal. A vigorous exchange of even heated opinions helps a group better understand the issues, gather new information, and explore the potential consequences of even seemingly minor decisions. Conflict generated from outside the group can forge group identity in ways that might not have happened without the external threat. Both research and experience have shown that when the facilitator is afraid of conflict and the group tries to please each other at all costs, the group arrives at lower-quality decisions compared with groups in which controversy and disagreement are properly facilitated.[16]

Effective facilitators have a number of specific techniques they can try when a group is being disrupted or paralyzed by conflict:

- Help the group articulate its ground rules, proactively defining its own norms and standards for group interaction. Ground rules should specify the importance of mutual respect, the unacceptability of personal attacks, the validity of multiple perspectives, and the centrality of personal safety and mutual trust. Once adopted, the group's ground rules can be made into a banner or colorful poster that is displayed at each meeting, written into the meeting packet, and articulated at the beginning of each meeting.

- Hold firm to the ground rules. Once the rules have been established, it is the facilitator's responsibility to keep them visible and fairly enforce them. This is much easier when the ground rules are known to all, formally adopted by the group, and reinforced by the facilitator and group leaders.

- Explore what the conflict is really about. It is not uncommon for persistent conflict to be about something other than the subject at hand. The effective facilitator watches, listens, and explores with key individuals what might be really going on. Getting to the real issue will help the facilitator and members approach the conflict, and the individual(s) involved, with greater insight and compassion. It will also suggest strategies that might not have been thought of before understanding the issues at that deeper level.

- Check in with key individuals. Sometimes, the facilitator's best process ally is the person "causing" the conflict. Talking quietly and nonjudgmentally outside of the meeting can often change the dynamics of an angry or hostile participant. An effective facilitator also checks in with others who observe or participate in the meeting, looking for insight and perspective to help defuse or reframe interpersonal conflicts when they again emerge.

- Have a plan for what can be done the next time conflict arises in the group. The response, what might be said to the group, and the range of reactions to draw from (depending on the degree and timing of the conflict) should be contemplated. A good facilitator might even role play possible responses with colleagues or key group members (e.g., opinion leaders, staff) in order to be calm and confident at the next meeting.

- Use good judgment. Some conflicts are healthy and move the group to new levels of awareness and response. But nonconstructive conflict can cause real harm. Physical and emotional safety are basic needs that must be met if a group is to be able to work together. The effective facilitator needs to listen carefully to participants' expressions of fear or vulnerability. Even if a facilitator does not feel threatened, responding proactively to the felt needs of group members may lead to important logistical changes such as moving the meetings to a different location, changing meeting times, arranging for security, or rearranging seating.

Facilitators vary in their own personal experience of conflict, which results in various approaches to facilitating groups when conflict arises. In general, the facilitator who withdraws from disagreement out of personal discomfort adds another burden to an already stressed group. The emergence of conflict requires quiet and consistent leadership on the part of the facilitator, for he or she is now modeling respectful engagement under trying circumstances. The confidence to facilitate in the presence of conflict comes from experience, the ability to "breathe" through dissonance, and an active commitment to the group's ability to be enriched by appropriate use and resolution of the conflict that has emerged.

What is the optimal method for handling conflict? Facilitators need to believe that there are a number of strategies they can use, that they can adapt their strategies to fit the group, and that conflict can be an opportunity for growth. The facilitator's attitude of inquiry can make the conflict inherently interesting rather than frightening or destructive. Exploring the various perspectives represented in the conflict, being willing to listen and learn, promoting the integrity of those who have differing opinions, and, above all, protecting the integrity of the group and its process will lead the facilitator to the strategies and tactics that appropriately manage any conflict that emerges.

Did You Know?

The American Psychological Association publishes a quarterly journal entitled *Group Dynamics: Theory, Practice, and Research.* This is a very helpful resource for facilitators.

Avoid Burnout

Both facilitators and group members get tired. Too many meetings, too many discussions, and too many challenges can exhaust even the most committed participant. Effective facilitators understand the emotional demands of the art of facilitation and proactively nourish their own hearts and minds. A facilitator cannot facilitate well when tired, stressed, or burned out. A few simple techniques help a facilitator keep the batteries charged.

- *Try not to rush.* Allowing adequate time to get to the location, get to the room, assemble the materials, and settle in before others arrive can make all the difference. Taking a few minutes at the end of the meeting to make notes about what went well and what one might try differently next time similarly helps end the facilitation calmly. This kind of beginning and ending serves a facilitator well.

Community connections 5

Near the middle of the second year, Jade and Justin encountered a kind of group conflict they were not sure how to handle. A group of activists in the community had been increasingly critical and vocal of the health department—one of the project's primary sponsors. They disrupted public meetings, staged demonstrations at government buildings, lobbied the media, and generally stopped work for a variety of county-sponsored projects. By the time their attention turned to the project with which Jade and Justin were working, they were fairly well discredited in the community. But their actions were increasingly unpredictable and their demeanor aggressive and threatening. Members of several of the project groups were concerned about their safety or comfort if they came to meetings—and yet the meetings must continue if they were to make progress on the project. This posed a significant facilitation challenge.

"I knew I might be nervous when facilitating, but I never thought I'd be downright scared," exclaimed Jade after a particularly hostile encounter with one of the activists during a public meeting. "I think I'm in over my head. Maybe we should think about giving notice."

"I know what you mean," Justin responded. "But facilitation is really all about helping groups find their voice, articulate their visions, and organize themselves to make the things happen that they believe in. What message would we be giving if we back out when it gets rough?"

"Good point. But what are we going to do? This is some pretty serious stuff, and it's getting so bad that people aren't coming to meetings anymore. When they do, they just sit there in silence, afraid to say anything for fear of being jumped on by the activists."

"I think you need some help," said their friend Cameron, who had been listening in.

- *Remember why one does this kind of work.* Most facilitators do the work because of deeply held values. Consciously remembering those values helps a facilitator see the bigger picture when the details are trying. Facilitation is an art form—a set of skills that are applied to an emerging and creative process. Consciously linking the day-to-day experience of facilitation to one's deeper purpose and commitment to life can be a powerfully grounding experience.

- *Talk with others.* If you find yourself losing enthusiasm for the task or burdened by expectations, talking with others can help cast the experience in a new light. Colleagues who know the group facilitator but are not part of the group may be able to offer important perspectives. Trusted friends can help put a facilitation challenge in a larger context. Sometimes, just expressing feelings of exhaustion, frustration, or stress helps relieve the pressure and reawakens one's more hopeful energies.

- *Seek out experts.* Resources and learning opportunities abound for facilitators. The local library or bookstore will have plenty of books on leadership, meeting facilitation, and group motivation. The professional

"Just because the group looks to you for process expertise doesn't mean you have to know it all."

Over the next week, Justin and Jade spoke with Valerie, Tracey, and Cameron—people who had experience with this particular group of activists—and others they knew who were experienced at conflict management and communication. They checked in with key group members, and they pulled out their old group process texts. Cameron offered to do an online literature review for them, and Jade flipped through back issues of *Health Promotion Practice* and other practitioner-oriented publications for related articles and advice. Justin consulted his friend, Ed, an organizational development expert. All of these different perspectives gave them ideas and insight into the situation they were facing and the unique roles and responsibilities of the facilitators.

In the end, they decided to try the following: At the request of many group members, they recommended the meetings be held in a secure building with security personnel nearby. This would allow Jade and Justin to return to the role of facilitation and not be responsible for group safety and security. They reviewed the group's participation ground rules and made them into a large banner easily read by all in the room. They adjusted the agenda to allow a few moments at the beginning of each meeting to clearly state the ground rules and the consequences of breaking them. They developed a carefully worded introduction to the meeting that welcomed all who were there and articulated the importance of an open, participatory process, and they brainstormed and prioritized their responses to a wide range of disruptive actions that might occur at the next meeting. And although they were still pretty nervous, they agreed to come to the meeting rested, refreshed, and relaxed, for, as Ed reminded them, "If you don't take care of yourselves, you won't be able to do the work the way you want to."

journals frequently feature articles and commentaries on facilitation and group dynamics. Workshops, conferences, continuing education, and professional development events may provide opportunities to observe, consult with, or learn from experts in the art and skills of facilitation.

- *Take care of yourself.* Do what would be advised to another: Get adequate rest, eat well, exercise, remember what is important, and live life in balance. These basic self-care techniques help a facilitator remain grounded, flexible, focused, and creative.

Expected Outcomes

If members were asked what they like about group involvement and group meetings, they might identify the characteristics listed in Table 11-3. Having satisfied group members is important, but satisfaction alone does not ensure group success. An effective group works collectively and productively to meet a common goal. This common goal should always be the forefront of planning, deliberating, and evaluating the group's efforts. By remembering and attending to the common purpose of the group, successful outcomes will more likely be obtained.

Table 11.3	**Characteristics of Effective Group Meetings**

- *Careful time management.* Time is a vital and carefully guarded commodity. Starting and ending on time is extremely important if the facilitator wants members to continue to attend meetings. Enough time should be allowed to finish the work and no more. Some facilitators designate a timekeeper to help with this, or rotate timekeeping responsibilities among members.

- *The facilitator and members are sensitive to each other's needs and expressions.* All members listen to and respect others' opinions. The environment is safe for expression, exploration, and multiple realities.

- *Goals and objectives are clearly defined.* All members understand the group's agenda, time frame, budget, planning, and evaluation procedures.

- *Interruptions at meetings are not allowed or are held to a minimum.* When the meeting is in progress, it has priority.

- *The facilitator is prepared.* Materials are ready and available, both prior to and at the meeting.

- *The atmosphere is engaging.* Even when the format is formal, there is an unassuming ambiance.

- *Members are qualified and have a vested interest in the group's purpose.* People who are there want to be there.

- *Accurate minutes or records are maintained.* The printed record of decisions and actions, and sometimes discussions, is available in a timely fashion well before the next meeting, and is able to provide direction for action between meetings as well as accurately documenting what took place.

- *Members feel validated.* Recognition and appreciation are given for contributions. Everyone has a role and everyone's participation is acknowledged.

- *The group's decisions or recommendations are actually used.*

Conclusion

Facilitation is almost second nature to community health educators. Both formal training and on-the-job experience prepare them to participate in the work of individual, group, and community change. Facilitation—making change easy and simple—is a bedrock skill. It is no wonder that health educators are often called upon to serve as the formal facilitators of all kinds of groups. From communication and decision-making groups to task-specific groups and oversight and advisory groups, health educators can bring their belief in the power of groups, genuine interest in others and attitude of inquiry, open and respectful communication styles, commitment to capacity development, and sense of humor to any group with which they are invited to work. Facilitators are stewards of individual hopes, weavers of context,[17] and agents of community change.

Community connections 6

As Jade and Justin entered the last quarter of the project, they decided to take a look back at all of the meeting evaluations they received over the three years. Early on, Valerie had hired Jay and Christina, two process evaluation consultants, to develop a method of evaluating the short- and long-term effectiveness of the group meetings, including facilitation. Their monthly reports and process memos provided Jade and Justin with a wealth of information from which to continuously analyze and improve their facilitation skills.

"Look at how excited participants were in the first months," exclaimed Jade as she flipped through surveys from the early meetings. "People really had a lot of hope for this project."

"They sure did. I think it really helped to have the goals and objectives of the project, each working group, and each meeting clearly defined. Look at how the average ratings went up once we made that standard procedure," said Justin. "Ratings, and attendance, also went up last year when we moved the meetings to a location that felt safer."

"That was a really hard time. I was scared, but I'm glad we stuck with it," said Jade.

"Look at these ratings, Jade—they really like your color overheads and the way you begin and end the meetings."

"And they appreciate the way you really listen," said Jade, looking over some comments from the past year. The evaluations also showed that participants appreciated the snacks, valued getting the agenda in advance, felt comfortable with the decisions that were made, and were proud of being part of the project. "But you know what seems to make the most difference?" she asked. "That what happened in the groups made a difference in their community. Vince, an experienced community activist and leader in the group, even reports that his experience in our group has strengthened his facilitation style and effectiveness in his own work. Groups working together, learning together, and making changes that support community health—that's what this was all about!"

KEY TERMS

action items: Items on a meeting's agenda that require a decision or action by the group.

agenda: A meeting's blueprint, indicating, at minimum, the items to be covered and the order of events.

Bobby's Rules: A more relaxed version of Robert's Rules of Order, in which questions are asked more informally and discussion flows more freely; however, decisions are still made through formal procedures and majority vote.

consensus: Agreement within a group on an action or principle that allows the group to go forward, even though there may be differences of opinion on some aspects of the issue.

facilitation: The act of making a meeting easier.

facilitator: The individual accepting the role of facilitation.

minutes: A brief, impartial account of what happened at a meeting. At a minimum, minutes record the date and location of the meeting, participants, topics covered, and decisions.

parliamentary procedure: A particular way of running a meeting, using a chair or facilitator to order discussion and decision making.

Robert's Rules of Order: The most typically used parliamentary protocol in the United States, involving a structured set of rules and a process for majority-vote decision making. Booklets describing Robert's Rules can be found at most bookstores and libraries.

REFERENCES

1. Guralnik, D. B. (1978). *Webster's new world dictionary of the American language, second college edition.* Cleveland: William Collins, World Publishing.

2. Fetterman, D. M., Kaftarian, S. J., & Wandersman, A. (1996). *Empowerment evaluation: Knowledge and tools for self-assessment and accountability.* Thousand Oaks, CA: Sage Publications.

3. Gibb, J. (1960). Defensive communication. *The Journal of Communication, 10,* 141–148.

4. Hackman, R. (1990). *Groups that work (and those that don't).* San Francisco: Jossey-Bass.

5. Schein, E. (1987). *Process consultation.* Reading, MA: Addison-Wesley.

6. Hart, L. (1992). *Faultless facilitation.* London: Kogan Page.

7. Heron, J. (1993). *Group facilitation: Theories and models for practice.* London: Kogan Page.

8. Jensen, A., & Chilberg, J. (1991). *Small group communication: Theory and application.* Belmont, CA: Wadsworth.

9. Phillips, L., & Phillips, M. (1993). Facilitated work groups: Theory and practice. *Journal of the Operational Research Society, 44,* 533–549.

10. Keltner, J. (1989). Facilitation, catalyst for group problem solving. *Management Communication Quarterly, 3,* 8–32.

11. Doyle, M., & Straus, D. (1976). *How to make meetings work.* New York: Jove Books.

12. Robert, H., III, & Evans, W. (1990). *Robert's rules of order.* New York: Harper Perennial.

13. State of California. (1996). *Statewide HIV prevention plan.* Sacramento, CA: AIDS Office, Department of Health and Human Services.

14. Ajzen, I. (1991). The theory of planned behavior. *Organizational Behavior and Human Decision Processes, 50,* 179–211.

15. Broome, B., & Keever, D. (1989). Next generation group facilitation: Proposed principles. *Management Communication Quarterly, 3,* 107–127.

16. Tjosvold, D. (1982). Effects of approach to controversy on superiors' incorporation of subordinates' information in decision making. *Journal of Applied Psychology, 67,* 189–193.

17. Casey, C. (1998). *Making the gods work for you.* New York: Harmony Books.

ADDITIONAL RESOURCES

Print

Bobo, K., Kendall, J., & Maxwell, S. (2001). *Organizing for social change: Midwest Academy manual for activists.* Santa Ana, CA: Seven Locks Press.

Costigan Lederman, L. (1995). *Asking questions and listening to answers: A guide to using individual, focus group, and debriefing interviews.* Dubuque, IA: Kendall/ Hunt Publishing Company.

Pfeiffer, J. W., & Ballew, A. C. (1998). *University Associates Training Technologies.* San Diego, CA: Pfeiffer & Company.

CHAPTER 12

Building and Sustaining Coalitions

Frances D. Butterfoss, Ph.D., M.S.Ed.

Author Comments

Developing and sustaining coalitions for health promotion is both challenging and rewarding. Working with local- and state-level coalitions over the past 18 years has enabled me to forge new insights about community organizing, local and state politics, interagency collaboration, and media relations. By collaborating with people and agencies in coalitions, my professional networks have been expanded and enriched. I have learned firsthand that coalition efforts reach many more people and reap much greater benefits than individual health educators could hope to achieve by working alone.

My past personal experiences, ideas from coalition practitioners, research findings, and the wisdom and advice of national experts help inform this chapter. I hope that this information will help guide you in your efforts to develop and sustain productive community coalitions. I have not developed a foolproof formula to build and sustain the ideal coalition. Each community provides a unique context in which a coalition can grow and realize its potential. Some ideas in this chapter are designed to help newcomers mobilize community partners to focus on a particular health issue, whereas others are designed for seasoned activists who are concerned with keeping existing coalitions on track. No matter what stage you are in, I expect that you will discover tips that make sense for your coalition.

Nurturing coalitions to achieve their aims is a long-term endeavor. Invite diverse groups and individuals to join your coalition effort, and create daring visions about what the coalition might accomplish. Above all, remember that coalition work is demanding—keeping a good sense of humor and celebrating every "win" along the way is essential.

Introduction

Strategic relationships are fundamental to modern society. Organizations, businesses, and even nations form alliances, joint ventures, and public-private partnerships. Coalitions develop when different sectors of the community, state, or nation join together to create opportunities that will benefit the entire organization. A **community coalition** is defined as a group of individuals representing diverse organizations, factions, or constituencies within the community who agree to work together to achieve a common goal.[1] Coalitions are characterized as formal, multipurpose, and long-term alliances.[2] The size of its membership may vary, but a community coalition usually involves both professional and grassroots organizations. A coalition is different from other types of groups in that a structured arrangement for collaboration between organizations exists in which all members work together toward a common purpose. If the group is composed solely of individuals and not groups, then it is probably an organization or network and not a "coalition" in its truest form.

As an action-oriented group, a coalition focuses on reducing or preventing a community problem by (1) analyzing the problem, (2) identifying and implementing solutions, and (3) creating social change. More specifically, coalition functions include planning, advocating, delivering services, promoting public awareness, promoting risk reduction, conducting professional education, networking, building partnerships, and creating community change.[3]

Coalitions promote community change by serving as effective and efficient forums for the exchange of knowledge, ideas, and strategies. Through coalitions, individuals and organizations may become involved in new, broader issues without being solely responsible for them. Additional benefits of a coalition include the following:[3]

- Demonstrating and developing community support or concern for issues
- Maximizing the power of individuals and groups through collective action
- Preventing the reinvention of the wheel
- Improving trust and communication among community agencies
- Mobilizing talents, resources, and strategies
- Building strength and cohesiveness by connecting individual activists
- Building a constituency

A coalition can be a very effective means of instituting social change. Central to this effectiveness is the ability for many organizations to work on a problem from a number of fronts. No single approach for community change is as effective as a broad-based coalition effort that provides the means for multiple strategies and involves key community individuals.[4] Because coalition building is a process that involves a long-term investment of time and resources, however, a coalition is not needed if a simpler, less complex structure will get the job done or if the community opposes the concept.

This chapter is intended for those who are called to develop or manage coalitions for health promotion and disease prevention. It focuses on issues regarding community organizing and development of coalitions, qualities and characteristics of successful coalitions, steps to building effective coalitions, and tips and techniques for managing and sustaining coalitions. After exploring strategies for overcoming barriers, the chapter culminates with expected outcomes for coalitions.

Community Organizing and Involvement

Traditional health education is just one piece of a comprehensive community campaign. Health education has typically focused on health educators as teachers and agents of change for individual health behaviors. The process may involve organizing educational events, teaching classes, and counseling individuals and often takes place within schools, health departments, community-based organizations, and health care systems.

In contrast, coalitions attempt to alleviate community problems by organizing the community to bring about change. The general focus of *community organizing* is on changing systems, rules, social norms, or laws to ultimately change the legality and social acceptability of behaviors. The venue for community organizing is the policy arena and often involves elected officials, businesses, community groups, media, and local and state legislatures. Community organizing is an ongoing process that involves identifying the many facets of a problem in a community and implementing a comprehensive plan to address the issue through established community channels and systems.

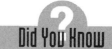
Did You Know

Coalitions exist that address every conceivable health issue, such as alcohol, tobacco, and other drug abuse, immunization promotion, asthma management, cardiovascular health, HIV/AIDS prevention, cancer detection and control, and improvement of nutrition.

Although coalitions usually operate in community settings, not all of them take advantage of communities' inherent power. When real community involvement exists, coalitions can address community health concerns while empowering or developing capacity in those communities. Health coalitions can foster local involvement and ownership that emphasize local assets and advocates for fair distribution of public resources and complementary activities to meet community needs.[5]

Development of Coalitions

The development of coalitions has escalated over the past 25 years. Coalitions form for many reasons. Local health organizations may form or join coalitions to augment their limited resources of staff, time, talent, equipment, materials, contacts, and influence. Joining with other agencies and individuals can benefit an organization by providing expanded access to printing and postage services, media coverage, marketing services, meeting space, community residents, influential people, personnel, community and professional networks, and expertise.[3] For example, health, civic, and faith-based groups develop coalitions to ensure adequate housing for the elderly and health insurance for the poor. Coalitions of health-related agencies, school districts, and community-based action groups form in response to an opportunity, such as new funding. For example, tobacco settlement funds helped support coalitions in their efforts to eliminate tobacco use among youth. Coalitions may also form because of a threat, such as a national story about rising asthma prevalence or a local event such as an outbreak of meningitis on a college campus. Thus, concerned advocates rally to highlight their issue or enable favorable policies and legislation.

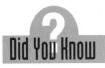

Did You Know

If you build them they will come. However, community coalitions are usually easier to build than they are to sustain over time.

The best of these coalitions are vehicles that bring people together, expand available resources, focus on a problem of community concern, and achieve better results than any single group or agency could have achieved alone. Not every coalition has been successful, however, and not every successful coalition has achieved its results without having its organizations pay a rather high price.[6] Even though coalitions are usually built from unselfish motives to better communities, they may experience the same challenges that are common among other voluntary organizations. With the initiation of a new coalition, new frustrations arise. Promised resources may not be made available, conflicting interests may prevent the coalition from having its desired effect in the community, and recognition for accomplishments may be slow in coming.

Successful coalitions display certain qualities that allow them to accomplish difficult tasks. They tend to be diverse, both in their organizational membership and in the individuals who represent these groups; formal in their working relationships and role expectations; flexible in considering new approaches to health problems; efficient in their group response to community issues; and collaborative in working toward a common goal by sharing risks, responsibilities, and rewards.[6] Regardless of their reason(s) for formation or focus, successful coalitions have certain factors in common, as highlighted in Table 12-1.[3,7]

Table 12-1 **Characteristics of Successful Coalitions**
■ Continuity of coalition staff, in particular the coordinator position.
■ Ownership of the problem by coalition members and community.
■ Community leaders support the coalition and its efforts.
■ Active involvement of community volunteer agencies.
■ High level of trust and reciprocity among members.
■ Frequent and ongoing training for coalition members and staff.
■ Benefits of membership outweigh the costs.
■ Active involvement of members in developing coalition goals, objectives, and strategies.
■ Development of a strategic action plan rather than a project-by-project approach.
■ Consensus is reached on issues instead of voting.
■ Productive coalition meetings.
■ Large problems are broken down into smaller, solvable pieces.
■ Steering committee of elected leaders and staff guides coalition.
■ Task or work groups of members design and implement strategies.
■ Rules and procedures are formalized.
■ Local media are actively involved.
■ Coalition and its activities are evaluated continuously.

Steps for Building Effective Coalitions

No two coalitions are alike or operate in the same way. Not every coalition needs to be community based. A coalition can be composed and take direction from a state agency, a hospital, or any organization. The structure of the coalition should fit the goals and resources of the organization. A statewide organization with a considerable budget might develop a formalized structure with bylaws, multiple committees, and a professionally developed communication plan. A local coalition without much funding and with part-time staff can be effective with less structure.

Even though providing services and developing programs are more exciting than focusing on internal coalition development, this aspect of coalition building cannot be ignored. Research shows that one of every three organizations or activities based on partnership fails, and up to half of all coalitions fail within their first year of operation.[8,9] Thus, whatever structure is created should be logical, simple,

Table 12-2	Steps for Building an Effective Coalition
1. Analyze the issue or problem on which the coalition will focus.	
2. Create awareness of the issue.	
3. Conduct initial coalition planning and recruitment.	
4. Develop resources and funding for the coalition.	
5. Create coalition infrastructure.	
6. Elect coalition leadership.	
7. Create an action plan.	

and help members accomplish their goals. Table 12-2 summarizes the steps for building an effective coalition, which are described in detail in this section. The steps provide a basic overview to the process, but local circumstances must be considered so that coalitions respond to community needs.

Analyze the Issue

The first step in forming a coalition is to analyze the issue or problem in the community. This can be accomplished by identifying and studying resource documents and collecting data (both local and state) relative to the issue. Many local health departments have conducted in-depth analyses, surveys, focus groups, and community assessments of health-related issues. These data are available for public use. City, university, and state health department libraries have excellent resources, including books, journals, and other documents. Many health-related statistics are available through state vital statistics offices, state agencies, community-based organizations, and community and state Internet sites. Centers for health promotion and chronic disease prevention at state health departments also offer free resources, statistics, and consultation on health-related issues.

Community connections 1

Natasha is a health educator who works in a local health department. Her supervisor has tasked her to develop a regional childhood obesity prevention program. She has a minimal budget and resources, a part-time administrative aide, and a constituency that includes a medium-sized city surrounded by a rural farming community. Considering the paucity of resources and the magnitude of the problem, Natasha soon realizes that the only way to develop interventions that will prevent overweight and obesity in school-aged children is to collaborate with other community agencies and groups. She decides to investigate the possibility of forming a community coalition to address this issue.

Create Awareness of the Issue

Creating public awareness of an issue helps to raise public concern and support for the coalition and its strategies, recruit coalition members, and obtain funds for the coalition.

Making the public aware of a health issue can be accomplished by providing information to the local media, including newspapers, radio, and television. A relationship with the media can be established by calling and introducing one's self to local health reporters, newspaper editors, and other media personnel. Media networking may help in maximizing media coverage on the issue and increase the likelihood of the coalition becoming a future resource for the media. Providing presentations to community groups and local officials on an issue and how it affects community members can also create awareness, garner support for coalition development, and secure funding. Coalitions should be aware that promoting community awareness of an issue is an ongoing process.

Some coalitions emerge because public awareness and concern about an issue already exists and funding is made available to help alleviate the problem. The legislature often will designate funding to allow for community prevention and control efforts on specific issues such as violence, tobacco, and diabetes.

Conduct Initial Coalition Planning and Recruitment

Coalition planning can be conducted in different ways. In most communities, an initial planning meeting is organized. Local voluntary agencies (such as the American Lung Association), health departments, medical personnel, and elected officials should be invited. The purpose of this meeting is to discuss the feasibility of developing a coalition. The following should be addressed in the planning meeting.[1]

- *Establish the coalition.* Is it worth the effort? Are there other established human service coalitions or groups that might consider either broadening their interests to include the issue or establishing a subcommittee that would, in essence, become a coalition in itself? Some effective community coalitions are actually subcommittees of established broader human service collaborating bodies.

- *Brainstorm who should be invited to join the coalition.* Potential coalition members should be identified by using member contacts; phone books; local government listings; and human service agency, business, school, and other community directories. Agencies and other groups that currently focus their efforts on the same issue as that of the proposed coalition should be included in the list of potential members. Parent groups, local voluntary associations, religious associations, youth groups, personal acquaintances, representatives of the target population(s), and representatives of the media should also be recruited. A coalition with a membership that reflects the diversity of the community is more likely to be effective.

- *Choose a date, time, and place for the first coalition meeting.* The initial meeting should be scheduled at least one month in advance in order to reduce scheduling conflicts. If possible, this meeting should coincide with another meeting at which some of the potential members are likely to be in attendance (e.g., a human service coordinating council meeting). The best way or ways for inviting potential members (e.g., phone, mail, media, or personal visits) need to be determined. Follow-up phone calls are likely to increase the number of people who attend the first meeting.

- *Decide who should lead the coalition.* A lead agency or individual needs to be identified who will continue to take responsibility for initially leading the coalition effort. After the coalition is well established and some funding has been secured for the group, leadership should be elected.

- *Develop an agenda for the first coalition meeting.* The first coalition meeting is crucial. Individuals will likely decide at the first meeting if they will become members of the coalition or if their time could be better spent elsewhere. The agenda should include an overview of the issue, coalition mission and goals, work or task group formation, meeting dates and times, and time for networking.

- *Contact the media.* Someone with prior experience in dealing with the media, or someone who is well versed on the issue and coalition plans, should be selected to contact the media regarding the establishment of the coalition. Press releases should be developed and distributed prior to the first coalition meeting.

- *Develop funding for the coalition.* Attendees at the initial meeting should explore all potential funding sources that may exist in their professional and personal networks.

Develop Resources and Funding for the Coalition

Coalitions must have or obtain the human and financial resources to do collaborative work. However, funding itself does not ensure longevity and effectiveness. Some coalitions have succeeded in accomplishing their goals with little or no outside funding, and other, well-funded coalitions have failed. A coalition must constantly ensure that its agenda is driven by its mission and goals and not by its funding. A coalition can do some activities with minimal funding, as long as member organizations are willing and committed to its vision and work. Diversity of funding is the key to coalition stability. Funds can come from membership dues, line items in the lead agency's budget that

Natasha's immediate concern is what community groups might be interested in this health issue and how she can engage them. Using a snowball recruitment technique, she contacts agencies that are likely to have an interest in childhood overweight and obesity. During each call, she asks the responder to suggest additional groups that might be interested. In this way, she recruits an active core of participants that includes the local hospital, social services, public schools, pediatric and family practices and clinics, nutritionists, a parent advocacy group, the YWCA, parks and recreation sports programs, Boy and Girl Scout troops, a local bicycle shop, the Red Cross, the Kiwanis and Rotary Clubs, a nondenominational minister's group, and the mayor's Health Council. They agree to hold a meeting to plan their approach.

pay for staff and basic operating expenses, donations from civic groups and businesses, partner financial and in-kind contributions, grants, contracts, and fund-raising events.

Generally, coalitions do not need vast amounts of funding to be effective. Coalitions are often successful when they work through established community events rather than spending time and money initiating new ones. For example, many communities hold regular events such as health fairs and breast cancer screenings. By capitalizing on these events to disseminate educational messages, coalitions can contribute with minimal cost. In fact, a large coalition budget can cause problems, such as focusing too much time and energy encumbering funds, debating how to spend the money, and paying bills. If one agency contributes most of the funds for the coalition (through a grant or other source), contributions from other member organizations may decrease, which could ultimately diminish teamwork, involvement, and support from other members. In addition, if one agency contributes the bulk of the funding for the coalition, it may feel the need to control the coalition agenda. A lack of shared input can be detrimental to the development of the coalition as a true partnership. Coalitions that involve a broad spectrum of people from the community as equal partners are most successful at building support and locating funding sources within their communities.

Grants are often available through state and federal agencies, private foundations, local community agencies, and businesses. They usually have very specific guidelines for activities, may involve significant reporting requirements and other paperwork, and come with certain restrictions on how the money can and cannot be spent, which may force a coalition to narrow or broaden its focus in order to qualify. Before applying for a grant, a coalition needs to consider whether the benefits of receiving a grant outweigh the responsibilities, requirements, and restrictions.

Effective coalitions are usually successful at seeking and securing donations from local businesses and community organizations due to their visibility in the community and public awareness of their accomplishments. Many businesses and community groups look for opportunities to be associated with a positive venture and may give money in exchange for their business's name being listed as a sponsor. Businesses that often contribute services to coalitions in exchange for recognition include printers, office supply stores, public relation firms, hospitals and other health care organizations, and restaurants. Community groups that would be likely to contribute funds to community coalition efforts include service groups such as the Lions Club, Rotary Club, Kiwanis International, Junior League, and Urban League. Requests for funding involve delegating specific coalition members to make phone calls, attend meetings, and conduct presentations about the coalition, its goals, and needs for financial assistance.

Other funding methods may include membership dues and fund-raising events. Some coalitions collect annual membership dues from each individual member and organization. Dues should be no more than needed to cover expenses, and since they may discourage people from participating, should be used with caution. Similarly, fund-raisers (e.g., bake sale, car wash) can be very time-consuming, divert the coalition from its mission, and generally have a low rate of returns on time invested.

Coalitions should be supported by and institutionalized within the communities that they serve. When grant funding ends, the coalition is more likely to sustain itself if it is not dependent on outside funding. Similarly, if the organizational members of the coalition feel that they own the coalition and are responsible for its success, they are more likely to support its meetings and activities. The exception here is funding for staff, research positions, and infrastructure (rental of space, office equipment, and supplies), which is more costly than most organizations can support. For example, coalition meetings may be sponsored by member organizations, with different members providing meeting space, parking, and lunch each quarter. In this way, the meeting site rotates, which gives the sponsoring agency visibility, educates coalition members about their peer organizations, and makes travel time to sites fair for all. Thus, each organization gives what it can in terms of cash, in-kind material support, or volunteers to implement activities. The formula is simple, and the results are empowering and often more than one expects.

A resource development team may be formed to obtain resources to help the coalition thrive, ease the transition from one source of funding to another, and help find money or goods from various sources. This group generally creates a development plan of objectives, strategies, and action steps to obtain financial resources for the coalition.

Sometimes coalitions decide that they need more autonomy from their lead agencies, or independence to pursue other goals. They may decide to apply for tax-exempt status as a 501c(3) organization. Careful consideration of the pros and cons of such a move is recommended.

Create Coalition Infrastructure

The **infrastructure** of a successful coalition should be formalized and supported by bylaws that are reviewed and revised on an annual basis. The bylaws include rules of governance as well as descriptions of the roles of officers and coalition members. Organizational structure is critical to coalition management. This is especially true because many coalitions are large and have members who are on the roster but not necessarily active. Therefore, the work of the coalition is conducted through smaller committees rather than through large membership meetings. Such subgroups are often called work, action, or task groups to connote their action orientation.

Community connections 3

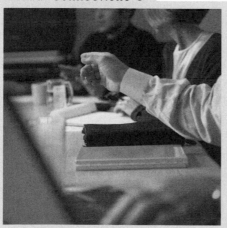

Because funds and resources are low, the newly formed Coalition for Food and Fitness agrees that each member organization must contribute to the effort in order to enact their action plan. The health department offers part of Natasha's time and clerical support, the hospital agrees to provide media and marketing expertise to develop a logo and print brochures, the ministers provide refreshments and meeting space in local churches, the Kiwanis and Rotary Clubs agree to raise funds for the prevention strategies, and the Boy and Girl Scouts offer volunteers to staff health fairs and stuff informational bags for parents. The pediatric and family practices agree to assess promising parent education methods and strategies that might be offered in their clinical settings to change eating and exercising behaviors. The social services representative agreed to help Natasha write a grant to obtain more funds for the coalition.

A sample work group structure and its functions are presented in the following list. All work groups serve the priority population as identified by the coalition. For each work group, task subgroups are developed as needed to carry out specific activities.

- *Assessment and Evaluation.* Provides needs assessment and evaluation as the basis for community planning and action to promote health and prevent disease and injury.
- *Community Empowerment and Education.* Reaches out to communities through public awareness to ensure appropriate education and access to health services and programs to improve health outcomes.
- *Health Care Providers.* Improves the knowledge, attitudes, and practices of health care providers to reduce barriers in the health care delivery system that contribute to the health problem under consideration.
- *Special Support Team.* Developed as the need arises. For example, a Media Advocacy team may develop in order to provide technical expertise and assistance in promoting newsworthy coalition activities.
- *Resource Development.* Provides expertise in identifying and securing material and in-kind resources for the coalition and its work groups.

In addition to work groups and task subgroups, a *steering committee* should be established to set the coalition agenda, coordinate the activities of all committees, and serve as a fast response team for the coalition when immediate or emergency action is required. The elected coalition leadership, coalition coordinator, and other honorary representatives from the lead and key agencies make up the steering committee. This committee ensures representative decision making and coordination among all components of the coalition. The steering committee meets a few times per year, usually prior to regularly scheduled membership meetings.

Elect Coalition Leadership

Capable leadership is integral to the success of a coalition. Leadership can be elected or appointed, formal or informal. Often the key to successful coalition leadership is the ability to delegate tasks to the membership, negotiate when differences of opinion arise, and communicate openly and effectively with members and the community.

Coalition leaders should know how to motivate members, but not push them too far. Effective leaders give their time and expertise, share credit for successes, concentrate on coalition strengths rather than weaknesses, know members well enough to be able to determine who can be counted on for extra support, realize that coalition members' time is equally important, and realize community needs are great in many areas.[3]

Coalition leadership generally consists of a coalition chairperson and vice-chairperson, work group chairperson and vice-chairperson, and coalition coordinator, as described in the following subsections. In order to elect leaders, a nominating committee may be appointed by the chair and coordinator to present a slate of officers for the steering committee to consider and announce to members prior to the first coalition meeting of the year. Qualifications and statements from the candidates are distributed to members, who are given the opportunity to add names to the slate. Election of work group chairs occurs at their first regular meeting by nominations from the floor and consensus voting. The term of office for all positions is usually one year, although consecutive terms are allowed.

Coalition Chairperson

Many coalitions opt to elect a chairperson for a one- or two-year period. The chairperson's responsibilities include facilitating meetings, public speaking, media relations, and directing projects. The chairperson should work closely with the coalition coordinator to do the following tasks:[1]

- Set meeting agendas
- Ensure that each meeting is well organized
- Encourage member discussion and input
- Delegate responsibilities to members
- Bring the coalition to consensus on issues
- Conduct follow-up with members
- Recruit and recognize members for accomplishments
- Appoint a media spokesperson
- Deal with difficult people and personalities
- Set up training for members

Coalition Vice-Chairperson

Given the busy schedules of health professionals and community volunteers, the vice-chairperson represents the chairperson during his or her absence. In addition, the vice-chairperson is mentored by the chairperson to promote development of leadership traits and provide future transition of leadership.

Work Group Chairperson and Vice-Chairperson

The work group members elect these leaders from within the group. Leader characteristics and responsibilities are similar to those described for the coalition chair and vice-chair. Work groups are smaller, more focused, and are good training grounds for those who will assume greater responsibility for the coalition later. Meeting facilitation and task delegation are critical skills at this level.

Coalition Coordinator

The coalition coordinator, a job that can often be demanding and time-consuming, is integral to the success of a coalition. The coordinator often works behind the scenes to organize the meetings, complete all necessary paperwork, recruit

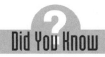

Did You Know

Evaluation of coalitions comes in threes. Evaluation must focus on (1) short-term outcomes such as member satisfaction and participation, (2) intermediate outcomes such as improved access to health care and quality of services, and (3) long-term outcomes such as improved health status.

members, organize member orientation and training, and coordinate membership recognition. The success of a coalition often hinges on the coordinator's energy, commitment, persistence, and credibility. Frequent co-ordinator turnover has been found to be detrimental to the success of many coalitions.

The lead agency of the coalition generally is responsible for selecting or hiring the coalition coordinator. This individual should not be the same person who is elected to serve as coalition chair, but rather someone who helped initiate the formation of the coalition. A health educator with community organizing interests and experience would be a natural fit for the coalition coordinator role.

Create an Action Plan

After the coalition has been formed, a mission statement, goals, objectives, and strategies need to be developed. Coalitions often start by formulating the mission statement, which is usually one sentence that describes what the coalition hopes to achieve, how it plans to accomplish its goals, and for whose benefit the coalition exists. A sample mission statement might read: "The Tri-County Cardiovascular Disease Prevention Coalition will reduce the incidence of cardiovascular disease among county residents through networking, education, and advocacy efforts."

The coalition should also develop short- and long-term goals, which are broad statements of purpose. For each goal, objectives (which are short-range, specific outcomes of a program or project) should be written. Objectives can be either process-oriented (i.e., outlining who will perform the activity, what exactly will be done, and when the activity will take place) or outcome based (i.e., providing quantifiable, measurable courses of action that can be evaluated).

Involving members in creating **action plans** builds coalition capacity. For example, one coalition reported that after planning together, 76% of members rated their planning ability as high, and 71% agreed that the resulting action plan accurately reflected their earlier needs assessment.[10] The same members reported that their capacity to plan in other arenas was increased as a result of their coalition experience. To increase the likelihood of success in the implementation and evaluation phases, the action plan must capture the voice of the people in the community whom the coalition program intends to reach. Having a coalition plan that represents the community makes this outcome more likely.

Strategic plans can help focus a coalition's limited resources and time on developing strategies that affect outcomes. Strategies for achieving coalition objectives should be realistic, built on the experience of others, flexible, respectful of organizational cultures, and designed to enhance coalition unity. Effective strategies often are educational and take into account that people learn as much from the process as from the end result.[11] Subcommittees of the coalition often implement strategies. This may mean that several ongoing strategies are implemented by the coalition simultaneously. Examples of successful strategies include organizing a cardiovascular disease conference for health care providers that focuses on developing a standard system to counsel patients on heart disease risk reduction, and conducting a media event (e.g., press conference) to highlight the success of the community mall walking project in lowering blood pressure rates and body fat ratios of the participants.

In the beginning, coalitions are recommended to pursue strategies that are both noncontroversial and "easy wins." These strategies could include booths at community events to promote community awareness about an issue, youth poster contests in community schools to promote health behaviors, and providing awards to individuals and businesses that have made an impact on the problem on which the coalition is focusing. Small successes are critical to building confidence and unity among members. However, even the best-planned strategy is not guaranteed to be successful. As coalitions mature, members will learn from their mistakes and successes, resulting in easier and more effective strategizing.[11]

Tips and Techniques for Managing and Sustaining Coalitions

The previous section on the steps for building an effective coalition should serve as a road map to get communities started in the coalition-building process. As multifaceted as this process is, nurturing and sustaining the coalition beyond its first few months or first year can be even more challenging. Government agencies, nonprofit organizations, and grassroots groups usually are enthusiastic in their support of coalitions that form to address a common need, threat, or opportunity. The real challenge lies in harnessing that enthusiasm and participation over the long haul. The following section provides some tips and suggestions on how to effectively manage and sustain coalitions by paying attention to stages of development, cultural competency, criteria for membership, recruitment, internal and external communication, marketing, and evaluation.

Understand Coalition Stages of Development

Coalitions move through a sequence of stages as they establish themselves to meet their goals. In general, these conform to the chronological stages of formation, implementation, maintenance, and accomplishment of goals or outcomes.[2] Understanding the developmental stages of coalitions gives practitioners critical insight to make strategic decisions. Table 12-3 illustrates these stages of development, with approximate time frame estimates and tasks to be accomplished during each stage.[10] The stages are presented in sequential order, but overlap of tasks occurs between stages. Coalitions are dynamic organizations. They may cycle through formation, implementation, and maintenance stages as new members are recruited and as old strategies are revised or new ones initiated.

Sometimes coalitions that form in response to the availability of outside funding are able to engage in a *preformation stage* in which needs assessments and other planning tasks may be accomplished. Healthy Start infant mortality initiatives, Allies Against Asthma initiatives, and ASSIST tobacco control coalitions had the advantage of this early stage of preparation. Most coalitions, however, begin with the *formation stage*. Key tasks to be accomplished during formation include clarifying the mission, recruiting members, and creating rules, roles, and operating procedures for the coalition.

During the *implementation stage*, coalitions move from formation tasks to planning the strategies designed to achieve the coalition's goal or goals. Raising community awareness about the problem and the coalition, assessing needs, and planning action are central to this stage. Implementing, refining, and

Table 12-3   Stages of Coalition Development

Stage	Time Estimate	Tasks
Formation	3–6 months	Identify community problem Recruit members Set mission Create rules and roles Collaborate Train on goals and issues
Implementation	9–12 months	Assess needs Collect, analyze, and feed back data Develop action plan
Maintenance	12–18 months	Initiate and monitor strategies Support and evaluate coalition processes
Outcome	18 months to 3 years	Begin to accomplish goals Progress toward results or impact from community-wide strategies

expanding coalition strategies take place during the *maintenance stage*. At this time, generating coalition funds and resources is essential.

During the *outcome stage*, coalitions begin to measure accomplishment of goals and objectives. Further community actions and community change should result in positive health outcomes. Coalitions need to work with funders to develop realistic expectations about the time needed to reach these outcomes.

The lifespan of a coalition should be tied to the accomplishment of its goals and objectives. When goals are measurable, then an end date tied to accomplishing those goals is implied. If goals are broad or indefinite, the coalition should revisit long-term goals at least every three to five years and determine whether to disband or whether more time or expanded goals are needed.

Consider Cultural Competency

To be most effective, coalitions need to be culturally competent. Research shows that members of effective coalitions tend to represent the diversity of the community under consideration, cite more benefits than costs of membership, and participate often in coalition meetings and activities.[12] Diversity in coalitions refers not only to race and ethnicity, but also to age, gender, sexual orientation, education, and socioeconomic and work status. Members need to be actively recruited from all segments of the community. Individuals who either directly or indirectly suffer from disease or hardship relative to the issue should also be encouraged to join, as they are excellent resources for better understanding the issue. If a coalition is multicultural, diverse social and cultural groups interact to shape the coalition, plan, make decisions, create a unique organizational culture, and guide all actions. It defines itself as a result of the interaction of people with diverse values, perspectives, and experiences and celebrates the contributions of culture. Coalitions also must ensure that their programs and interventions are culturally competent.

Coalition members should be involved from the start in planning, implementing, and evaluating interventions with a focus on cultural competency. Members will then appreciate that organizational and personal styles and communication and language differences must be accommodated. For example, planning must proceed at a pace that is comfortable for all, with enough time for members to question decisions. In meetings and activities, coalitions must be sensitive and aware of the different religious/cultural holidays, customs, and food preferences of the members and priority groups they are trying to reach. Finally, during intervention and evaluation phases, materials and communications must appropriately reflect the language, reading levels, and content for the targeted populations.

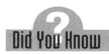

Did You Know

The average meeting attendance rate for coalitions is about 50%.

Create Criteria for Membership

Coalitions should develop written criteria for participation to determine who should be members. This strategy is not intended to exclude members, but rather to build a goal-oriented coalition. Potential coalition members can be asked to share volunteer and communications networks and demonstrate organizational support for the coalition's major issues. Ties to the media and relationships with elected and appointed officials are also valuable member resources. Specific criteria for member organizations include the following:[13]

- Designate a specific individual as liaison to the coalition
- Participate in meetings and activities
- Place key coalition issues on agendas of their respective organizations
- Communicate information to their members through newsletters, mailings, or other means
- Take formal, organizational positions on issues consistent with policies developed by the coalition
- Provide in-kind contributions of volunteer time, financial resources, and material resources to the coalition

Both organizations and individuals representing those organizations should be recruited. Even though an organization may be admired for the work it does for the community, it may actually be a poor partner for a coalition. An individual may not reflect the strong characteristics of the organization, and a marginal organization may be chosen because of a particular individual who represents it. Good coalition partners have certain traits in common. They usually follow a plan, make and fulfill all commitments, act in an egalitarian manner and support all members of the coalition, communicate well, and provide and respond to leadership.[6]

Recruit Partners

The most critical component of any health promotion coalition is its membership. The ultimate success of the coalition depends on how well its members are invested in and committed to the process of collaboration. While a loyal core of member organizations is enough to start a coalition, more members are usually needed to effect real change. From the outset, core members must be involved to expand and strengthen membership. To that end, a few principles of recruitment stand out: (1) Recruit about twice as many volunteers as needed, (2) develop specific criteria for members, with "job descriptions" that outline duties, and (3) find out why volunteers want to be involved, while stressing the benefits that the coalition offers to them and their organizations.

Turnover of coalition members, new people arriving in the community, changing needs, and new ideas for including groups and individuals in the coalition make membership recruitment a constant process. Persuading people to join the coalition and invest their time and energy will take some effort, especially because potential members usually already participate in other committees and coalitions.

Some coalitions have had great success recruiting members by organizing membership drives. Successful approaches have included staging a widely publicized special event or mass meeting; doing phone or in-person interviews to identify persons and organizations who might be interested; marketing the coalition by providing information at community events; placing ads in local newspapers; requesting that businesses and human service organizations appoint a person to represent their organization on the coalition; presenting information to religious groups, PTA groups, and community associations about the issue and coalition plans to alleviate the problem; appealing to area schools for students who are looking for community service opportunities; and approaching other volunteer groups for assistance on projects.

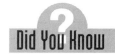

Did You Know

Approximately one-third of coalition members on the roster form the active core of the coalition.

Personal contacts are generally more successful in recruiting members than mass mailings. Members can also be recruited through invitation letters from top administrators of lead organizations involved in the coalition-planning group. Each organization that receives an invitation should be asked to appoint a representative to the coalition. Often a follow-up phone call is needed to establish who will represent the organization.

Local chapters of associations related to the coalition issue are likely prospects. For example, relevant organizations for a tobacco coalition might include the American Heart Association, American Lung Association, and American Cancer Society. Staff and volunteers associated with these organizations work to improve the health of their community and may be interested in serving on relevant coalitions.

Local policymakers and other influential individuals in the local community may be interested in membership because of their commitment to the community and the coalition's potential to provide personal recognition and visibility. Coalitions should try to achieve a balance, however, between the "doers" and those who only lend their names and voices to the effort.

Coalitions should enlist the support of volunteers interested in providing community service. Volunteers can often be located through a local volunteer action center, university or community college, high school, or voluntary association. Offering potential members something in return for participating can be helpful in recruiting. For example, an organization may need assistance with media training or contacts to attract attention to its cause. Someone with media experience from the coalition could assist it in that area in return for their commitment to work on a coalition project.[14]

Another segment of the population from which to recruit members is youth. Organized youth groups such as 4-H Clubs, church groups, peer-to-peer counselors, local chapters of Students Against Destructive Decisions (SADD), environmental youth clubs, and youth athletic clubs may be enlisted to join the coalition or support specific coalition projects. Existing youth groups may be willing to adapt their mission statements to include the coalition issue. For example, a SADD chapter might consider including other drugs, such as tobacco, in its mission and work on specific tobacco coalition projects. Youth groups welcome suggestions for activities.

No matter which segment of the population is being recruited for the coalition, personal motivation should be considered. Generally, individuals will participate in coalitions because of their commitment to alleviating a problem. Other members participate because they gain a sense of satisfaction from volunteering and working with other professionals. Becoming active in a coalition may help individuals to overcome the sense of powerlessness that can discourage even the most committed advocates. Experience shows that individuals are motivated to become members of coalitions based on the need to[15]

- Fulfill a shared interest
- Improve community services and the health of community members
- Share resources, including money, staff, and materials
- Be visible in the community and demonstrate civic responsibility

Marketing efforts that consider why potential members might be motivated to join the coalition will likely improve recruitment and retention. A six-step member recruitment process called the *buddy program* has proved successful for many coalitions. By following the process outlined in Table 12-4, new members enter their first coalition meeting having reviewed relevant coalition documents, and leave knowing at least two members of the work group and feeling more fully engaged. They are likely to return to the next meeting and participate fully.

Promote Internal and External Communication

Coalitions are valued because they bring different people and organizations together in a collaborative approach. This strength in diversity, however, is often a challenge to communication. Research shows that communication at every level between staff and members is beneficial. Clear and frequent

Table 12-4	The Buddy Program for Coalition Member Recruitment

Step 1. Each time a new strategy is introduced, the work group chair asks members to consider this question: "Who is not at the table that might help us enact this strategy or idea?"

Step 2. For each identified organization, a work group member who has the best connection to that organization is asked to begin the recruitment process and volunteer to be the "buddy."

Step 3. The buddy contacts the prospective member and asks him or her to join the coalition effort. The buddy encourages the recruit and answers any immediate questions about participation or the coalition. Successful contact information is forwarded to the work group chair and coordinator.

Step 4. The coordinator follows up with a phone call, and sends an orientation packet to the new member. The packet contains the coalition brochure, member roster, bylaws, minutes of the last full coalition and work group meetings, a map and calendar of meetings, recent program materials, and press coverage.

Step 5. As soon as the buddy receives notice of the next work group meeting, he or she phones the recruit, makes sure that the notice was received, and encourages the new member to attend. Babysitting or transportation needs are attended to as well.

Step 6. At the meeting, the buddy introduces himself or herself to the new member, helps acclimate the member to the surroundings and meeting protocol, and introduces the new member to others. The new member is given an opportunity to introduce himself or herself to the group. A personal welcome and offer of assistance by the chair occurs at some point during the meeting.

communication concerning the action plan and its level of implementation is especially crucial.[16] Coalitions can take concrete action to promote communication:

- Create an environment where people can have open discussion and input.

- Distribute member rosters and meeting minutes in timely fashion.

- Use basic forms of communication, such as telephone chains, fax, or email alerts about meetings and events.

- Follow up by telephone if members miss meetings.

- Expect members and staff to produce formal or informal reports after tasks are completed.

- Set up expectations about how communications will take place and evaluate the effectiveness of communications.

- Use newsletters, mailings, and email to keep organizations' leaders involved even if program staff usually attends the coalition meetings.[6]

Coalitions must also learn how best to communicate with the world outside the coalition. To produce open, positive external communication, develop materials that explain the coalition and its position on relevant issues. Then contact every organization likely to be involved, especially those that have a real stake in the issue, and continue to stay in touch.

Market the Coalition

A coalition is affected by the same dynamics as every other profit or nonprofit organization. To sustain its momentum, a coalition needs to engage in marketing. Marketing is not directed at sales promotion, but rather at making someone want the service or product offered. Marketing can help build a positive image, recruit members, promote awareness, obtain funding, build morale, and gain support from influential people.[6] Additionally, marketing helps a coalition present itself as so valuable that other organizations and individuals are willing to make an exchange of time, material goods, or services in order to be a part of it.

Evaluate Coalition Success

Evaluation is critical to a coalition's development and maintenance. Evaluation helps provide accountability to members and funders (Did the program achieve results?) and improves programs or develops better approaches (What programs work well?). Linking coalition efforts to empirical end points is complicated because coalitions often work on long-term projects (e.g., changing community policies) that may ultimately affect personal behaviors. A long period of time may lapse before the behavior change takes place and can be measured. For instance, it is difficult to measure if a coalition project designed to encourage parents to quit smoking actually affects whether children will initiate smoking. Evaluation also is compromised because the data needed to evaluate coalition efforts are often not collected. Funding is usually spent on intervention rather than evaluation, making it difficult to evaluate coalition effectiveness.

Given these challenges, three types of evaluation are appropriate for coalitions:[7]

- *Process evaluation*. Documents what was done and how many people were reached by coalition interventions. With this form of evaluation, record keeping of coalition efforts is essential. An annual report, highlighting coalition accomplishments and number of people served, can be used to report process results. Process evaluation can also be used to document whether the coalition itself is functioning optimally or as originally intended. Attendance records, types of organizations that make up the membership, minutes of meetings, satisfaction and participation of members in coalition activities, and costs and benefits of membership are examples of process measures that may be used to document the coalition's structure and function.

- *Impact evaluation.* Documents accomplishments of specific objectives. This type of evaluation determines the extent to which the coalition efforts were effective. These measures can be determined by recording whether objectives within the action plan were achieved, partly achieved, or not achieved. Impact evaluation results can be helpful for recruiting organizations and raising funds for coalition activities.

- *Outcome evaluation.* Assesses long-term results and measures the changes brought about by the coalition and its activities. This type of evaluation involves measuring the effect coalition efforts have had on key community indicators, such as immunization rates, teen pregnancy, and drug and alcohol use. An outcome evaluation focuses on all changes (positive and negative) brought about by coalition activities, not just those that were intended. Because of inability to control extraneous variables, however, accurately determining the long-term effect of coalition efforts is challenging.

Coalitions must conduct regular evaluation in order to justify refunding, gain additional support, demonstrate the effectiveness of various programs, and provide a basis for future planning.[6] The coalition and its member organizations implement activities that are developed through the strategic planning process. Each of these activities is related to specific educational or behavioral outcomes and ultimately to health status outcomes. Without participation and significant effort by members and member groups, these activities will not be achieved.

The data that measure the participation of coalition members and efforts of the coalition itself are generated by (1) self-report in member surveys (e.g., role and number of hours devoted to specific coalition activities); (2) structured interviews with key stakeholders outside the coalition regarding specific contributions of the coalition in addressing the health problem; (3) process evaluation data about the participation of the intended priority groups in planned activities and concomitant changes in knowledge, attitudes, behaviors, and health status of those groups; and (4) pre- and post-intervention data on outcomes from emergency rooms, inpatient facilities, clinics, schools, and other community settings. The first two types of data are obtained and managed by coalition staff with developmental input and feedback from coalition members. Process data and outcome data are gathered by coalition member organizations (e.g., Head Start centers, health departments, hospitals, and schools). Data from state agencies (e.g., health departments) are managed by those institutions and accessed by the coalition with their permission.

Overcoming Challenges to Coalition Success

All coalitions face problems or barriers that hinder their ability to achieve goals and objectives. These problems could seriously affect the effectiveness of the coalition and set back community efforts to address the issue. Table 12-5 lists common problems that coalitions face. The suggestions that follow can assist coalitions to avoid barriers known to impede success.[11]

Recognize Member Efforts

Member recognition and retention should be high priorities. Pay attention to the six Rs of participation: recognition, role, respect, reward, relationship, and results.[17] According to the six Rs, members need to

- Be recognized publicly for their coalition efforts
- Have clear expectations of the role(s) they will play in coalition operations and strategies
- Be respected for their culture, religion, race, and educational level
- Be rewarded for their contributions
- Develop meaningful relationships with other members and leaders
- Find that their efforts will lead to measurable results

Paying tribute to members for their efforts in the coalition is paramount. Through public and personal recognition, members feel their efforts are worthwhile and appreciated. Activities for member recognition may include hosting a recognition breakfast, sending letters of appreciation to members and their supervisors at work, publishing a program newsletter that includes highlights of members' involvement, presenting certificates of service, and soliciting area businesses to provide complimentary tickets for community events.[1]

Table 12-5   Common Problems That Coalitions Experience

- Too many planners and not enough "doers"
- Difficulty engaging local policymakers in the cause
- Not enough high-level administrative support from the coalition organizations to implement strategies
- Lack of funding or inadequate funding from local sources
- Difficulty coming to a consensus about what should be done
- Failure to plan or failure to act
- Membership burnout and turnover
- Lack of training among coalition members and staff
- Inadequate time allocated for coordinator to effectively manage the coalition

Obtain Member Organization Commitment

Top administrators of lead organizations should demonstrate their commitment by communicating regularly to the coalition and the general public. Ask members to sign an annual letter of commitment that outlines the expectations of membership regarding participation in coalition meetings and activities and contribution of time, talent, and resources (either monetary or in kind). Ask groups that remain uncertain and uncommitted to the cause to consider leaving the coalition.

Link with Other Community Coalitions

A coalition that advances the work of its partners and sister coalitions gains credibility in the community. The coalition must constantly define and redefine its mission and the role it plays in promoting the health of the community. A fine line must be drawn between promoting a coalition's self-interest and letting go to enhance the work of other groups. For example, by agreeing to contribute volunteers and resources to established events such as the American Heart Association's Great American Smokeout, the March of Dimes's WalkAmerica, and the American Cancer Society's Relay for Life, the coalitions and the collaborating agencies all win. Such collaboration and selflessness will eventually pay dividends by building a respectable coalition image. When members of the community outside of the coalition seek out the opinions, advice, and contributions of coalition members, the coalition's future is further assured.

Maintain Equal Member Representation

The coalition coordinator must discover and respond to the hidden agendas of its members. While coalitions should attempt to meet individual agendas, the overall common mission must not be lost. Domination by one or more powerful groups in the coalition might deprive other groups of their sense of equal participation. Institute open communication and a "one-vote rule" for each organization, regardless of size or financial contribution to the coalition.

Address Expectations of Staff and Members

Because of the diverse nature of coalitions, both staff and members approach coalitions with different expectations. Members want to know how much time away from job and family duties will be required. They want to know what their role is in the coalition and how their time and talents can best be used. Staff are often concerned about whether they will be able to handle the demands of a job where most of the work is done by volunteers, as well as how to motivate volunteers who have varying degrees of understanding and commitment to the coalition. They may be concerned about their skill and success in obtaining funds and resources for the coalition. Finally, they are concerned about how to coordinate the many activities the coalition engages in over a reasonable time frame.

To encourage realistic expectations, coalitions should develop job descriptions for volunteers and staff that carefully outline the prerequisite skills, time commitments, and expected duties. Both staff and volunteer leaders should have formal performance appraisals that show whether they are exceeding, meeting, or not meeting expectations as outlined in their job descriptions. Biannual staff and member surveys can help determine whether personal expectations are being met by coalition work. Providing varied opportunities for training, technical assistance, and networking with other coalitions can also increase satisfaction and commitment.

Delegate Tasks

Delegation is the process of transferring the following to coalition members:

- *Responsibility*. The obligation to carry out an assignment
- *Authority*. The power necessary to ensure that the end result is achieved
- *Accountability*. The responsibility for results

Delegation is essential because the coalition staff cannot, and should not, do all of the coalition work. Delegating tasks promotes a sense of ownership for the coalition among its members—the coalition is not one agency's initiative but a shared initiative among all members. Engaging many members in coalition efforts will have more impact than utilizing the energy of only one or two people.

In order to effectively delegate tasks, the goals for the coalition and its projects should be clearly stated. Volunteer workers should be actively recruited and trained in skills needed to accomplish coalition objectives. Coalition members should be provided with tasks that fit their area of interest or expertise. Working on issues in which members are interested increases member ownership and commitment. The key is to get to know each of the members personally and to find common interests that will benefit individual members and the coalition. Additionally, leaders must be able to release control of the process and details associated with coalition activities and encourage ownership and mutual input on expected outcomes, strategies, and the like. Finally, an environment that fosters initiative and rewards results should be cultivated.[18,19] In contrast, certain characteristics are likely to hinder the coalition leader's successful delegation of tasks (see Table 12-6).

Reduce Conflict

Conflict is normal and inevitable when working with people who are trying to agree upon and achieve mutual goals. Conflicts are frequently the basis for defensiveness, reduced communication, and the termination of relationships among members of a group. Sources of conflict include differences in values and goals; allocation of scarce resources such as money, facilities, and time; perceived threats to autonomy, rights, or identity; and differences in relation to

Table 12-6 **Characteristics That Hinder Task Delegation**

- Unclear goals and objectives
- Attitude of "doer"—doing things by self versus working with others to accomplish tasks
- "I can do it better and faster" syndrome
- A desire to engage in enjoyable tasks alone
- Unwillingness to transfer the responsibility/authority to untrained or inexperienced staff
- Insecurities
- Poorly organized to provide directives and ensure they are enacted
- Unwillingness to let others determine project methods and details
- Perfectionism
- Aversion to risk
- Concerned with performing several tasks instead of managing the coalition
- Organizational instability
- Lack of resources
- Poorly defined accountability

how desired ends should be achieved. If not addressed and minimized, conflict can cripple a coalition. Conflict can, however, be resolved in constructive ways that will likely enhance future collaboration and creativity. Table 12-7 contains suggestions to help reduce conflict within coalitions.[1]

Table 12-7 **Strategies for Reducing Conflict**

- Rotate leadership at least every two years to address conflicts that arise from unequal sharing of power.
- Separate individuals from the problem. Let individuals express their differences and work together to resolve them.
- Use formal group process techniques to address conflict arising from lack of full participation in meetings or from the overparticipation by some.
- Distribute information relative to the coalition or its issue as it becomes available.
- Rotate meeting sites to reduce "turf" battles.
- Do not allow "either-or" thinking. Require that dissenting parties generate an alternative to "my way" or "your way."
- Rule out the use of "you" messages and personal accusations. Instruct members to suggest a joint effort to locate the source of the problem.
- Change seating arrangements. Creatively seat parties next to (as opposed to across from) each other. Rotate seating to promote or reduce communication.
- Search for areas of agreement and trust.
- Take a break from the topic until emotions have cooled.

Expected Outcomes

A number of outcomes are associated with community coalition efforts. One would expect that in order to be embraced and supported by its community, a coalition must show that it has an effect on the ultimate health behaviors and health status indicators that it seeks to address. Thus, over a reasonable time period, one would expect to see positive coalition outcomes, such as reduced rates of youth smoking, increased immunization rates, reduced hospital and emergency room admissions of chronic asthmatics, and earlier detection of breast cancer. Some coalition outcomes, however, are related to the *process* of coalition building and maintenance. Examples of these are identified in the following list. Most outcomes result from increased commitment, collaboration, and participation by community groups.

- *Partnerships and relationships are established among community agencies, individuals, and influential people.* These relationships are developed through networking and collaboration and may be useful in focusing on other community issues in the future.

- *Relationships are developed with the media.* As coalition staff and members strive to accomplish their goals, they may have frequent contact with reporters, write letters to the editors of local papers, and speak on local radio or television. A relationship is built in which the coalition and members become recognized by the media as experts on the issue. As a result, the media will often take the initiative to contact someone from the coalition the next time the issue is referenced.

- *Public awareness is raised and community and social change is initiated.* Creating community awareness of an issue often leads to changes in individual beliefs and personal habits, as well as in public policy. Many times, changes in public policy precede changes in personal habits. For example, businesses that establish smoke-free policies may influence employees to quit smoking.

- *Legislators and local policymakers become aware of the coalition and its potential influence.* Coalitions tend to be highly visible in communities and can easily draw the attention and interest of legislators and local policymakers. These individuals are interested in having their names associated with initiatives that lead to positive changes in their communities.

- *Coalition members and community members are empowered from their experiences.* The process of implementing coalition strategies creates a sense of accomplishment and a "can do" and "can make a difference" attitude for coalition members, priority audiences, and the whole community.

- *Each person, or organization, within a coalition becomes part of a greater whole.* They now speak to the problem with a combined power and a unified voice.[7] This combined power is much greater than what each organization could accomplish alone. Issues are solved because individuals and agencies in the community begin to talk with each other and take ownership of the community problem.

- *A community standard of acceptability is developed.* A coalition that addresses an issue and creates awareness of the risks, benefits, and possible solutions can help change a community norm of what is and is not acceptable. Coalition efforts become a process of setting the community standard of beliefs and behavior.

A coalition also serves as a catalyst to engender community involvement and build **community capacity.** Innovative strategies that are carefully planned, executed, and evaluated by a diverse, collaborative group usually have a strong chance of success. Coalitions should pride themselves on the fact that they do not develop new programs with the intent of owning them. Instead, these programs are developed to help empower the community to solve its own health problems. Programs should be based within community organizations and agencies. The material and personnel resources the coalition brings serve as seeds to generate future ownership of these and other spin-off programs.

A coalition's job is to use resources fairly and wisely so that it is seen as a partner in the change process and not as the owner. Ultimately, traditional health care providers and grassroots groups will have to see that this collaborative approach is effective in changing behaviors and health status before they will embrace these programs and activities. The best compliment a coalition can receive is to see that a program it started within the community is still thriving or has been adapted to fit changing circumstances. For example, partners who help develop new standards of care for managing pediatric asthma should feel real ownership of the process and product. If so, the standards will be easily embraced as routine for institutions, such as schools and hospitals, instead of being imposed by an outside authority (i.e., the coalition).

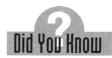

Did You Know

When coalitions *exceed* the expectations of both their members and the community, success in reaching outcomes is inevitable.

Conclusion

Coalition building can be challenging and time-consuming. Most often, however, the benefits to communities and health professionals far outweigh these drawbacks. Community benefits that derive from coalitions are numerous, including the ultimate reduction of the community health problem or issue. As reinforced in this chapter, the skills required to build or maintain a coalition can be learned. A variety of manuals, textbooks, and Web-based references and tools are available (see the Additional Resources list). Many foundations and professional organizations offer technical assistance and training opportunities for health educators. Serving on coalitions can expand professional networks, enhance personal knowledge and experiences in community organizing, and assist in achieving professional goals concerning health promotion and disease prevention. It is no longer a question of whether you will be asked to join or form a health coalition, but when. Preparing for that opportunity will be well worth the effort.

KEY TERMS

action plan: The written strategic plan for how the coalition will carry out its mission. It includes goals, objectives, strategies, resources, responsibilities of members, and budget and evaluation elements.

coalition barriers: The inherent problems within a coalition that hinder it from achieving goals and objectives (e.g., member burnout and turnover, difficulty reaching consensus).

coalition benefits: The inherent positive factors that result from participating in coalition activities (e.g., sharing resources, promoting a sense of civic duty, and improving health outcomes).

coalition infrastructure: The formal structures within a coalition that organize its operation (e.g., mission statement, bylaws, committees, and leadership).

community capacity: A community's ability to sustain a level of action needed to accomplish coalition goals.

community coalition: A formal, long-term alliance among a group of individuals representing diverse organizations, factions, or constituencies who agree to work together to achieve a common goal.

REFERENCES

1. Feighery, E., & Rogers, T. (1990). *How-to guides on community health promotion: Guide 12. Building and maintaining effective coalitions.* Palo Alto, CA: Stanford Health Promotion Resource Center.

2. Butterfoss, F. D., Goodman, R. M., & Wandersman, A. (1993). Community coalitions for prevention and health promotion. *Health Education Research, 8,* 315–330.

3. Whitt, M. (1993). *Fighting tobacco: A coalition approach to improving your community's health.* Lansing, MI: Michigan Department of Public Health.

4. McLeroy, K., Kegler, M., Steckler, A., Burdine, J., & Wisotzky, M. (1994). Community coalitions for health promotion: Summary and further reflections. *Health Education Research, 9,* 1–11.

5. Eisen, A. (1994). Survey of neighborhood-based comprehensive community empowerment initiatives. *Health Education Quarterly, 21,* 234–252.

6. Dowling, J. D., O'Donnell, H. J., & Wellington Consulting Group. (2000). *A development manual for asthma coalitions.* Northbrook, IL: The CHEST Foundation and the American College of Chest Physicians.

7. Merenda, D. (1986). *A practical guide to creating and managing school/community partnerships.* Alexandria, VA: National School Volunteer Program.

8. Berquist, W., Betwee, J., & Meuei, D. (1995). *Building strategic relationships.* San Francisco: Jossey-Bass.

9. Kreuter, M. W., Lezin, N. A., & Young, L. A. (2000). Evaluating community-based collaborative mechanisms: Implications for practitioners. *Health Promotion Practice, 1,* 49–63.

10. Butterfoss, F. D., Morrow, A. L., Rosenthal, J., Dini, E., Crews, R. C., Webster, J. D., & Louis, P. (1998). CINCH: An urban coalition for empowerment and action. *Health Education and Behavior, 25,* 215–225.

11. Pertschuk, M. (1988, March 18). Smoking or health: The coalition as giant killer. Keynote address to the Michigan Coalition on Smoking or Health Training Conference for Volunteers, Lansing, MI.

12. Butterfoss, F. D., Goodman, R. M., & Wandersman, A. (1996). Community coalitions for prevention and health promotion: Factors predicting satisfaction, participation and planning. *Health Education Quarterly, 23,* 65–79.

13. Sutton, C. D., & Brown, J. (1996). *Community coalitions: A how-to manual.* Philadelphia: Onyx Group.

14. Stop Teenage Addiction to Tobacco. (1992). *Community organizers' manual* (pp. 35–36). Springfield, MA: Author.

15. Minnesota Department of Health. (1988). *A guide for promoting health in Minnesota: A community approach.* St. Paul, MN: Author.

16. Kegler, M. C., Steckler, A., McLeroy, K., & Malek, S. H. (1998). Factors that contribute to effective health promotion coalitions: A study of 10 Project ASSIST coalitions in North Carolina. *Health Education and Behavior, 25,* 338–353.

17. Kaye, G., & Wolff, T. (1995). *From the ground up: A workbook on community development and coalition building.* Amherst, MA: AHEC Community Partners.

18. Wolff, T. (2001). A practitioner's guide to successful coalitions. *American Journal of Community Psychology, 29,* 173–191.

19. American Stop Smoking Intervention Study. (1991). *Orientation manual.* Washington, DC: National Cancer Institute.

ADDITIONAL RESOURCES

Print

Amherst H. Wilder Foundation. (1977). *The collaboration handbook: Creating, sustaining and enjoying the journey.* St. Paul, MN: Author.

Bobo, K., Kendall, J., & Max, S. (2001). *Organizing for social change: Midwest Academy manual for activists* (4th ed.). Santa Ana, CA: Seven Locks Press.

Bracht, N. (Ed.). (1990). *Health promotion at the community level.* Thousand Oaks, CA: Sage Publications.

Brownson, R. C., Baker, E. A., & Novick, L. F. (1989). *Community-based prevention: Programs that work.* Gaithersburg, MD: Aspen Publications.

Butterfoss, F. D. (2007). *Coalitions and partnerships in community health.* San Francisco: Jossey-Bass Publications.

Centers for Disease Control and Prevention, Division of Partnerships and Strategic Alliances, National Center for Health Marketing. (2006). *Partnership tool kit.* Atlanta, GA: Author.

Fetterman, D., Kafterian, S., & Wandersman, A. (1996). *Empowerment evaluation: Knowledge and tools for self-assessment and accountability.* Thousand Oaks, CA: Sage Publications.

Kretzmann, J. P., & McKnight, J. (1993). *Building communities from the inside out: A path toward finding and mobilizing a community's assets.* Chicago: ACTA Publications.

Kreuter, M., Lezin, L., Kreuter, M., & Green, L. (1998). *Community health promotion ideas that work: A field-book for practitioners.* Sudbury, MA: Jones and Bartlett.

The National Network for Collaboration. (1996). *Collaboration framework: Addressing community capacity.* Fargo, ND: Author.

Turning Point Social Marketing National Excellence Collaborative. (2003). *Social marketing and public health: Lessons from the field.* Seattle, WA: Turning Point.

W. K. Kellogg Foundation. (1998). *W. K. Kellogg Foundation evaluation handbook.* Battle Creek, MI: Author.

Internet

The Advocacy Institute. (2005). *Empower the coalition: Making partnerships and collaborations that work.* Available: http://www.advocacy.org/coalitions/.

Civicus. (2005). *Promoting your organization.* Available: http://www.civicus.org/new/media/Promoting%20your%20organisation.doc.

The Democracy Center. (2002). *Citizen action series: Developing an advocacy strategy.* Available: http://www.democracyctr.org/resources/manual/curricula/doc1.htm.

Mosaica. (2005). *Boards of directors and private-sector fundraising: Getting started.* Available: http://mosaica.coure-tech.com/resources/brdfdr.pdf.

Mosaica. (n.d.). *Preparing effective competitive grant applications.* Available: http://mosaica. coure-tech.com/resources/preapps.pdf.

The National Campaign to Prevent Teen Pregnancy. (2003). *Breaking ground: Lessons learned from the community coalition partnership programs for the prevention of teen pregnancy.* Available: http://www.dhs.state.or.us/children/publications/tpp/breaking ground.pdf.

University of Kansas Work Group on Health Promotion and Community Development. *The community toolbox.* Available: http://ctb.ku.edu.

Foundations and Agencies That Fund Coalition Initiatives

American Legacy Foundation. Washington, DC. Youth Empowerment Tobacco Control Coalitions.

Centers for Disease Control and Prevention (CDC). Atlanta, GA. Coalitions to promote immunizations; 5-a-Day nutrition programs; diabetes control; asthma control and management; HIV/AIDS community planning; breast, cervical, and prostate cancer control; and unintentional childhood injury prevention, among others.

Centers for Substance Abuse Prevention (CSAP). Bethesda, MD. Community Partnerships for Alcohol, Tobacco and Other Drug Abuse Prevention.

Health Care Finance Administration (HCFA). Bethesda, MD. New Horizons Adult Immunization Program.

Health Services Resource Administration (HRSA). Bethesda, MD. Healthy Start Initiative to Reduce Infant Mortality.

Robert Wood Johnson Foundation. Princeton, NJ. Allies Against Asthma Grant Program.

W. K. Kellogg Foundation. Chicago, IL. Healthy Community coalitions, among others.

13

Using Advocacy to Affect Policy

Sue Lachenmayr, M.P.H., CHES

Author Comments

As a government employee whose job is implementing public policy, I recognize how important it is to hear from frontline people who are delivering programs, from the individuals who are receiving services, and most important, from the people who are not able to access the services they need. Whether you are happy with current programming and services or you think changes need to be made, your advocacy efforts make a difference. When you speak directly to your elected officials or testify at a public hearing, sharing your personal experiences can have a tremendous impact. If you don't speak out about what makes good public health policy, legislators will assume either that no one cares about the program, so funding can be cut, or that no changes are needed. If special interest groups want the funding for another cause and they are the only ones who speak out, legislators may assume there is only one point of view. *Healthy People 2010*, the comprehensive planning document for ensuring the health of the public, provides an advocacy call to action and challenges all health educators to help "increase quality and years of healthy life" and "eliminate health disparities."[1]

Introduction

For too long, health educators and other public health professionals have been followers rather than leaders in the crafting of public health policy. Advocacy is an essential component of the Code of Ethics for the Health Education Profession[2,3] and a required competency for health educators[3,4] of health education programs. Learning how to use local, state, and national issues to develop laws and regulations will help support individual and community health promotion. Health educators have a personal right and a professional responsibility to become effective policy advocates—and it is not all that difficult.

Becoming involved in the political process has been identified as a key function of health educators since the late 1970s.[5] Practitioners need to be involved in the legislative process in many ways, not only to influence the kind and amount of resources allocated for health education programs, but also to affect the larger policy framework that defines all of public health. Advocacy is a critical skill needed by health educators as well as the public health education workforce[6] and should be an integral part of every health agency. When it comes to shaping policy, nothing is more effective than a well-educated, unified voice. Effective advocacy and affecting policy is a long-term commitment. Building relationships with policymakers at every level is essential for success.

Health educators possess certain skills that policymakers need in crafting legislation and gathering support for an issue. Specifically, health educators can support issues with data, are experts in assessing individual and community needs, and have skills in consensus building and in planning, implementing, and evaluating programs. In addition, health educators are experts at defining the problem using the facts and impact, as well as personal stories about the people who are affected. This expertise can assist policymakers in moving an issue from idea to **law**.

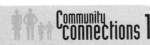

Community connections 1

Erica is a Master's of Public Health student who works part-time for a community hospital. She was unfamiliar with the word *advocacy* until one of her professors gave a lecture on advocacy and the political process. When she learned that an advocate is someone who speaks on behalf of others, Erica recognized that she had acted as an advocate for her classmates when she protested about increased university parking rates. She realized she enjoyed the process of advocating for change.

Advocacy, Lobbying, and Grassroots Activities

Often, practitioners are unclear about steps they can take to influence public health policy. Advocacy, lobbying, and grassroots activities are tools to use to influence policy. Practical advocacy strategies that health educators can use are readily available.[7] Both *lobbying* and *grassroots activities* are legal strategies frequently utilized by for-profit and nonprofit organizations to support or change policy. **Legislative advocacy** can be defined as contact made with a policymaker or legislator to discuss a social or economic problem on behalf of a particular interest group or population as long as no specific bill number is mentioned.[8] Nonprofit organizations need to follow specific guidelines as defined in the U.S. tax code, but as a private citizen, anyone has the right to engage in these activities without restrictions.

For some people, sharing their opinion about a social or economic problem with their elected official or advocating for an issue they believe in seems natural. For most people, however, the initial reaction to the term *lobbying*, or *lobbyist*, is often negative. But lobbying is a very effective way to ensure an issue becomes a law. **Direct lobbying** can be defined as communication about specific legislation with a legislator, or communication about a specific position on that legislation. In other words, asking a legislator to support (or veto) a specific bill is considered lobbying. **Grassroots lobbying** is when a group or organization appeals to the general public and asks them to take action to influence specific legislation. For example, a letter to parents of schoolchildren asking them to call or write their congressperson to support a bill to increase funding for a new school program is considered grassroots lobbying. In this instance, instead of a direct appeal to a legislator, all the people in the community are asked to take action and tell their legislator to support the bill. Providing a policymaker with factual, nonpartisan information on an issue or sharing information with the public without asking them to urge their legislator to vote in a certain way is *not* considered lobbying.

Did You Know

Even a busy person, or a beginner, can be an advocate. All it takes is. . .

- 1 minute to leave a telephone message for your legislator
- 3 to 5 minutes to copy and share an article of interest with a legislator or colleague
- 5 to 10 minutes to send a letter or email message to your legislator
- 10 to 15 minutes to visit a Web site for the latest information on bills or advocacy issues

Source: Coalition of National Health Education Organizations. (2007). *Making your advocacy efforts count* [Brochure]. Available: http://healtheducationadvocate. org/Advocacy%20brochure.pdf.

Be prepared by answering the question, Why should the government be involved in the solution? Many legislators prefer to let private industry address the problem. If the best solution is for government (at any level) to take an active role, advocates need to be able to make the case that private industry has not and cannot address the problem and why government action is needed.

Steps for Advocating Legislation

Understanding the legislative process will increase the likelihood of success. Six crucial steps to legislative involvement are (1) identifying the issue and developing a fact sheet, (2) understanding the steps needed to enact legislation, (3) identifying potential partners and forming or joining coalitions to strengthen the likelihood of success, (4) building grassroots support, (5) using the Internet for advocacy, and (6) working with policymakers.

Identify the Issue and Develop a Support Fact Sheet

Start by defining what the problem is and who is affected by the problem. How many people are affected? Are some more affected than others (or at greater risk)?

What is the cost if the problem is not addressed? What policy or law could help resolve the problem? Who else might be concerned about the problem? Answering these questions can help clarify the issue and determine where to start.

Develop a fact sheet about the issue that can be given to potential advocates and to legislators. Include the key points identified above: a statement of the problem, the number of people affected, the cost of the problem, and strategies to lessen the problem. Include a personal story about a community member who has experienced the problem (or been helped by a program that needs more funding). Many nonprofit organizations and federal agencies have examples of fact sheets. The Centers for Disease Control and Prevention (CDC) and the nonprofit organization Research!America have examples of effective public health fact sheets on their Web sites.[9,10]

Most issues can be addressed at several different levels. *Voluntary policies* are implemented without government direction. *Local ordinances*, or regulations, are enacted by township or county governmental entities. *State laws* are enacted by the vote of state legislators and the governor. Senators and representatives at the federal level pass bills that are then signed into *federal law* by the president. Often policies may start as voluntary practices, become local regulations, and then become state or federal law. For example, in many communities, organizations established no-smoking policies. These policies gained favor and some communities made public buildings smoke free, which in turn influenced enactment of state and federal policies banning smoking in public places.

Policies can be implemented at worksites or in community settings by choice rather than by law. For example, a magazine publisher can enact a policy not to accept alcohol or tobacco advertising. Governmental bodies such as township committees, local boards of health, local school boards, boards of chosen freeholders, or boards of county commissioners or supervisors enact ordinances at the city, township, or county level. For example, a county board of commissioners may mandate smoke-free buildings in private worksites for businesses registered within the county. Elected **legislators** enact state and federal laws. For instance, a state may enact specific penalties for drunk driving. In general, state and federal laws are more difficult policies to influence, so identifying influential partners and increasing media attention can increase success.

Groups or organizations that have never engaged in advocacy efforts should begin with a "winnable issue." A small success, or several small successes, can build confidence to tackle more difficult issues. This strategy also enables members to work together to develop advocacy strategies. Encouraging adoption of voluntary policy, such as encouraging restaurants to go smoke free on their own rather than advocating for a city ordinance to ban smoking in restaurants, could start the process. Encouraging voluntary policy can gain allies who will support the issue at the regulatory level, especially if they have benefited from a voluntary

Table 13-1	Choosing an Advocacy Issue

- Why is this issue important? Who is affected?
- What will be gained or lost by supporting or opposing the issue?
- What is the experience and level of commitment of the advocacy group?
- Are there sufficient staff and volunteers to implement a legislative campaign?
- What funding is available to support the campaign? (Some funding agencies and grant funds have specific guidelines about legislative involvement. This should be determined beforehand in case alternative funding is needed.)
- What community resources (e.g., money, space, materials) are available?
- Who are the advocacy group's allies and adversaries on this issue?
- Who else (groups or individuals) shares this problem?
- What would those groups who share the problem gain or lose by joining the campaign?
- What laws, if any, already exist to deal with the issue of concern?
- What are the rules and regulations that govern involvement in legislative advocacy?
- What stories, metaphors, and facts can be used to make your case?

policy. For example, the restaurant owner whose business increases as a result of being smoke free may encourage other restaurants to adopt similar policies. If there are large increases in health care costs for employees in a smoking restaurant, the owner may be more supportive of regulation that requires restaurants to become smoke free. Table 13-1 includes a number of questions a group should consider prior to choosing an issue to pursue.[11]

Understand the Steps Needed to Enact Legislation

Health educators can educate policymakers about an issue or, even better, persuade a legislator to **sponsor** (or author) a bill to address the problem. Identifying **bipartisan** sponsors (sponsors from each major political party) can increase the likelihood that a bill will gain broad support. A legislator who sponsors a bill can be a champion for the issue. Steps must occur, however, before a bill actually becomes law at the local, state, or federal level. In most states, only about 10% of the bills introduced each year actually make it through the process and become law. Persuading a legislator to sponsor a bill is only the start. Advocating for action at each step in the process increases the likelihood for success.

Local policy issues are fairly easy to introduce. Begin by contacting a member of the local governing body in which the policy is to be introduced to determine the best approach. Table 13-2 outlines the process that is normally followed once a policy issue (in this example, at the county level) has been introduced.[12]

Table 13-2	Steps for Passing a County Regulation

1. Advocacy group raises an issue to the health department of the county government. (Include background information about the issue, anticipated benefits, and need for new regulations.)
2. Health officer or other community leader introduces idea to the Board of Health.
3. Regulation language (how the bill will be written) is researched (e.g., find examples of laws about similar issues).
4. Language is drafted and reviewed by the county attorney.
5. Regulation language and data are presented to the Board of Health.
6. The Board of Health holds meetings or hearings to discuss the proposed regulation.
7. Once passed by the Board of Health, the regulation is presented to the county Board of Commissioners (or Freeholders) for approval.
8. A task force may be appointed to research the regulation, table it, or refer it to another committee for their recommendation.
9. Public hearing dates are set (normally three dates).
10. Notification of public hearing dates is published in the local newspaper.
11. Public hearings at which the community has the opportunity to present arguments for or against the proposed regulation are held.
12. Commissioners vote on the regulation.
13. If passed by the Board of Commissioners, the local health department has authority to adopt the regulation.

Note: This process may vary depending on locality and individual issues.

At the state level, the policy issue must be introduced to the legislature. This occurs either in the House of Representatives (or State Assembly), the Senate, or both simultaneously. A member of the advocacy group, or the group's **lobbyist**, proposes the issue to a legislator, who then introduces the issue to the legislature. The president of the Senate or Speaker of the House (or Assembly) must agree to have the bill introduced (also known as *dropped* or *posted*).

Once introduced, the issue will be processed as a bill. The bill is then referred to all committees that have jurisdiction over the issues presented in the bill. For example, if the bill requests a new health screening and funding to cover the health screening, the bill must be heard by both the Health Committee and the Appropriations Committee. A bill passed by committee is then marked up to be heard by the full house. If passed by both the House and Senate, the bill goes

Did You Know

Ninety percent of the letters, telephone calls, or visits received by policymakers are about taxes, guns, or abortion. All other issues, from education and the environment to highways and health, make up the remaining 10% of visits. You have a real opportunity to educate legislators about your issues if they are about anything other than the top three issues.

before the governor. When the governor signs the bill, the bill becomes a law. The process for passing a bill into law at the federal level is similar. Table 13-3 outlines the general steps of how a bill becomes a law.[13]

Table 13-3	**How a Bill Becomes a Law**

1. A bill is introduced in either the Senate or the House. Sometimes identical bills are simultaneously introduced. The bill receives *first reading* (which means it is recognized as an issue and given a title and number). The majority leader of the Senate or the Speaker of the House then refers the bill to an appropriate standing committee (e.g., Education, Commerce, and Health). If the bill is a budget bill or has fiscal implications, it will be referred directly to the Appropriations Committee (a joint committee of the Senate and House) or to an appropriate standing committee and then to the Appropriations Committee.

2. In the standing committee, the bill is discussed and debated. Public hearings may be held. Not every bill before the committee will be considered. The committee may take one of several different actions:
   - Report the bill with favorable recommendation.
   - Add amendments and report the bill with favorable recommendation.
   - Replace the original bill with a substitute.
   - Report the bill with adverse recommendation.
   - Report the bill without recommendation.
   - Report the bill with amendments but without recommendation.
   - Report the bill with the recommendation that the bill be referred to another committee.
   - Take no action on the bill.
   - Refuse to report the bill out of committee.

3. If a bill is reported out favorably or a substitute is offered, the bill is returned to the Senate or House, where it receives a *general orders* status in the Senate and *second reading* status in the House. The Senate resolves itself into the committee-of-the-whole (the entire Senate sitting as a committee and operating under informal rules), and the House assumes the order of second reading. At this time, committee recommendations are considered and amendments may be offered and adopted. The bill then advances to *third reading* (the final stage of consideration of a legislative bill before a vote on its final form).

4. Upon third reading in the Senate, an entire bill is read unless unanimous consent is given to consider the bill read. In the House, the bill is read in its entirety on third reading unless four-fifths of the members consent to consider the bill read. At third reading the bill is again subject to debate and amendment. At the conclusion of third reading, the bill is either passed or defeated by a roll call vote of the majority of members elected and serving, *or* one of the following options may be used to delay final action:
   - Refer bill back to committee for further consideration.
   - Postpone bill indefinitely.
   - Make the bill a special order of business on third reading for a specific date.

(Continued)

Table 13-3	How a Bill Becomes a Law (Continued)

- Table the bill.
- Following either passage or defeat of a bill, a legislator may move to have the bill reconsidered. In the Senate the motion must be made within the next two session days; in the House, by the next day.

5. If the bill passes, it goes to the other legislative branch (i.e., House or Senate), where the same procedure is followed. If both houses pass the bill in the same form, it is ordered *enrolled* in the house in which it originated. It then goes to the governor (or president) for signature.

6. If the second house passes the bill in a different form, the bill is returned to its house of origin. If this house accepts the changes, the bill is enrolled and sent to the governor (or president). If the changes are rejected, the bill is sent to a conference committee that tries to resolve differences. If the first conference report is rejected, a second conference committee may be appointed.

7. The governor (or president) has 14 days after receiving a bill to consider it. The bill may be

   - Signed. The bill becomes law 90 days after the legislature adjourns at the end of the year or at a later date as specified in the bill. The bill can take effect immediately by a two-thirds vote of the members elected and it becomes law upon the governor's (or president's) signature.
   - Vetoed (can be overridden by a two-thirds vote by both houses).
   - Neither signed nor vetoed, in which case the bill becomes law 14 days after reaching the governor's (or president's) desk, unless the legislature adjourns at the end of the year within the 14 days. In that case, the bill does not become law.

8. If the governor (or president) vetoes a bill while the legislature is in session or recess, one of the following actions may occur:

   - The legislature may override the veto by a two-thirds vote of the members elected and serving in both houses.
   - The bill may not receive the necessary two-thirds vote, and thus the attempt to override the veto will fail.
   - The bill may be tabled pending an attempt to override the veto.
   - The bill may be re-referred to a committee.

Note: In general, this process is the same throughout the United States. However, health educators should research their state's legislative processes.

Each step that is taken to affect legislation should also be used to target the executive branch of government, regardless of whether the goal is to enact new legislation, establish regulations, or implement and enforce the new law.

Identify Potential Partners

People usually feel more confident and willing to tackle legislative issues when they are part of a group in which members have similar beliefs. Forming a group to advocate for or against an issue can be more effective than an individual voice because a group can share responsibilities and complete more tasks. For example, when groups like the American Cancer Society, American Lung Association, and American Heart Association join forces in Washington, DC, they are representing hundreds of thousands of individual voices. Policymakers listen because they know that some of their constituents are part of these groups.

Identifying nontraditional allies and partners can significantly strengthen the likelihood of success. Looking for common ground among unlikely groups, such as mothers opposing gun violence in schools and gun retailers, or public health professionals and tobacco farmers, has led to strong coalitions with expanded resources. Understanding the values, needs, and concerns of perceived opponents to an issue and identifying areas of common ground can result in broader, more realistic options that will create additional advocates.

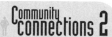

Community Connections 2

Erica realized that a nursing shortage affected the quality of care in the hospital where she worked. Erica tried to encourage nurses to sign a letter to legislators that outlined some of the issues. Many of the nurses were too busy to talk with Erica about her ideas, and others thought they might lose their jobs if they complained about conditions at their hospital. Erica was stumped—she was just one person and only a student. How could she make a difference?

Erica was a member of a student public health association. She took her concerns to them and they agreed to help her write a letter and sign it. Some members of the student association were members of professional organizations; they took the letter to those organizations and received even more signatures.

Build Grassroots Support

Grassroots movements are alliances of local people, usually volunteers, working together toward a common goal. Mobilizing local support for an issue greatly increases the likelihood that a policymaker will be interested in the group's position. Through grassroots initiatives, health educators have the opportunity not just to advocate for those who need better policies, but also to empower members of the public to become their own advocates. When current services are not available, the people who are directly affected can be the most powerful advocates for change.

Motivating individuals for a grassroots movement is more likely if the issue affects many community members. Helping new advocates articulate the issues will increase their confidence when they have the opportunity to voice their concerns before policymakers. Increase the confidence of grassroots advocates by providing facts about the issue and giving examples of the experiences of others. Encourage

Did You Know

When you ask a legislator to sponsor new legislation or support a bill that is already introduced, the worst that can happen is that the legislator will say no. If you are a constituent, the legislator is likely to say yes to your request because your vote in the next election is important.

advocates to share their stories by providing a guide for the type of information they should share, and ask them to practice their stories to increase their confidence.

Organizing a grassroots legislative action follows many of the same steps as organizing a coalition (see Chapter 12). Even a grassroots effort that is loosely organized requires a leader and a shared decision-making process. Key community leaders, organizations, and community members who have the ability to create change should be recruited. These individuals often have the skills and resources (e.g., experience and political connections) to help make the initiative a success.

A grassroots group can formulate either a short- or long-term legislative initiative. The goals of the group will help determine the strategies needed for success. Activities might include developing an information campaign, polling policymakers to identify potential legislative support, contacting government offices to determine the procedure to introduce policy issues, creating a media campaign, or developing a budget. Each group member's previous experience with legislative committees, reputation in the community, personal or professional experience with the issue, and association with the group should be considered. For example, in introducing a policy on maintenance and safety checks for park equipment, a parent of a child injured in a poorly maintained playground would be an effective spokesperson.

Review the group's progress to determine (1) whether objectives are being met, (2) whether members feel satisfied with their involvement, (3) what barriers continue to exist, and (4) the future direction of the initiative. Asking members about their achievements and challenges, listing policymakers' stands on the issue, assessing changes in policy or community opinion, and identifying what still needs to be done and what is not working all provide important information about the potential success or failure of the grassroots campaign.

As suggested earlier, policy issues should reflect the problems identified by the local community or coalition. If the issue will have great impact in the community, ask others to identify people affected by the issue who are not part of the legislative efforts and invite them to join. Suggestions for recruiting advocates can be found in Table 13-4.

Use the Internet for Advocacy

The Internet has revolutionized how people and organizations engage in advocacy. The Internet can be used for recruiting, educating, and mobilizing advocates concerning a specific issue. A public service site that can be used to

Table 13-4	How to Recruit Grassroots Advocates

- *Meet with or write to potential advocates.* Ask for their help and outline the issue, describing how new legislation can benefit members of the community or group.

- *Ask volunteers to write, fax, or phone their legislators.* Provide fact sheets and sample letters to use as a guide. Include information about how to ask legislators for services. Share examples of personal stories and how the impact of personal stories can help change legislation.

- *Provide support for first-time advocates.* Identify others who have had similar experiences and ask them to describe their contact with legislators.

- *Share effective stories from other advocates as a model.* Legislators respond to personal stories of constituents. Including personal stories with information sent to new advocates will illustrate how someone's personal experiences can influence policymakers.

fax or email members of Congress via the Web is www.congress.org. Other Internet services help advocates track the positions and votes of their elected officials. Several organizations, such as MoveOn.org (www.moveon.org), a mobilization campaign founded in 1998, now have more than a million members who can be mobilized to take action on political issues. Television programs, newspapers, university research groups, and nonprofit organizations all make use of surveys or polls on timely issues. Advocacy groups can raise an issue or shape public opinion by utilizing online "voting" in polls or surveys.

Internet advocacy tools include chat rooms, which allow real-time electronic communication among participants; **Usenet newsgroups** that focus discussion around a specific topic; **blogs**, or Web logs, which are publicly accessible personal journals; and video-sharing Web sites, such as YouTube (www.youtube.com).

Work with Policymakers

Policymakers are the elected officials who enact policy, laws, and ordinances. At local, state, and federal levels, they are responsible for creating and enacting policies that guide and influence the activities and actions of individuals and organizations. Table 13-5 contains a list of typical policymakers at each level and how they can be reached.

Elected officials are often treated with a level of respect that seems to place them at a different level from the ordinary citizen, but their claims to the positions they hold are the result of the votes cast by ordinary citizens. Politicians are people, too. In fact, their primary job is to respond to the concerns of their **constituents** (voters and residents of their district). Although legislators listen to their party, special interest groups, and lobbyists, their greatest allegiance is to the residents of their district—those who voted them into office (or might vote for or against them in the next election).

Table 13-5	Levels of Policymakers

- *Local officials.* County, city, township, or village elected officials, such as commissioners, council members, supervisors, mayors, and village presidents. A list of local policymakers can be obtained from any city, township, or county office. The office addresses and telephone numbers, office hours, and committee assignments (e.g., budget and finance, health policy, transportation) of each elected official are also available.

- *State officials.* Elected individuals, such as the governor, members of the state assembly and state senate, and other elected or appointed government officials (e.g., judges, lieutenant governors, attorneys general, commissioners, assistant commissioners, deputy commissioners, and others). A legislative directory may be available from organizations such as the League of Women Voters. The directory includes state and federal legislators' mailing addresses, telephone and fax numbers, legislative aides, and committee assignments. The guide also lists addresses for state and federal executive branches. In addition to this type of directory, many legislators can be reached through the Internet via state or federal legislative Web pages.

- *Federal officials.* The president, vice president, members of the U.S. House of Representatives and Senate, and appointed policymakers, such as representatives of governmental agencies or cabinet members. Directories of federal elected officials are available from many nonprofit organizations and federal and legislative Web pages.

As a health educator, providing well-documented information will help policymakers develop or support good public health laws and regulations. The health educator's experience as a person who works in the community to improve the health of the community can be an asset to legislators.

Establishing a Relationship: How to Influence Policymakers

Developing a relationship with legislators requires more than an occasional meeting or letter about an issue. Building a relationship means a long-term commitment that involves an ongoing exchange of information, such as letters or phone calls congratulating legislators when they support important issues. Local officials are accessible and there are many opportunities to meet with them. For instance, many policymakers hold "coffee hours" at local establishments in their districts. This allows constituents to meet with their policymakers without an appointment. Knowing the civic groups in which the official is a member (e.g., Lions Club, Rotary Club) can provide insight into personal interests and community commitment and may help determine allies or opponents for legislative concerns. Attending hearings before local boards of health, township committees, and other local committees helps identify priority issues at the local level and provides the opportunity to meet policymakers prior to a formal appointment. Consider inviting legislators to visit one's place of work

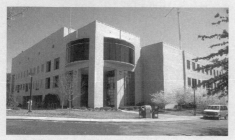

Community Connections 3

As part of a class assignment, Erica had to identify her state representatives and find out the type of government in her town. Finding out about her state representatives was easy—she went to her state's legislative Web page and put in her zip code, and the names of her two assembly representatives and her state senator appeared. Each of them had his or her own Web page, so she could find out their party affiliations, the committees they were on, and the bills they sponsored.

Identifying her city's governing body was just as easy. She just went to her city's Web page to learn the names of the council members and the mayor. One of her classmates made a trip to her town's municipal building, where all of the information was available to the public.

Table 13-6   Steps for Advocating Legislation

- Make a monetary donation. A financial contribution, even a small one, puts your name on the legislator's list of contributors. Consider contributing to two opposing candidates—this is what major corporations do to ensure they are seen as a "friend" regardless of who is elected. *Caution:* This is a good strategy for an individual or a for-profit organization; however, there are strict rules regarding nonprofit organizations and direct campaign contributions and electioneering (supporting or opposing a candidate for public office).[8]

- Provide policymakers with objective, factual information about key issues. Supply that information periodically (even when there is not an immediate issue for which a legislator's help is needed).

- Visit legislators when they are in the district, attend their town meetings or other public appearances, and make an appointment to visit them when they are at their government office. Let the legislator know you are a constituent of the legislator's district. If not a constituent, identify local residents to make the visit and discuss how this issue affects them. Always provide written information about the issue and the legislative action that should be taken.

- Invite legislators to a community site so they can see a program in action and meet people who are benefiting from the program. (*Note:* Nonprofit organizations that invite elected officials for a site visit near the time of an election should also invite opposition candidates for a site visit, so the organization is not seen as **electioneering**.)

- Recognize legislators when they introduce or vote for a bill on an issue that is important to you. Write letters of appreciation or send a press release to the local newspaper.

- Involve constituents and community members who have been directly involved with or affected by the issue.

- Criticism of, or opposition to, a bill is fine, but provide a solution so that the legislator can work to rectify the situation.

or attend a local event. Table 13-6 identifies actions to increase the likelihood of gaining a legislator's attention.

Find out when committee meetings and general legislative sessions are scheduled. Any official's office staff or legislative aide can assist with this information. Newspapers usually print committee and board meeting information a week in advance. These meetings are open to the public, and can provide an opportunity to meet policymakers before introducing a legislative issue.

State legislators usually divide their time between the state capitol and their individual districts. In Michigan, for example, legislators are typically in their respective districts on Monday and Friday, while the rest of week is spent at the capitol working on legislative issues. It is usually easier to speak with legislators when they are in their local districts. If you are at the capitol, however, do not miss an opportunity to meet legislators and their staff. Even though a scheduled appointment is best, one may visit an official's office without an appointment. If the official is not available, request a meeting or leave information with one of the legislator's staff members.

Which Policymaker Should Be Contacted?

The appropriate level for policy change (local, state, or federal) will help determine which elected official to contact. Staff and legislative aides of elected and appointed officials can be key allies, since all correspondence and appointments go through these individuals. In addition, it is the staff who provide background information that will shape the legislator's position on an issue. Do not be disappointed when meeting with a staff member rather than a legislator, because the aides listen carefully, gather pertinent information, and read the materials they are given.

Develop a plan for the legislative visits to increase support for an issue. To address state-level issues, start with your own Assembly or House representative. Being a constituent offers the greatest likelihood of success. Next, determine the committee that might hear the issue.

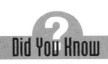

Did You Know

Rarely is any public health advocacy effort strong enough to compete against well-funded competing interests. Forming or joining a broad coalition with similar goals can increase success.

For example, if the issue is related to health and the legislator is not on the Health Committee, ask him or her to write a letter of support to the chair of the Health Committee. Plan to meet with the chair or another member of the Health Committee to discuss the issue. If the issue will need funding to implement (nearly every issue requires some funding), schedule a meeting with members of the Appropriations Committee. Whenever possible, identify members of the organization or coalition who are constituents, so

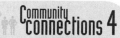

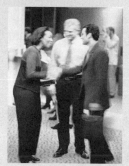

Erica and some of her classmates attended a free advocacy training session that was held on her campus. To her surprise, her own senator was one of the speakers. The senator talked about health care and encouraged attendees to visit their representatives. Erica was nervous, but with her classmates' encouragement, she introduced herself. She told the senator her concerns about nursing shortages and her letter-writing campaign. The senator asked Erica to send him a copy of the letter.

they can also attend. Each of these steps will need to be repeated to identify a legislative sponsor and gain support for that legislation in the legislature.

When the appropriate committee for the issue has been identified, consider meeting with officials from the state health department (or other agency) to enlist their support. This is an important step because the governor will want the department's endorsement before the bill will be signed into law (if a state issue). It is important to develop a positive working relationship with individuals in the state or local health department (depending on the level of the issue), because they may be able to provide supporting information about the need for the proposed legislation.

Meetings with staff members of the minority and majority legislative offices will identify support and opposition and will provide the opportunity to educate additional policymakers about the issue. Additional meetings with members of the governor's cabinet to discuss the legislation should also be considered. Do not forget to enlist the support of local officials; they can reinforce the need for legislation and describe how local citizens will benefit from the new legislation.

Introducing and Tracking Legislation

The steps required to introduce legislation are described in Tables 13-2 and 13-3. Remember, just introducing legislation does not ensure it will become law. Meet with various local and state officials to build support for the issue. When a representative agrees to sponsor a bill, seek both Republican and Democratic cosponsors from the appropriate committee so the bill will have bipartisan support.

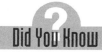

Did You Know

Elected officials serve you, whether you voted for them or not. You are a constituent and have the right to ask for their support or to take action on issues that matter to you.

Once a bill has been posted (or dropped), initiate letter-writing campaigns (described in the next section) to committee members, requesting the bill be heard and requesting support for the legislation. Maintain regular contact with staff of the sponsoring legislator to monitor the need for additional letters or visits.

Health educators should understand the legislative process and carefully monitor bills as they progress through the system. Recognize that amendments, which are a normal part of building support, can often weaken or strengthen legislation.

Tips and Techniques for Successful Legislative Advocacy

All too often legislation is enacted, changed, or dissolved without the public's knowledge. Elected officials need to know how their constituents feel about the issues. If policymakers do not hear from their constituency, their votes may not reflect the opinions of the community. This could result in passing laws that will hurt, rather than help, the people of their district. Providing useful ways for the public to get involved will increase the likelihood of success. Strategies for getting the public involved include legislative alerts, letter-writing and telephone campaigns, Internet advocacy, meeting with legislators, testifying at hearings, and media advocacy. These activities will educate the community and policymakers about the issue and move the public to action.

Develop Legislative Alerts

Legislative alerts are notices to a group's members about upcoming votes, needed action (e.g., letters or phone calls to officials), committee meetings, or hearings. An effective alert contains a summary of the issue, the position of the group, background information, and the action needed by the individual or group receiving the information. To make contacting a policymaker easier, the official's name, address, and phone number should be strategically placed on the alert. A simple message, accompanied by a specific action, will help ensure that the alert is understood. Include the specific time period needed for action, and request members to record the action they took. Legislative alerts can be distributed to members via mail, fax, or email (see Figure 13-1 for an example legislative alert).

Initiate Letter-Writing and Telephone Campaigns

Letter-writing campaigns are used to educate policymakers and urge them to take action. A successful campaign encompasses the information found in a legislative alert, but with more detail. It is important to find out how a legislator prefers to be contacted (i.e., telephone, direct contact, or letters). Some legislators view email as an acceptable method of communication, whereas others do not. All legislative offices, however, routinely tally issues mentioned by constituents, regardless of how the message is received.

ACTION ALERT

TO: Wai Ki Ki Surfers Association

FROM: Aloha, Inc.

RE: HB 2304

DATE: April 23, 2008

Aloha, Inc., urges you to contact (by phone, fax, letter, or e-mail) the following legislators, all of whom serve on the Water Safety Subcommittee, and urge them to vote against HB 2304, a bill that requires surfers to wear protective helmets during all water activity. This bill is currently in committee and expected to be reviewed on May 1, 2008.

Name	Phone	Fax
Rep. Matt Devoe (Chair)	(555) 123-3355	(555) 123-3352
Rep. Tom Broekma	(555) 123-4353	(555) 123-4354
Rep. Tim Turton	(555) 123-3272	(555) 123-3273
Rep. Perk Sonnega	(555) 123-5782	(555) 123-5783
Rep. Rodney Prahl	(555) 123-4456	(555) 123-4457

Letters may be sent to:

Honorable _____
House of Representatives
4040 Skylark
Honolulu, HI 91432

It is just a matter of time until all water activities are curtailed by legislation such as this. We believe it would be foolish to enact such legislation for the following reasons:

- Water helmets have been proven to increase serious injuries to the wearer, particularly in high wake situations.
- Water helmets currently have no regulations regarding safety specifications.
- The use of water helmets will greatly reduce the tourism to the Hawaiian Islands.
- Mandatory use of water helmets is an infringement of personal choice.

Thank you for your support in this important issue.

Figure 13-1 Example Legislative Alert

A letter-writing campaign can begin before or after the issue has been introduced as a bill. A sample letter to legislators should include opportunities for individuals to personalize the letter with their own thoughts. Often, community response to letter-writing campaigns is small because people are unaware of what to do. Names should be spelled out and the letter proofread prior to mailing. Letters from constituents that are individually authored have more impact than form letters. A personal letter shows that time and thought went into the letter. When time is of the essence, however, a signed form letter or email is better than no correspondence at all. Table 13-7 includes tips on how to write an influential letter.[6] Telephone or email campaigns should follow the same suggestions as letter-writing campaigns. It may be better to fax or email,

Table 13-7   Writing a Letter to a Policymaker

- *Address the letter properly.* Use the legislator's full name and the following format:

For a U.S. Senator	*For a State Representative*
The Honorable (full name)	The Honorable (full name)
United States Senator	State Representative
Address	District
	Address
Dear Senator (last name):	Dear Representative (last name):

- *Include your name and address and telephone number in the letter.* A letter cannot be answered if no return address exists or the signature is not legible.
- *Use your own words.* In general, legislators do not like form letters. These are identified as organized pressure campaigns and are often answered with form replies. As stated previously, however, sending sample letters to members helps organize thoughts. If time is of the essence, a form letter is better than no letter.
- *Timing is everything.* Write the legislator and the chair of the committee in which the bill is assigned while the bill is still in committee to request the bill be heard.
- *Identify the bill by number or by title.* For instance, "House Bill 2440" is a bill number, while "Healthy Michigan Fund" is a bill title. The Secretary of the Senate, Clerk of the House, or the sponsoring legislator's office will have information about the bill of interest.
- *Be brief and constructive.* State the facts and the group's issues, solutions, and personal positions on the matter. Keep the letter to one page, if possible. If you disagree with a bill or policy, be constructive and offer solutions, or state a better way to approach the issue.
- *Request a response.* Responses are not always sent. Asking for one in your letter, however, will increase the likelihood of receiving a response. Follow up with the legislator's office if a reply is not received.
- Fax the letter to the legislator's office, rather than mailing it. The speed associated with faxing ensures swift receipt.
- *Send a thank you.* If legislators have taken action requested, thank them. Legislating can be a thankless job, so recognizing a legislator's efforts is all the more important to maintaining good relations.

Community connections 5

After Erica sent her senator a copy of the letter about nursing shortages, she received a response from him, inviting her to meet with him about the issue. Although Erica was becoming more proficient as an advocate, being a health educator she knew she was not an expert on nursing shortages. She went to her student public health association to ask for help. They helped her identify nursing professionals who were willing to attend the meeting with the senator. They got together as a group to review the issues they wanted to present. Because Erica had made the initial contact, she agreed to introduce the nurses to the senator and let them tell their story.

rather than mail, letters to U.S. representatives and senators. Check with the legislator's staff to determine the most effective method for delivering letters.

Meet with Legislators

Contact by members of the policymaker's constituency is crucial. Policymakers are elected by their local residents to represent them in a larger arena (e.g., city, county, state, federal). Writing, calling, and meeting with legislators reminds them that local constituents support the issue. Legislators also learn that someone is concerned and watching their actions. Table 13-8 contains suggestions for an effective meeting with a legislator.[8]

Testify at a Legislative Hearing

The purpose of a committee hearing is to obtain written and oral testimony on a bill. Before the start of the hearing, audience members usually submit testifying cards, which include the individual's name, organization, and position on the bill. Even if not testifying, a card indicating support or opposition to the bill should be completed because all completed cards are filed and tabulated for the record. Table 13-9 consists of a number of suggestions for increasing the likelihood of delivering effective testimony.[14,15]

Use Media for Legislative Advocacy

The media can strengthen the public's desire to see changes made and can promote an issue. Media can educate policymakers, other members of the media, and the general public. Effective media campaigns require planning similar to the steps required to have a bill introduced. If possible, begin by establishing relationships with media personnel before providing information on an issue. Table 13-10 contains strategies for building media relationships.[16,17] See Chapters 10, "Working with the Media," and 14, "Using Media Advocacy to Influence Policy," for further skills on using media.

Table 13-8   Visiting a Policymaker

- *Look for advocates who have personal contacts with policymakers.* Being on a first-name basis improves access to officials, and personal and professional relationships with policymakers can be an advantage.

- *Know the facts.* Before contacting the policymaker, all sides of the issue should be researched for a clear understanding of the facts about the issue. If possible, find out the legislator's position on the issue ahead of time so advocates can argue persuasively. Although expertise is not required, the group should be well informed.

- *Know when and how to contact policymakers.* Advocates should be aware of when policymakers are at the capitol or in their respective districts prior to initiating a meeting. If the policymaker is unavailable, a meeting should be arranged with a legislative aide. Staff members are often more accessible, and they will share your concerns with the official.

- *Send a letter or fax, or telephone to request an appointment.* Submit your request to the district office or to the legislator's office at the capitol, depending on where you want to meet with your legislator. Identify yourself as a constituent.

- *Follow-up by phone or fax to confirm the appointment.* It may take several calls to arrange for a visit, but do not give up.

- *Be an expert.* Expertise on an issue should be shared with a policymaker. Policymakers cannot be experts on everything, so they will welcome additional information. Share your fact sheet on the issue.

- *Arrive on time.* If you are meeting with a staff member, be sure you have the correct contact name.

- *Send other advocates to talk with policymakers.* A crowd is not necessary to get a message across. A few advocates who represent the group can be effective. A primary spokesperson should be identified to keep the meeting focused on the issue.

- *Keep it simple.* Select pertinent information about the issue and present it to the policymaker during a face-to-face meeting. Be sure to ask the policymaker for a specific action (e.g., support for a bill, contacting a fellow policymaker, or sponsoring legislation). A cover letter providing a brief overview of the group's position and a business card for follow-up should be left for the policymaker.

- *Remain calm.* If the legislator disagrees with the group's position on an issue, advocates should remain calm and polite. Listen to arguments and take notes to help in developing counterarguments.

- *Be patient.* Once information is presented, give the policymaker a few days to review the issue. The bill or policy must be tracked as it moves through the legislative process, since legislators may need to be approached several times to increase support for the issue.

- *Follow up with a letter.* Thank your legislator for meeting with you; ask for a response to your request.

Table 13-9	Developing Effective Testimony

- *Prepare a written statement in advance.* Keep it brief. Usually, each person testifying is allotted two to three minutes. Comments should be practiced ahead of time. Before testifying, a person's name, organization, and position on the bill should be stated.

- *Use sound bites.* Legislators will remember sound bites, and the press will quote them. For example: "The number of tobacco-related deaths each year is equal to two jumbo jets crashing every day for a year."

- *Use personal experiences to enhance testimony.* For instance, personal insight on how drunk driving has affected families or how barriers to health care have diminished a child's health may be helpful. Avoid overly emotional testimony and inflammatory words that might alienate committee members.

- *Listen to prior speakers.* By taking notes, those testifying can avoid repeating previously stated facts. When it is time to speak, offer highlights of your prepared testimony and ask that the full written testimony be placed in record.

- *Observe the members of the committee.* Watch officials' body language and their comments to one another and other speakers. Change testimony if needed, or reinforce a previous point made with additional facts.

- *Do not be disappointed if members of the committee are not attentive.* Frequently members may talk during testimonies, or they may be called out of the session. In this situation, continue presenting the testimony. Those who did not hear it will receive a written copy or can listen to a recorded version.

- *Expect questions or comments.* When answering a question, do not improvise. This is not the time for misinformation. Offer to provide written comments later to avoid misinformation. If a hostile response is received from committee members, stay calm and cool. Stop and think about the appropriate answer before responding.

- *Testifying in opposition to a bill.* If a bill will be opposed, research the facts, consult with other professionals, and provide alternatives to the bill. Stay focused on solving the problem.

Overcoming Challenges in Advocating for Legislation

There are barriers to being an effective advocate; some are easier to overcome than others. Following are strategies for overcoming some of the more common barriers to legislative involvement and action.

Prepare for Opposition

It is important to be prepared for opposition to any issue, because opponents are just as determined as advocates to ensure that their voices are heard. Research the facts and become familiar with the plans of those who may not support the issue. Consider becoming a member of opposing organizations. For example, in the tobacco arena, many tobacco-reduction advocates are on

Table 13-10	Using Media Advocacy to Support a Legislative Advocacy Campaign

- Develop an effective message that identifies the problem, the solution, and who can make the solution possible (i.e., whose support is needed to make the solution happen). The message should be simple and clear; it should state why people should be concerned with the problem in persuasive and compelling terms.
- Identify a local person who has been personally affected by the problem and ask that individual if he or she would be willing to tell the story to the press. Help the person "rehearse" the story, and ask the individual permission to share his or her contact information with the press.
- Create a media list, including local papers and television and radio stations. Identify the audience a station or paper reaches. Create a list of media contacts and find out how reporters like to receive information (fax, email, or phone).
- Select a spokesperson who is comfortable with speaking to the media and answering questions and who is knowledgeable on the issue.
- Write editorials stating the issue and the solution. Meet with newspaper and magazine editors to ask for advice on editorials.
- Write news releases about the issue.
- Involve members of the media in training advocates about effective media communication. This strategy informs advocates how to utilize the media, and it provides an opportunity to educate the media about issues.

smokers' rights mailing lists to gather information. This tactic alerts the group to upcoming legislative initiatives the opposition will be proposing, so that effective strategies for countering their actions can be planned.

Mobilize Community Support

Lack of community interest is a barrier most groups must deal with at one time or another. Even the largest, best-facilitated groups struggle to keep the public aware of their issue. The group, organization, or coalition should continually strive to provide clear, concise information and identify tasks for members and the community constituency to perform. Too often, people are unaware of their elected and appointed officials and are unsure of how to communicate with policymakers. Continue to assess community needs and be certain those needs align with the issues. Provide updates on progress and recognize accomplishments of group members.

Did You Know

Even if a pro-health law is passed, the administrative rules and regulations can often greatly alter the law (and its intent). Health educators must be diligent in following the process through the regulatory stage once a bill is passed and signed.

Prevent Volunteer Burnout

Provide advocates with short, time-specific activities for involvement to combat volunteer burnout. Give them opportunities to improve communication skills for effective letter writing and testimony. People are more likely to get involved if they are educated about the process and have specific tasks to complete. Continue to recruit new members to replace those who are no longer active. Burnout is bound to occur, so look for new ways to encourage members. Celebrate small successes and recognize the hard work of advocates at every opportunity.

Deal with Internal Politics

Organizations may limit the types of activities and amount of resources that can be used for advocacy. If limitations exist, ways to participate in the legislative process other than advocacy or lobbying should be determined. For instance, an organization could write a letter of support to a policymaker. The organization might also identify individuals who support the issue and encourage them to bring the issue to the policymaker's attention. Adequate funding to promote legislative issues is often a major limitation for many organizations and coalitions.

Did You Know

Just five or six letters or telephone calls to a state policymaker can make a difference in how that legislator views an issue. At the federal level, as few as 20 letters can make an impact.

Keep the Bill Moving through the Legislative Process

Bills and policies are often stalled in committee or never brought up for a hearing. Tracking the bill is the best way to monitor the process. Frequently, legislation does not move because of partisan views. If bipartisan sponsors have been identified for a bill, contact both the minority and majority offices to enlist their aid in moving the bill forward. When a bill is stalled, request that the chair of the committee provide information about why the bill has not progressed. It may even be appropriate to request the Speaker of the House or Senate president to refer the bill to another committee for consideration. Bills that have not been referred to another committee may have to be reintroduced to the committee during the next session. It may even be possible to add a bill onto another bill that has already passed the committee. The bill's sponsor should be contacted to determine if this is a viable strategy. If both houses do not pass the bill during the current session, ask the bill's sponsor to refile the bill for hearing in the next session. If a bill has remained stalled, the upcoming election may change the balance of power and the bill can be reintroduced during the next session. Bills that are introduced often get caught up in the re-election cycle. If a bill is introduced late in an election cycle, there may be no follow-up. The best strategy is to plan to introduce legislation early and recognize that it may need to be reintroduced.

It is often difficult to predict the outcome of legislative involvement and action because many internal and external factors can influence the outcome. If the goal has been successfully achieved, there will be more work to do following the celebration. Any new policy should be continuously reviewed and enhanced, because legislation can be overturned or be made less effective by other policies.

If the policy was not adopted, review the original plan to determine areas for improvement. It is important to build on the positives of the effort, especially if community members were mobilized around the issue. Continue to identify additional advocates and build alliances with other groups who may have similar positions. There is strength in numbers.

Most important, do not give up! It can take two or three years to move a bill through committees, house votes, and eventual signing into law. Regardless of the outcome, the process itself provides invaluable experience that will be an asset when taking on the next issue.

Expected Outcomes

By following the suggestions in this chapter, health educators can increase their legislative advocacy skills. More important, they will find they have taken steps to affect public health policy. Just remember, the legislative process moves slowly: Often two or three years may pass before legislation is written, introduced, and passed into law. Be sure to celebrate interim goals. This can serve as inspiration for the additional commitment needed to reach the next level of success. New legislation should be monitored and reviewed to determine its effects. Be aware that any legislation can be overturned or watered down by other policies, making it much more difficult to enact changes in the future.

When the proposed policy is not adopted into law, reevaluate efforts, review the challenges encountered, and look for areas to improve. Use the experience as an opportunity to incorporate "lessons learned" and to identify legislators who will be more supportive in the future, and keep working to build broader community support for the issue. Continue to build on the successes achieved and keep community members mobilized by providing them with additional strategies.

Community connections 6

Erica and her friends told a compelling tale to Erica's senator. Many other groups came forward to express similar concerns, and the senator agreed to sponsor legislation to help address the nursing shortages. This was a complex issue that required several bills to address excessive overtime, salary scales, and funding for university nursing programs.

Conclusion

Advocating for personal and community health is an essential responsibility of health educators.[3,18] The efforts of advocates, health educators, and other health-related professionals have resulted in important legislative changes, such as seat belt and helmet laws and tobacco-control regulations.

Although health educators have not traditionally been trained to take a leadership role in policy development and enactment, they are uniquely qualified to provide input into public health policy. With an understanding of public policy, health educators can use their unique skills to help assess the needs of the community to determine key issues and motivate community members to action. Health educators have a clear understanding of the impact a particular issue has on constituents because they are in daily contact with community members directly affected by regulations or by the lack of legislation that provides protection or access.

The principles presented in this chapter can guide a community through the legislative process. Advocacy groups, facilitated by a knowledgeable health educator, should choose legislative issues important to the community and issues that can be improved by legislative advocacy efforts.

KEY TERMS

bipartisan: Supported by members of both major parties. Such support increases the likelihood that a bill will be posted into committee and passed into law.

blog: An individual's personal journal, usually a daily diary, that is publicly accessible on the Internet.

constituent: Any person who is entitled to vote for a representative of a specific district (a House member's district is a defined portion of a state, while a senator's district is the entire state).

direct lobbying: Support for, or opposition to, certain legislation; the attempt to influence specific legislation.

electioneering: any attempt by a nonprofit or public organization to influence an election by mentioning a candidate running for office (including such words as "vote for," "vote against," "elect," "defeat," "support," or "oppose").

grassroots lobbying: An initiative that reaches out to community members, members of an organization, or the general public and contains a call to action, such as asking people to call or write their legislators to urge them to support or reject specific legislation.

law: A principle governing action or procedure that has been approved by a legislative body, has been published to notify the general public, and is enforced by representatives of the local, state, or federal governments.

legislative advocacy: To speak for those who have no voice or representation. Effective advocacy works to create a shift in public opinion, money, and other resources and to support an issue, policy, or constituency.

legislator: A citizen who is elected to represent the local, state, or federal level and enact laws. Also referred to as a policymaker or official; includes commissioners, township supervisors, and so on.

lobbyist: A person who works to promote the passage of specific legislation by influencing public officials.

policymaker: Anyone who sets policy, such as Rotary committees, college administrators, and PTA members. Every institution makes policy, so every institution has policymakers.

policy initiative: An action, or set of actions, undertaken to change policy or put pressure on an institution to enforce existing policies.

sponsor: A legislator who writes or submits legislation is known as the prime sponsor or author of the legislation. Additional legislators, or cosponsors, may sign on to the bill to indicate their support.

Usenet newsgroups: Internet discussion groups that are topic specific. Followers post messages (articles) for others to read and respond.

REFERENCES

1. U.S. Department of Health and Human Services. (2000). *Healthy People 2010*. Washington, DC: Author.

2. Code of Ethics for the Health Education Profession. (2000). *Journal of Health Education, 31*, 216–218.

3. Tappe, M. K., & Galer-Unti, R. (2001). Health educator's role in promoting health literacy and advocacy for the 21st century. *Journal of School Health, 71*, 477–482.

4. National Commission for Health Education Credentialing. (1986). *A competency-based framework for the professional development of certified health education specialist*. Allentown, PA: Author.

5. Auld, M. E., & Dixon-Terry, E. (1999). The role of health education associations in advocacy. *Health Education Monograph Series, 17*, 10–14.

6. Allegrante, J. P., Moon, R., Auld, M. E., & Gebbie, K. (in press). Future training needs of the public health education workforce. *Health Promotion Practice*.

7. Galer-Unti, R. A, Tappe, M. K, and Lachenmayr, S. (2004). Advocacy 101: Getting started in health education advocacy. *Health Promotion Practice, 5*, 280–288.

8. Vernick, J. S. (1999). Lobbying and advocacy for the public's health: What are the limits for nonprofit organizations? *American Journal of Public Health, 89*, 1425–1429.

9. Centers for Disease Control and Prevention, Chronic Disease Prevention Programs and Campaigns. (2007). Available: http://www.cdc.gov/nccdphp/.

10. Research!America. (2007). Available: http://www.researchamerica.org/.

11. The Marin Institute for Prevention of Alcohol and Other Drug Problems. (1994). *Advocating for policy change.* San Rafael, CA: Author.

12. Michigan Department of Public Health. (1994). *Preparing your policy campaigns.* Lansing, MI: Author.

13. Michigan State Legislative Council. (1995). *A citizen's guide to state government.* Lansing, MI: Allied Printing.

14. Americans for Nonsmokers' Rights. (1994). *Tips for testifying.* Berkeley, CA: Author.

15. Americans for Nonsmokers' Rights. (1994). *Meeting with elected officials.* Berkeley, CA: Author.

16. ASSIST. (1993). *ASSIST training materials: Vol. VI. Media advocacy: A strategic tool for change.* Rockville, MD: ASSIST Coordinating Center.

17. American Public Health Association. (2000). *2000 APHA media advocacy manual.* Washington, DC: Author.

18. Wooley, S. J., Balin, S., & Reynolds, S. (1999). Partners for advocacy: Non-profit organizations and lobbyists. *Health Education Monograph Series, 17,* 45–48.

ADDITIONAL RESOURCES

Print

Altman, D. (1994). *Public health advocacy: Creating community change to improve health.* Palo Alto, CA: Stanford University Press.

American Public Health Association. (2000). *APHA advocates handbook: A guide for effective public health advocacy.* Washington, DC: Author.

Christoffel, K. K. (2000). Public health advocacy: Process and product. *American Journal of Public Health, 5,* 722.

Goodhart, F. W. (1999). Approaches to advocacy for health educators. *The Health Education Monograph Series, 2,* 26–28.

Kolbe, L. J., & Iverson, D. C. (1981). Implementing comprehensive school health education: Educational innovations and social change. *Health Education Quarterly, 8,* 57–80.

Smith, C. (2005). *Writing public policy: A practical guide to communicating the policy-making process.* New York: Oxford University Press.

Steckler, A., & Dawson, L. (1982). The role of health education in public policy development. *Health Education Quarterly, 9,* 275–292.

Steckler, A., Dawson, L., Goodman, R. M., & Epstein, N. (1987). Policy advocacy: Three emerging roles for health education. *Advances in Health Education and Promotion, 2,* 5–27.

Stone, D. (2002). *Policy paradox: The art of political decision making.* New York: W.W. Norton.

Wallack, L., Dorfman, L., Jernigan, D., & Themba, M. (1993). *Media advocacy and public health: Power for prevention.* Newbury Park, CA: Sage Publications.

Internet

American Public Health Association. *Tips for effective advocacy.* Available: http://www.apha.org/legislative/Writingtips.htm.

CDC community guide. Available: http://www.thecommunityguide.org/home_f.html.

Coalition of National Health Education Organizations. *Health education advocate.* Available: http://healtheducationadvocate.org.

Healthy People 2010. Available: http://www.health.gov/healthypeople.

National Conference of State Legislatures. Available: http://www.ncsl.org. Site to identify state legislators.

Research!America. Available: http://researchamerica.org.

THOMAS: Legislative information on the Internet. Available: http://thomas.loc.gov. Site for current federal bills.

U.S. Census Bureau. Available: http://www.census.gov.

U.S. House of Representatives. Available: http://www.house.gov/.

U.S. Senate. Available: http://www.senate.gov/.

The White House. Available: http://www.whitehouse.gov.

14

Using Media Advocacy to Influence Policy

Lori Dorfman, Dr.P.H.

Author Comments

Media advocacy is exciting because it is one of the few public heath education tools we have that allows us to work "upstream," on the overarching issues that perpetuate public health problems and unhealthy environments. Media advocacy, used as a tool to accelerate and amplify community organizing and policy advocacy, can direct public and policymaker attention to the policies that can reshape our social and physical environments so that people can make healthier choices.

We can learn a great deal from the successful development of media advocacy in the field of tobacco control. Since the first Surgeon General's report linking tobacco with cancer and heart disease, we have seen an incredible shift in attitude about smoking in public. Much of this is due to information on the toxicity of secondhand smoke, the health effects associated with smoking, and the emergence of the non-smokers' rights movement. News coverage of public debates about tobacco has contributed to the number of smoke-free worksites, restaurants, and public places by influencing institutional policy changes, local ordinances, and state and federal laws. As a result, we have seen a decrease in adult tobacco use in communities and states (e.g., California and Utah) that have policies restricting public smoking. Media advocacy has helped public health advocates enact policies on issues as varied as alcohol, firearms, nutrition, childhood lead poisoning, children's oral health, injury control, and other public health issues.

This chapter will help you think strategically about working with the news media. This means switching from thinking about using mass media solely as a tool for getting information to health consumers to thinking about the news media as a mechanism for informing citizens and pressuring decision makers. By learning the skills presented in this chapter and acting on them, you will help yourself and others focus on mass media in its most powerful form.

Introduction

The history of public health is clear: Social conditions and the physical environment are important determinants of health. The primary tool available to public health for influencing social conditions and environments is policy. Policies define the structures and set the rules by which we live. If public health practitioners are going to improve social conditions and physical environments in lasting and meaningful ways, they must be involved in policy development and policy advocacy. Furthermore, being successful in policy advocacy means paying attention to the news.

The reach of the news media is intoxicating. In society, the news media largely determine what issues we collectively think about, how we think about them, and what kinds of alternatives are considered viable, which, in turn, influences key policy decisions pertaining to health. The public and policymakers do not consider issues unless they are visible, and they are not visible unless the news has brought them to light. Naturally, public health educators want to take advantage of the vast audience the news media reach.

Nonprofit organizations and community activists often are unhappy with the way their issues are presented in the news, and typically respond by criticizing the media, ignoring it, or even becoming hostile. These responses are nonproductive because they cede power over the public portrayal of their issues to journalists and widen the gulf between journalists and advocates. Media advocacy addresses this problem. It is an approach to health communication that differs significantly from traditional mass communication approaches. Media advocacy helps people understand the importance and reach of news coverage, the need to participate actively in shaping such coverage, and the methods to do so effectively.

News portrayals of health issues are significant for how they influence policymakers and the public regarding who has responsibility for health. If public health–oriented solutions are to be given full consideration, then advocates talking to journalists, and journalists themselves, must understand how to frame issues from the perspective of shared accountability so news coverage is not focused exclusively on individual responsibility. This shared accountability recognizes that health and social problems will only be adequately addressed when all sectors of society—not just the individual—share responsibility for solutions. Media advocacy emphasizes social accountability, which typically receives less attention from the news than individually oriented solutions.

Public health practitioners tend to overlook the power of the news media to influence change. Journalists themselves, even when committed to covering social problems, often produce stories that emphasize individual behavior and treatment rather than social factors and prevention. Despite the media's enormous reach and potential as a tool for change, public health professionals rarely use mass media to its full advantage. Rather, they tend to use it in its least effective capacity: to convey personal health information to consumers.[1] By contrast, media advocacy harnesses the power of the news to mobilize advocates and apply pressure for policy change.

Steps for Developing Effective Media Advocacy Campaigns

Before public health advocates can harness the power of the news, they have to be clear and precise about why they want to use media advocacy. Four layers of strategy organize the approach to communications campaigns. The first is the *overall strategy*—the ultimate goal of the campaign. Next is the *media strategy*—chosen based on appropriateness for the overall strategy. This chapter focuses on one media strategy: *media advocacy*. Other chapters in this text offer communication tools that suit different goals. Once they have selected a media strategy, advocates need to determine the specifics of what they want to say, who will say it, and to whom. That is the *message strategy*. Finally, once the other layers of strategy are in place, advocates can figure out how to attract news attention—the *access strategy*. Unfortunately, many groups begin by trying to attract journalists' attention without figuring out first why they want that attention, and what they will say after they have it. This chapter is designed to prepare readers so they know when to call on journalists and are confident about what to say once they have their attention.

Develop an Overall Strategy

The most important part of a media strategy does not concern media at all. Rather, it is the clarification, articulation, justification, and operationalization of the desired change. The media advocacy *prime directive* is that "You cannot have a media strategy without an overall strategy." Advocates should begin by asking themselves, "What changes will improve the public's health?" It makes sense for advocates to develop a media strategy only after they know what needs to be accomplished overall and how it will be done. In practical terms, this usually means determining the policy that needs to be enacted, changed, or enforced. The following four questions can help guide the development of an overall strategy:

1. What is the problem or issue?

2. What is a solution or policy—the desired outcome?

3. Who has the power to make the necessary change?

4. Who must be mobilized to apply the necessary pressure?

The following subsections examine each question in detail.

What Is the Problem or Issue?

Defining the problem is often not as simple as it seems. It is a process rife with social and political tension because different stakeholders will offer competing definitions of the problem. This process is exceptionally important because the ultimate definition of the problem will fundamentally determine the solution. For example, recent increases in the incidence of type 2 diabetes among children might be explained by various factors related to nutrition and physical activity, such as too much time watching TV or playing video games; the $10.5 billion spent annually on sophisticated food marketing targeting children; eating encouraged in places it never was before, such as cars and bookstores; soda and fast food available in schools; a decline in physical education; urban "food deserts" where it's easy to find hamburgers but hard to find fruits and vegetables; and social conditions that have sped up contemporary life, putting a premium on time and creating a huge demand for fast foods that are high in salts and sugars. News attention to one or the other of these factors helps determine the saliency of various policies and, ultimately, which will prevail.

Articulating the problem is important because it will need to be conveyed concisely to a reporter. Public health is often very problem oriented. This means those from health departments or social service agencies can endlessly discuss the problem. Indeed, health officials often feel they have a moral and professional obligation to tell journalists everything they know any time they are asked about the problem because they know their issue is of such vital importance. The realities of news today, however, demand that health professionals identify only the most critical aspect of the problem and be able to describe it well in just a sentence or two.

Did You Know

Media advocacy has been applied to issues as varied as affirmative action, alcohol, childhood lead poisoning, disability rights, early childhood development and child care, exercise and nutrition, injury control, gun violence, juvenile justice, public housing, sexual assault, suicide, and, of course, tobacco.

Advocates must isolate the piece of the large public health problem that will be addressed specifically. For example, alcohol is related to more than 105,000 deaths a year in this country and is the number one drug choice for young people. One way advocates can narrow the problem is by focusing on how alcohol creates problems on college campuses, particularly when it is consumed in large quantities over a short period of time. The problem of binge drinking on college campuses might be narrowed further and defined in terms of price specials at bars nearby that encourage those who are drinking to get drunk. Cheap alcohol is certainly not the only factor leading to alcohol problems on campus, but it is probably an important one. It is also a problem that can be remedied by a clear policy solution that would affect the overall alcohol environment. Rather than

Community connections 1

Violence against women is a pervasive problem in the United States. While there are not enough programs to assist women trying to leave battering relationships, there are even fewer programs working to prevent the violence in the first place. Advocates seeking to change the environment that fosters violence against women have few options.

In 1990, the Trauma Foundation, the Los Angeles Commission on Assaults Against Women, the Center for Women's Studies and Services, and the Institute for Health Advocacy began the Dangerous Promises campaign, an effort to address the role of alcohol advertising in violence against women. The Dangerous Promises coalition sought mechanisms to remedy the social and cultural factors at the root of violence against women. Alcohol, they knew, was a risk factor for violence against women. Though it does not cause the violence, they maintained, its use and expectations about it "contribute to myths about sexuality, power, and control which in turn can reinforce a climate of violence against women." After much debate, the Dangerous Promises coalition defined the problem as alcohol advertising that contributed to sexist notions of men's power over women and reinforced or trivialized violence against women. They then developed a strategy to eliminate such advertising.

educating reporters about the extensive range of alcohol problems, public health advocates would be more effective by narrowing the focus of their discussion with reporters to the details relevant to a specific policy goal.

What Is a Solution or Policy—The Desired Outcome?

Sometimes advocates are so concerned about focusing attention on the problem they give inadequate attention to the solution. Or, they may not have identified a clear solution. Public health advocates need to identify a solution or policy—not necessarily one that will solve the entire problem, but something that can make a difference. Typical inadequate responses tend to be statements such as "This is a very complex problem with multifaceted solutions," "There is no magic bullet," "Children are our future and we must do something," or "The community needs to come together." Unfortunately, none of these responses provides any concrete direction. Public health advocates need to be clear about what they want to happen: Is a new law necessary? Is more enforcement required? Does the budget need to be changed? Does someone need to take responsibility to do something to protect the community's health? Who? What should they do? When should they do it?

In the example of problems related to alcohol on campus, one solution is to eliminate happy hour price specials that encourage quick consumption of large quantities of alcohol. Advocates may be working on only one salient part of the problem or one policy solution at a time, or more, depending on what resources are available.

Community connections 2

The goal of the Dangerous Promises campaign was to convince alcohol companies to eliminate sexist advertising and promotions. But the alcohol industry is large and powerful. The advocates needed to focus their limited resources and narrow their target strategically.

The brewers, vintners, and purveyors of distilled spirits have corresponding trade associations that maintain codes of advertising ethics for their members. While the associations and adherence to their respective codes are voluntary, they provide a mechanism for holding the alcohol industry accountable for its advertising practices. The codes describe limits on marketing to children, for example. The Dangerous Promises campaign wanted the advertising codes to be amended to include language stating that alcohol advertising and promotion shall not reinforce or trivialize the problem of violence against women; degrade, demean, or objectivize the form, image, or status of women or any ethnic or minority group; associate alcohol with adversarial, abusive, or violent relationships or situations; or suggest sex as an expected result of or reward for drinking alcohol. In November 1992, the Dangerous Promises campaign wrote to each association, the Wine Institute, the Distilled Spirits Council of the U.S. (DISCUS), and the Beer Institute, explaining the connection between alcohol advertising and violence against women, providing examples of pertinent alcohol ads, and asking them to adopt the code amendments.

In a surprising move, the Wine Institute agreed to adopt the codes. The Beer Institute and DISCUS were not so receptive. The Dangerous Promises coalition decided to launch a media advocacy campaign to put public pressure on DISCUS and the Beer Institute to adopt the codes.

Who Has the Power to Make the Necessary Change?

The next step is figuring out what person, group, organization, or body has the power to make the desired change. This question identifies the **focus audience**, but reflects a fundamental change in what that term means. In this context, there is a difference between traditional use of mass media in public health as a vehicle for public information campaigns to change personal behavior, and integrating media as an advocacy tool to change policy. In the former, the person with power to make the change is the one with the problem—for example, the person who drinks too much, smokes, does not exercise, or has a poor diet. When using media advocacy to change, implement, or enforce policy, the target is different because the power may reside with a legislator, other elected official, regulatory agency, small business owner, or corporate officer. In addition, the locus of power—or focus audience—is likely to change over time. For example, changing a regulation may require focusing on different targets depending on the stage of development of the issue.

The primary target for a media advocacy campaign to reduce alcohol problems on and around campus would not be the students who are drinking. Instead, it would be the alcohol vendors and those who regulate them. Eliminating happy hours, to use the policy example mentioned previously, is not in the power of the students. Once happy hours are gone, there will be a beneficial effect regardless of the knowledge and attitude of student drinkers—one avenue for the dangerous behavior would be closed. News coverage generated by media advocacy activities can describe the problem and articulate the demands for solutions so the city government and campus community can more easily move ahead. Advocates must articulate for reporters the reason for the policy and what it will accomplish. Thus, the public learns about the problems alcohol causes on campus via the news, which is perceived as a highly legitimate and credible source.

Who Must Be Mobilized to Apply the Necessary Pressure?

Public health–oriented policies are often hotly contested. Fluoridation of drinking water, distribution of condoms, mandating bicycle or motorcycle helmets, or limiting the availability of junk food, alcohol, handguns, or tobacco brings out intense opposition to public health goals. Many legislators and other policymakers are unlikely to support a controversial change unless constituency groups put pressure on them. The pressure can consist of telephone calls, letters, demonstrations, media coverage, and office visits. The role of news coverage here is twofold. First, media coverage of the issue will let the policymaker know that his or her vote or position is being watched and will be part of the public debate. Second, media coverage can help mobilize constituency groups to contact the policymaker or get involved in other ways, thus applying pressure.

Mobilizing supportive groups is important because public health policy efforts can often be prolonged struggles. The media can only provide periodic coverage, placing the spotlight on the issue at key times. Constituency groups need to apply pressure on a continuing basis. For example, students and local merchants around campus can put pressure on bar owners directly to change their policies about pricing alcohol. They can also put pressure on campus administration, city government, and alcoholic beverage regulating agencies to take actions that will reduce the problems related to alcohol use. They can strengthen and amplify those efforts by garnering news coverage at key moments, such as prior to a policy decision.

Paying attention to these four questions is a good start to creating an overall strategy. Once advocates have defined the problem, selected and developed a realistic and achievable policy objective, conducted an analysis to identify the locus for change, and identified and mobilized groups to apply pressure, then they can determine the media, message, and access strategies.

Develop a Media Strategy

Traditional forms of mass media interventions emphasize the "information gap" or "motivation gap," which suggests health problems are caused by individuals with the problem or at risk for the problem who lack either information or sufficient desire to behave in a more healthful manner. Health educators then attempt to provide information to fill that gap. When people have the information and "know the facts," it is assumed they will adopt a positive attitude toward the health behavior and then act accordingly, and the problem will be solved. The role of the media, in this case, is to deliver the solution (knowledge) to the millions of individuals who need it. Media advocacy, on the other hand, focuses on the "power gap," viewing health problems as arising from a lack of power to create change in social and physical environments.

Media advocacy can be defined as the strategic use of mass media to advance public policy by applying pressure to policymakers.[2] The use of media advocacy has evolved as the definition of health problems has shifted from the individual level to the policy level. What distinguishes media advocacy from traditional health promotion and educational efforts is the goal of the effort (see Figure 14-1).[3]

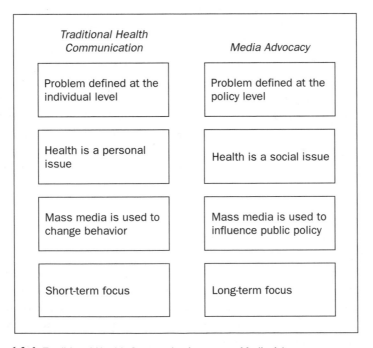

Figure 14-1 Traditional Health Communication versus Media Advocacy

Media advocacy differs in many ways from traditional public health campaigns. It is most marked by an emphasis on

- Linking public health and social problems to inequities in social arrangements rather than to flaws in the individual
- Changing public policy rather than personal health behavior
- Focusing primarily on reaching opinion leaders and policymakers rather than on those who have the problem (the traditional audience of public health communication campaigns)
- Working with groups to increase participation and amplify their voices rather than providing health behavior change messages
- Having a primary goal of reducing the power gap rather than just filling the information gap[1]

In practice, media advocacy uses some of the same media relations techniques that practitioners of social marketing or public information campaigns might use: sending out news releases, pitching stories to journalists, monitoring the media and keeping a list of media contacts, and paying attention to what is newsworthy. But these practices alone are not media advocacy, though they are frequently used by media advocates and may be the most visible part of a media advocate's process. Because media advocacy's target is the power gap, it attempts to motivate social and political involvement rather than changes in personal health behavior.[3] It is the best media strategy choice when the overall strategy involves changing policy.

Develop a Message Strategy

The message is what is said to the target. The overall strategy determines the focus audience: a single person or a small group, perhaps the CEO of a company, or a legislative committee. The message is delivered to the target by selected messengers through the news media. Other mechanisms for delivering the message are used at the same time because media advocacy is used in combination with community organizing and policy advocacy. Media advocacy adds power and amplification to those strategies by harnessing the news media's reach. It is a mechanism for thrusting the discussion with the target into the public conversation.

Framing: What It Is, Why It Matters

Because media advocacy messages are transmitted through the news media, it is useful to examine how the news media typically represent issues. This process is called **framing**. Framing, in general, is about how people interpret and integrate information they receive from the outside world with the understanding they already possess about the topic. People are only able to interpret words, images, actions, or text of any kind because their brains fit those texts into an existing conceptual system that gives them order and meaning. Just a few cues—a word, an image—trigger whole frames that determine meaning.[4] The information might come from pictures, words, sounds, or actions people witness. People's brains organize the information so they can make sense of the world around them. Various disciplines, from cognitive linguistics to social psychology, describe framing slightly differently, but all the explanations concern how people extract and absorb meaning from experience and information. Frames help people integrate new information into their existing understanding of how the world works, which helps them determine what is important and how to act.

The default frame.   Social psychologists have shown that a pervasive frame people use to understand the world emphasizes personal motivations, not the situations influencing personal decisions. Over the years, hundreds of experiments have demonstrated that people tend to "see the actors and miss the stage." When explaining others' behavior, people in the United States tend to emphasize personal attributes such as skill, desire, or work ethic; their explanations tend to ignore the influence of the situation surrounding the person. Much like a spotlight illuminates an actor onstage but leaves the rest of the set in shadows, this tendency to focus on people's motivations renders the surrounding elements almost invisible, reinforcing the idea of personal responsibility and minimizing the role of larger structural forces. This default frame—that people's behavior is determined by personal motivation, not by the situations in which they find themselves—makes advocating for health policy challenging, since many policies are designed to change the conditions or situations surrounding individuals.

The default frame taken to its logical conclusion gives us "rugged individualism," a popular cultural ideal in the United States. The frame reinforces the value of personal responsibility for overcoming harsh odds, as in the Horatio Alger "pull yourself up by your bootstraps" myth. It is one of the most common stories Americans tell about themselves. Former Labor Secretary Robert Reich calls it the story of the "triumphant individual." The personal responsibility frame includes the idea that you can accomplish anything you put your mind to. But, at the same time, the frame includes the reverse idea: that if you do not succeed, it is your own fault. Both of these ideas come together in the default frame. If you evoke rugged individualism you also evoke personal responsibility and self-sufficiency. The default frame gets reproduced in many exchanges of information, including through the media. Journalists are subject to the default frame as much as any other group in society. In fact, because they are high media consumers, journalists may have even greater exposure to the default frame.

The special case of news frames.   News frames are one particular type of framing that have evolved from the routine practices of journalism. Any message that media advocates have will be filtered through the news frame. News is organized, or framed, to make sense of infinitely sided and shaded issues. Framing is the process of identifying how the issue will be depicted; it is "the package in which the main point of the story is developed, supported, and understood."[5] Inevitably, some elements of a story are left out while others are included. Similarly, some arguments, metaphors, or story lines may be featured prominently, while others are relegated to the margins of the story. News frames are important because the facts, values, or images included in news coverage are accorded legitimacy, while those not emphasized or excluded are marginalized or left out of public discussion. The coverage will significantly contribute to how the issue is "felt" and talked about by the public.

Traditions and routines exist in journalism that result in consistent frames, almost like story lines or scripts that reporters gravitate toward, such as heroes and villains, overcoming adversity, and the unexpected or ironic twist of the protector causing harm. Stories have characters, characters have roles, and characters carry out their actions on location in recognizable circumstances within a range of predictable outcomes. Television, in particular, with its two-minute storytelling, uses compact symbols to tell a familiar story. By studying the patterns of news storytelling, advocates can determine the implications for public health.

Portraits versus Landscapes: Typical News Frames and the Challenge for Framing Public Health Issues

Most news, especially television news, tries to "put a face on the issue." The impact of an issue on an individual's life is often of more interest to news reporters than the policy implications of an issue, in part because they believe readers and viewers are more likely to identify emotionally with a person's plight. News stories tend to focus on specific, concrete events, using good pictures to tell a short, simple story. Unfortunately, research on television's effects has shown that when viewers see individually focused, event-oriented stories and then are asked what should be done about the problem depicted, the viewers will respond in ways that tend to blame the victim.[5] Stories about isolated episodes do not help audiences understand how to deliberate and solve social problems beyond demanding that individuals take more responsibility for themselves. "Following exposure to episodic framing," notes researcher Shanto Iyengar, "Americans describe chronic problems such as poverty and crime not in terms of deep-seated social or economic conditions, but as mere idiosyncratic outcomes."[5] Alternatively, when stories are more issue-oriented, audiences respond differently—they include government and social institutions as part of the solution. That is usually the type of response sought by public health advocates.

A simple way to distinguish between the two story types is to think of the difference between a portrait and a landscape. In a news story framed as a portrait, one may learn a great deal about an individual or an event, with great drama and detail. But it is hard to see what surrounds that individual or what brought him or her to that moment in time. A landscape pulls back the lens to take a broader view. It may include people and events, but must connect them to the larger social and economic forces. The challenge for media advocates is to make stories about the public health landscape as compelling and interesting as the portrait.

To focus attention on the landscape, media advocates try to frame the *content* of a news story, or the message in that story. **Framing for content** shifts the individual problem to a social issue. For example, attention to problems related to childhood nutrition has prompted calls for parents to make good nutrition choices for their children. But parents don't choose what is stocked in grocery stores. Parents don't control pricing strategies that make 20 ounces of soda cheaper than 20 ounces of milk. Parents don't decide whether a grocery store will be located in their neighborhood. Parents don't blazon cartoon characters on sugary cereals and salty snacks. Personal responsibility matters, but so does the environment in which those decisions are made, and it is the involved industries and the policymakers who support them who largely determine the nature of that environment. Framing for content makes the industry's role in causing the problem better understood, and then advocates can articulate why it is reasonable to assign responsibility for changing practices to the industry.

Did You Know

Television news stories that focus on individuals or events alone may do more harm than good. Experiments have demonstrated that people use explanations of personal responsibility as their default. That is, in the absence of an explanation that explicitly involves forces outside the individual, audiences will blame the victim. News stories that focus on the plight of individuals without bringing in the larger social or environmental context distance viewers from the problem. From a public health perspective, a news story framed this way may be worse than no news story at all.

Components of a Message

The message is what is to be said to the target audience—those who have the power to make the change being sought. But the message is going to be delivered in the context of a news story, so it must conform to the needs of journalists for clear, concise statements. Therefore, it is important to keep it simple.

To improve reporting from a public health perspective, advocates will need to be well versed in social factors and other contextual variables related to their issue so they can inform journalists of those links. They should be able to fill in the blanks in the following statement. Similarly, advocates should understand how typical news stories might connect to particular health issues and be able to complete the reverse of the same statement.

Every time there is a story on _____, *it should include information about* _____.

For example, asthma rates began rising in the late 1980s, and studies began to define risk factors such as outdoor pollutants and secondhand smoke.[6] Advocates working to prevent asthma need to determine whether news stories reflected this understanding. If they do not, advocates will know how to focus their discussions with journalists. Given what is now known from epidemiologists, it is reasonable to expect that whenever there is a story on children's health, it mentions rising asthma rates. Similarly, whenever there is a story on asthma, it should mention children's rates going up, prevention measures for parents, potential environmental policy protections, and the health department as a community resource. It would also be appropriate to include an angle on asthma in stories on environmental tobacco smoke or air quality. Think of it this way:

Every time there is a story on <u>asthma</u>, it should include information about <u>secondhand smoke</u>.

Every time there is a story on <u>secondhand smoke</u>, it should include information about <u>asthma</u>.

Advocates can use the same formula to think through other public health issues, their risk factors, and important aspects of prevention that should be included regularly in news stories. So, for example, if advocates' policy goal is focused on reducing air pollution from idling diesel trucks, as was the case for asthma prevention programs in Long Beach, California, they might think of the message in news stories this way:

Every time there is a story on <u>asthma</u>, it should include information about <u>diesel trucks and air pollution</u>.

Every time there is a story on <u>diesel trucks or air pollution</u>, it should include information about <u>asthma</u>.

Advocates can collect the materials that clearly and simply make their point to have on hand to send to reporters on short notice when an article on the topic appears. They will need to have data and examples at the ready to explain why the reporters should include this information in their story.

The message an advocate delivers is often in the context of an answer to a journalist's question. Journalists will usually ask at least two questions: "What is the problem?" and "What is the solution?"[7] It is common for public health professionals and their community allies to spend about 80% of their time talking about the problem and 20% talking about the solution. Strategically, it is important to reverse the ratio. Advocates should identify the problem briefly, but emphasize more what needs to be done to solve it.

A practical rule of thumb is that a good message uses concise, direct language to convey at least three elements.[8] One component is the clear statement of concern—for example, the fact that there are too many alcohol-related problems on campus. The second component represents the value dimension, such as the threat to healthy student life and a nurturing learning environment. The third component elucidates the policy objective, for example, the elimination of happy hours in bars near campuses. The components need not always fall in that order, but they are usually all present.

For example, when the latest study was released on drinking on college campuses, reporters sought comments from those who were directly concerned or affected by the problem. At the University of Iowa, a coalition had formed to try to reduce alcohol problems on and around campus. The coalition had several specific policy goals as its prime directive and had been trained in media advocacy. When the time came to respond to the study, Mary Sue Coleman, then president of the university, told reporters, "Of course, students who drink too much must be responsible for the problems that they cause. But students are not responsible for manufacturing and marketing alcoholic beverages. Students are not responsible for the excessive number of bars within walking distance of our campuses. Students are not responsible for the price specials that encourage drinking to get drunk."[9] In that statement, Dr. Coleman was able to acknowledge the personal responsibility of students but also paint a picture of the landscape surrounding those students that helps illustrate why the policies she seeks are both necessary and reasonable. She cannot say everything in one small media bite, but her example goes a long way to define the problem, illustrate the landscape surrounding the problem, and effectively point to the solution.

Media advocates can develop all the story elements reporters need to tell the public health side of the story. Media bites, like Dr. Coleman's, are essential. In addition, media advocates can prepare compelling visuals to help illustrate their point of view, calculate "social math" so large numbers can be made meaningful, identify "authentic voices"—those advocates who can effectively "put a face on the issue," as reporters might put it—and identify and use evocative symbols in their descriptions of the problem and solution (see Tips and Techniques for Successful Media Advocacy). Having ready story elements that portray the public health frame will make it easier for journalists to cover the story.

Develop an Access Strategy

After advocates have determined an overall strategy, selected a media strategy, and crafted the message, then they are ready to attract journalists' attention. At this point, they must think of what parts of the issue will make a good story. By emphasizing those elements, advocates will be **framing** the issue **for access**.

Journalists are not likely to think of the public health aspects of the stories they write, but they are always eager for a new and interesting angle. Public health practitioners can offer ideas to journalists by suggesting stories directly on the topic on which they work, and by thinking about how the public health angle fits into the news of the day.

Monitoring the News and Building Relationships with Journalists

In order to work well with journalists, advocates need to understand how they define and report news. Advocates can do this by carefully watching television news, reading newspapers, and listening to the radio. Advocates should regularly scan all sections of the local newspaper for articles that directly or indirectly relate to the advocacy issue. For instance, the sports page may cover a rodeo that is tobacco sponsored. This may provide an opportunity for a group working on a policy to ban tobacco-sponsored sporting events. Members of the group could respond to the article with a letter to the editor or an invitation to the reporter who covered the event to learn more about sponsorship. Copies of the article can be sent to other community activists and appropriate legislators.

Monitoring means listing and paying attention to the local and relevant national media outlets. For each of the outlets, advocates will have to determine how often they cover the issues that are of concern. To monitor means that they will notice what the coverage says about the issue. Does it tell the whole story? Advocates need not do a detailed study of the media, but they need enough information to inform the media advocacy efforts. To do this, they should read and watch the news critically from a public health perspective. When reading the newspaper, they can ask themselves: Does the article include everything it should given the topic it covers? Are there important aspects missing? Is there a public health aspect to this story that should have been included? These questions can

Community connections 3

The Dangerous Promises campaign got news attention in San Diego, Los Angeles, and the San Francisco Bay area, all major California media markets. In each city, the coalition members were careful to focus consistently on a concise message to communicate that (1) sexism is a root cause of violence against women, (2) sexist alcohol ads reinforce myths that contribute to violence against women, and (3) alcohol companies should stop making dangerous promises to promote their products. Advocates provided the visual images reporters needed to tell the story, including pictures of alcohol ads that made their point, and used social math and localized data to illustrate their case. As a result, most of the coverage reflected the Dangerous Promises message and reiterated the policy goal.

After the news coverage put alcohol advertising's connection to violence against women on the public agenda and increased the credibility of the Dangerous Promises coalitions and the legitimacy of their demands, the coalitions got a better response from the lagging industry associations. In a meeting with coalition members, the Beer Institute agreed to reexamine the proposed code. In 1995, DISCUS adopted two of the three points in the proposed code and a modified version of the third.

help advocates evaluate the comprehensiveness of a news story and determine the specifics to bring to the attention of the journalist, who may do similar stories in the future.

By carefully paying attention to news stories about an issue, advocates can identify which journalists are most interested in a specific topic, and what aspect of the topic interests them the most. Advocates will also start to see how different symbols and journalistic conventions are used to tell the story. This is the foundation from which they can approach journalists about the aspects of the story that are not receiving attention.[8]

Advocates will have greater success attracting journalists to the story if they have built a relationship with them. The first step is to compile a list of local media contacts. Each entry on the list should include (1) the name of the reporter; (2) telephone and fax numbers; (3) email and mailing addresses; (4) the name of the newspaper, magazine, or television or radio station; (5) the best time to be reached; (6) sections, or *beats*, in which the reporter writes or reports (e.g., sports, columnist, lifestyle, health); and (7) any notes pertaining to interactions to date. Advocates should meet with the reporters who may have an interest in their issue, or those whose beats intersect with the issue. The advocate should introduce herself or himself, explain why she or he has an interest in meeting, and get to know them. Advocates need to update the media list regularly because there is a high rate of turnover in the news business. It is therefore important to keep track of contacts as they move on to other news outlets. A relationship at a local television station today may be a relationship at a national news program tomorrow.

Newsworthiness

Framing the issue for access involves making the issue newsworthy. The following questions can help determine newsworthiness:[3]

- Is the issue controversial (e.g., freedom of choice versus restricting the sale of sweetened beverages in schools)?

- Is there a milestone event (e.g., the Institute of Medicine's report on childhood obesity)?

- Is there an anniversary (e.g., the date the first school district in the country banned the sale of sodas in schools)?

- Can irony or outrage be used (e.g., schools "pushing" soda on students in the face of a rising obesity rate)?

- Can a local issue be connected with a larger, national event (e.g., local school district efforts to improve nutrition in schools tied to state or federal policy campaigns)?

Identifying newsworthy components can help turn an issue into a story. Stories have action, plot, and characters. What are they in relation to the topic of interest? Why is it a story *now*? Why does it matter to the people who read that newspaper or watch that television station?

General Strategies

There are four general strategies for getting in the news: creating news, piggybacking on breaking news, paying for advertisements, and editorial strategies. Each is detailed in this section.

Creating news.   Tobacco control advocate Russell Sciandra said, "To gain the media's attention, you can't just say something; you have to do something."[8] That "something" need not be elaborate, but it must be newsworthy. Creating news can be as simple as releasing new data or announcing a specific demand. The important part is that it be done publicly, that someone alerts the news media, emphasizing why the story is newsworthy. For example, if advocates know that an important document will be released, they could plan a briefing for journalists so they will be prepared, or issue a statement with the group's reaction to it.

Piggybacking on breaking news.   When advocates identify a connection between an issue and news of the day, they should make the story known to journalists. Tobacco control advocates used the occasion of President Clinton's perjury hearings to highlight the fact that tobacco company executives had lied under oath to Congress. Family planning advocates used news hype about Viagra to point out that health insurance plans were not covering contraceptives for women, though they covered Viagra. Piggybacking on breaking news can be achieved in a letter to the editor, with a news conference, or by other actions.

Paid advertising. Buying space is sometimes the only way to be sure a message gets out unadulterated. In San Francisco, children's advocates used paid advertising to highlight a positive policy change that the news media were ignoring. The job market was tight in San Francisco in 2000, and that meant a crisis for child care. Childcare workers, typically paid less than $7 an hour—less than parking attendants—were leaving the field for more lucrative jobs. Families that qualified for subsidized care could not get it because the childcare centers did not have the staff. Working with Coleman Advocates for Children and Youth, among others, Mayor Willie Brown took an unprecedented action: He allocated $4.1 million to increase the wages of 1,000 childcare workers serving low-income families. Never before had the city subsidized the salaries of noncity employees. The advocates were thrilled and immediately alerted the local news media. The reporters, however, refused to cover the story. They did not want to "toot the mayor's horn."

The advocates thought it was a legitimate story and were frustrated by the nonresponsive reporters. They decided to tell the story themselves in a full-page ad in the west coast edition of the *New York Times*. The ad ran on August 7, 2000, during the Democratic national convention, which was being held in San Diego that year. The ad proclaimed: "Childcare History in the Making—San Francisco Mayor Willie Brown Sets National Standard for Quality, Affordable Childcare!"[10] It suggested that readers challenge their own mayors to take the same action in their home towns. Mayor Willie Brown was still talking about the ad six months later when he signed the next budget allocations for child care.

Editorial strategies. Letters to the editor, editorials, and "op-eds" (opinion editorials, or opinion pieces found opposite the editorial page) provide other opportunities for bringing attention to a policy solution. Letters are usually 200 words or less and can be written, faxed, or emailed to the editor of the newspaper. They are usually in response to a specific article or editorial the paper has published, offering a concise statement of support or objection.

Editorials (sometimes called *masthead editorials*) are unsigned and written by the editorial board of the newspaper. Advocates can make an appointment to talk with the editorial board to ask them to take a position and make a statement about an issue or a pending policy. The meeting is usually attended by the newspaper staff responsible for writing the editorial and those who will make the decision about whether the newspaper will take a position on the issue. The advocates may have two or three people there who can speak to various aspects of the issue or represent different perspectives.

If the newspaper decides not to do an editorial, the advocates can ask if the paper would publish an op-ed. An op-ed is an opinion piece that appears opposite the editorials. Op-eds are usually 600 to 800 words, written from a personal point of view. They describe the problem, solution, and its relevance to the readers. Monitoring should include reviewing op-eds, both to keep tabs on how an issue is being argued and to identify the style the news outlet prefers.

Newspapers often publish on the editorial pages the contact information and instructions for submitting letters and op-eds. Some radio stations and television news programs allow audience members to record commentaries that function like op-eds, though they are usually short (i.e., no more than a few minutes).

Tips and Techniques for Successful Media Advocacy

Several techniques can enhance media advocacy's effectiveness: calculating social math, localizing stories, cultivating authentic voices, and reusing the news.

Calculate Social Math

Social math is the art of making large numbers meaningful, usually by breaking them down and making a relevant, vivid comparison. Calculating social math can illustrate a message. Raw numbers assume that the audience already knows something about the issue and why the numbers are important or revealing. Comparisons, on the other hand, can highlight a specific point of view at the same time they deliver basic information.

To calculate social math, restate large numbers in terms of time or place, personalize numbers, or make comparisons that help bring a picture to mind. Consider these simple facts, stated with effective comparisons.

- A children and youth advocacy group wanted to increase county spending on prevention of violence. To make their point they said, "In San Francisco, there is one police officer for every 18 young people and only one school counselor for every 500 kids."[11]

- The Institute of Medicine noted that the food and beverage industry spends $10.5 billion dollars annually marketing food of poor nutritional quality to children.[12] Advocates pointed out that that amounts to more than $1 million of junk food ads targeting kids every hour of every day.

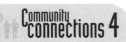

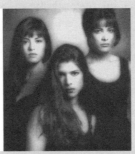

Reprinted with permission from the Los Angeles Commission on Assaults Against Women.

Dangerous Promises coalitions in both Northern and Southern California used a paid advertising strategy to attract news attention. They designed black-and-white billboards with a headshot of three models looking directly into the camera. The copy read, "Hey Bud—Stop using our cans to sell yours." In Los Angeles, no billboard company would agree to run the image, even though the coalition was prepared to pay and was not asking for free space. Instead, the Dangerous Promises coalition there was forced to hire

- Newspaper columnist Ellen Goodman noted that a worker who helps bury people makes more than one who helps them learn: The median wage for a funeral attendant is $7.16 an hour, while the median wage for a childcare worker is $6.17 an hour. Goodman feels that childcare workers are being paid based on what mothers are paid—nothing—and on what professional teachers earn.[13]

- Public health education professor Meredith Minkler noted, "In a single year one company spent more than $30 million advertising a single sugar-coated cereal. During the same year, the amount spent by the U.S. government on nutrition education for school children was just $50,000 per state."[14]

- A reporter in the *Wall Street Journal* illustrated the amount of chewing tobacco being consumed by writing, "Cigarette sales are down; dip sales are up. Laid out tin-to-tin, the dip sold last year would stretch between New York and Los Angeles 11 times. So there is quite a bit of furtive spitting going on."[15]

- A victim's right's advocate used irony to point out society's skewed priorities and illustrate the need for more resources when he said, "We have more shelters for animals than we have for human victims of abuse."[16]

a "mobile billboard," a vehicle that drove around the city with the billboard attached to its sides. In San Diego, the Dangerous Promises coalition purchased several billboards using a revised image with the "Hey Bud" removed. The coalition held a news conference to announce the campaign in a parking lot below one of the billboards. Local television and newspaper stories could easily include the image of the billboard in their coverage. In the San Francisco Bay area, the Dangerous Promises campaign took a more confrontational stance. The image for its billboard was a parody of the Budweiser logo that said "Bloodweiser, King of Tears—Selling Violence Against Women." No billboard company would accept that image.

The controversy regarding the ads was part of the access strategy. The groups held news conferences in each locale launching the campaign, lauding the Wine Institute's action, and criticizing the Beer Institute and DISCUS for not doing the same. Advocates highlighted the controversy when they pitched the story, inviting journalists to see "the anti-violence campaign so controversial that local billboard companies refused to run it."

Localize Stories

Every day there is a multitude of news from which to choose. News outlets are tuned in to satellite broadcasts from around the world that operate 24 hours daily. Assignment editors, city desk editors, reporters, and producers read several newspapers every morning, listen to news radio and police scanners, and monitor wire services. One way advocates can break through that clutter is to alert their news contacts about the local relevance of a story. Questions they can consider include "Why does this story matter to people who live here?" and "Why would it matter to the listeners at this radio station, the viewers of this local television news, or this newspaper?" When advocates know the answers to those questions, they will know what to tell the reporter. Every reporter has to convince his or her boss why to select one story over another. If the story has local relevance, it is much more likely to be pursued.

Elevate Authentic Voices

Reporters populate their stories with characters. A common character in health stories is the "victim"—someone who has suffered from or who has direct experience with the problem, whatever it might be. If the story is about binge drinking on college campuses, reporters will want to talk to students. If the story is about gun safety in the home, they will want to talk to a parent whose child was hurt or killed by a gun in the home. If the story is about immunizations for children, they will want to show a toddler getting injected.

Reporters do this for two reasons. First, the reporter needs to present evidence in the story that what happened was real, that it happened to a real person. Showing someone with direct experience in the story makes that clear. Second, reporters feel that their audience will connect more with the emotion than the facts of a story. People who actually endured a trauma or other experience can be more compelling because they are speaking from experience. They qualify as a "real person," in journalists' parlance.

Besides the usual questions—"What is the problem?" and "What is the solution?"—reporters will ask victims another question: "How do you feel about the tragedy?" The problem, of course, is that if the story does not move much beyond the "victim"—if it is a portrait rather than a landscape—when audiences see the story they are likely to distance themselves from the individual and say, "That won't happen to me," or, in some cases, even blame the victim. Journalists cannot tell stories without characters, and victims can be powerful spokespeople for public health. However, a better approach is to change the dynamic and think of victims as survivors or *authentic voices*. Authentic voices are survivors who have become advocates. They bring personal experience to the story, just like a victim, but they understand their role as advocates. When an authentic voice gets the question, "How do you feel about this tragedy?" he or she responds, "I feel angry because this tragedy could have been prevented," and then explains how.

Victims become authentic voices with training and experience as they move through their grief and put it to work for prevention. There are many authentic voices to thank in public health for opening up their lives to the public and becoming leaders for change in breast cancer, HIV/AIDS, tobacco control, and other diseases. For example, in 2000 Mary Leigh Blek became the first chair of the board for the Million Moms March; she lost her son Matthew to a "Saturday night special" handgun and has been advocating for reasonable gun laws ever since. In 1980, Mothers Against Drunk Driving was created by a small group of women in California after a drunk driver killed Candy Lightner's 13-year-old daughter. Survivors have joined with public health advocates to advocate for safer baby cribs, drowning prevention, pedestrian safety, motorcycle helmets, mandatory CPR training, and auto safety, including interior trunk release latches.[17] All of these authentic voices have selflessly shared their stories and been willing characters in news stories to help further policies that can save lives.

"Reuse the News"

Media advocacy uses mass communication to reach a very small target— sometimes just one person. The power comes from the fact that a vast audience has been privy to this conversation between the advocates and the target. It is a public conversation, not a private conversation. To ensure the target understands this, advocates can "reuse the news." If their op-ed is published, advocates can clip it, copy it, and send it to the target. They can have the target's constituents copy and send news stories and letters to the editor that have been published. They can also reuse the news to educate reporters who are just coming to the issue or use it to educate new advocates. They can share clippings and discuss them in order to become better at framing issues and anticipating the opposition's questions and challenges. News, simply by virtue of its having been published, confers legitimacy and credibility on issues. Media advocates reuse the news to remind the target that the public is paying attention and knows what it wants done.

Overcoming Challenges in Media Advocacy

The biggest barrier to successful media advocacy is in the development of a clear overall strategy, even before getting access to reporters is considered. Other barriers include institutional constraints, not staying "on message," and being distracted by the opposition. This section discusses strategies for overcoming these barriers.

Avoid Having a Murky Strategy

The most important part of media advocacy is developing strategy. If the strategy is not clear and the target has not been well defined, the media advocacy effort will be diffused and ineffective. Public health advocates sometimes resist the simplification necessary to carve out a viable strategy. Public health problems are complex, and that complexity needs to be addressed. Yet at the same time, not everything can be done at once. Public health problems need to be prioritized into manageable chunks that can be addressed in specific time periods. The alternative—strategies that remain too large or overly vague—will be ineffective. Goals such as "raising awareness" are not specific enough for media advocacy campaigns. Instead, clear objectives must be stated that identify who must do what to create or change the rules that will ensure healthier social and physical environments.

Advocates must translate general principles into substantive demands. For example, in San Francisco, a campaign to seek justice for a man who unnecessarily died in police custody was transformed into a campaign to change police practices. Demanding justice was too vague and left the action up to others. So the advocates asked themselves: What would justice look like? They decided that the offending police officer should be fired and safeguards put in place to avoid future hires of officers with similar records of brutality. Advocates had then defined justice in tangible terms that could be put into practice, and used media advocacy to put pressure on the mayor and the police commission to enact the policy changes they desired.

Media advocacy strategies and targets can change over time. In fact, they *should* change. Targets and strategies will shift in response to circumstances and after the advocates achieve their objectives. Advocates can use the strategy development questions discussed earlier to refocus their efforts and evaluate their strategies. With every new activity, they should ask themselves: How will this help us achieve our objectives? And will this make a clear, positive change in the environment surrounding the people whose health we are concerned about? The answers to those questions can guide strategy and decisions throughout the media advocacy effort.

Alter Perceived Institutional Constraints

Media advocacy is about raising community voices to demand change. In most cases, policy change is the desired outcome. Sometimes this will require lobbying that public agencies and some nonprofits are prohibited from conducting. In most cases, however, there is a lot those in both public and nonprofit agencies can do that is not considered lobbying. Unfortunately, advocates often stop short of what is allowed and limit their effectiveness needlessly. Organizations such as the Alliance for Justice provide training and consultation to nonprofits to help them maximize their ability to participate legally in the policy process. Constraints are often not as prohibitive as some in the agency perceive.

Still, media advocacy can be confrontational. Thus, public health practitioners in health departments or other institutions may not be comfortable being "out front" on media advocacy campaigns. Some have a preference for consensus when, instead, conflict is what is needed. In these cases, individuals can find roles for themselves in the media advocacy effort that place them more in the background than the foreground. For example, health departments can provide data, resources, meeting space, technical assistance, and other supports without compromise.

Avoid Being Distracted by the Opposition

While media advocates need to construct thoughtful, succinct answers to the questions their opponents will raise, their goal is not to convince the opposition. Media advocates can be distracted by the arguments their opposition puts forward, and may be tempted to answer those arguments point by point. Sometimes that is necessary, but often it is a ploy by opponents to frame the issue on their own terms. Instead, media advocates' goal is to motivate and mobilize their supporters so those voices will be heard and attended to by policymakers. Everyone does not have to be convinced that the proposal is worth supporting—only those who have decision-making power must be convinced. Media advocacy employs the mass media to make private conversations public, so decision makers can be held accountable for their decisions and the impact of those decisions on the public's health. Advocates should use the media to give credibility and visibility to their own arguments so those who agree with them will know they are not alone.

Stay on Message

Media advocates need to be vigilant when defining the problem and the solution and focus their attention on the clear and consistent articulation of what they want. Thus, articulating a clear message and staying on message are extremely important. Staying on message means that whatever advocates may be asked, they do not stray from the key message they are trying to deliver. Staying on message is a skill that can be honed with practice. It is especially helpful to practice aloud, with colleagues. That way, advocates can anticipate what questions they might receive from reporters, decision makers, or the opposition, and craft answers that lead logically from the question to the outcome they seek. Practicing aloud is important because speaking is different from writing or thinking. The right words will flow more easily if they have been said before. At the same time, advocates should not memorize a script—that can sound stiff and forced. Instead, frequent practice and feedback sessions will help advocates prepare for staying on message.

Expected Outcomes

When media advocacy is done well, healthy public policy is enacted and implemented. Enacting policies that benefit the public's health is a long-term process, however, with many contributing factors. Media advocacy cannot achieve that end alone but can certainly amplify advocates' voices and accelerate the process. Properly applied, media advocacy can punctuate the advocacy process, add urgency to a campaign, and create visibility. Media advocacy does this by increasing the salience of issues for the public and policymakers through agenda setting and framing. Practicing media advocacy will also increase the capacity of local groups to influence the rules that govern their environments.

Increased Skills and Power

Because policy advocacy is usually a long-term endeavor, it is useful to identify some interim effects and outcomes of media advocacy. The most immediate interim effects of media advocacy are the increases in skills and power of the groups using it. By developing and adapting strategy, advocates can gain skills in critical thinking. By talking with journalists and others about the solutions they seek, advocates develop the confidence necessary to speak effectively in public. They become skillful at framing for content and understanding news-worthiness so they can frame for access. By participating in the policy process, either by meeting with decision makers or mobilizing supporters, advocates exercise their democratic power. These skills build on one another and transfer as advocates work together in a community setting to demand change.

Better Relationships with Journalists

An important outcome advocates can expect from media advocacy campaigns is better relationships with journalists. This tangible benefit develops over the course of a media advocacy campaign—and from one campaign to an-other—because advocates bring good information and interesting stories to reporters. The mutually beneficial relationship helps reporters get what they need to do their job and eases advocates' access to and responsiveness from journalists. Simply, an expected outcome of media advocacy is that certain reporters and advocates end up in each other's contact list or email address book. For example, after their concerted media advocacy effort to generate news that reframed alcohol as a policy issue, staff at the Marin Institute for the Prevention of Alcohol and Other Drug Problems, located in California, were frequent sources for journalists. Eventually, reporters would call the Marin Institute for comments on stories that had been generated elsewhere. The Marin Institute was now a required source on alcohol policy issues.

Increased Visibility and Influence

Advocates' increased skills and power, along with their better relationships with reporters, lead to increased visibility for the issue and more influence from the advocates on how that issue is interpreted. If they are successful, advocates will have generated news that put their issue and solution on the policymaker's agenda. Advocates can expect to see their examples used in debate by them-selves and eventually by others, shifting the debate toward the advocates' de-sired outcomes. Advocates' influence will increase with the increased visibility because news coverage confers legitimacy and credibility.

Conclusion

Public health educators can harness the power of the news media to advance healthy public policy. They can increase their effectiveness by developing an overall strategy, learning about how the news media operate, developing a spe-cific media strategy, developing a message that frames the issue from a public health perspective, and understanding how to attract journalists' attention.

The news media are too important a resource to ignore. If health educators are serious about serving the public and improving its health, they need to be serious about the news and about learning how to better integrate it into prevention efforts.

Media advocacy, however, is not appropriate in every instance. The strategy requires a clear and precise plan for policy change and a constituency that can carry it out. It is a public strategy—on the record. Media advocates bring public attention to specific individuals. At times they may need to be confrontational and adversarial, depending on the situation. The policies being advocated for are usually controversial. If they were not, then there would not be a need for a pressure tool and publicity via media advocacy. Advocates should be clear with themselves and their colleagues about what is at stake when choosing to use media advocacy.

Media advocacy is the right choice when public demands must be made and pressure brought to bear on decision makers to protect and promote the public's health.

KEY TERMS

focus audience: The person or body (e.g., CEO, school board, city council) who has the power to enact or enforce the policy or change being sought.

framing: How an issue or idea is explained and interpreted.

framing for access: Focusing on what is newsworthy about an issue.

framing for content: Focusing what is said about an issue on the desired outcome, the solution or policy goal being sought. Framing for content focuses on institutional accountability rather than personal responsibility.

media advocacy: The strategic use of mass media to enhance the effectiveness of community organizing and policy advocacy.

REFERENCES

1. Wallack, L., & Dorfman, L. (2001). Putting policy into health communication: The role of media advocacy. In R. E. Rice & C. K. Atkin (Eds.), *Public communication campaigns* (3rd ed.). Thousand Oaks, CA: Sage Publications.

2. Wallack, L., Dorfman, L., Jernigan, D., & Themba, M. (1993). *Media advocacy and public health: Power for prevention.* Newbury Park, CA: Sage Publications.

3. Wallack, L., & Dorfman, L. (1996). Media advocacy: A strategy for advancing policy and promoting health. *Health Education Quarterly, 23,* 293–317.

4. Dorfman, L., Wallack, L., & Woodruff, K. (2005). More than a message: Framing public health advocacy to change corporate practices. *Health Education and Behavior, 32*(4), 320–336.

5. Iyengar, S. (1991). *Is anyone responsible?* Chicago: University of Chicago Press.

6. California Center for Health Improvement. (2000, December). Joining forces to fight childhood asthma: A Prop 10 opportunity. *Field Lessons, 1*(5).

7. Dorfman, L. (1994). *News operations: How television reports on health.* Doctoral dissertation, University of California at Berkeley.

8. Wallack, L., Woodruff, K., Dorfman, L., & Diaz, I. (1999). *News for a change: An advocate's guide to working with the media.* Thousand Oaks, CA: Sage Publications.

9. Wilgoren, J. (2000, March 15). Effort to curb binge drinking in college falls short. *New York Times,* A16.

10. Paid advertisement. (2000, August 7). *New York Times,* West Coast Edition, p. A19.

11. Coleman Advocates for Children and Youth. (n.d.). *Youth time* [Brochure]. San Francisco: Author.

12. Institute of Medicine. (2006). *Food marketing to children and youth: Threat or opportunity?* Washington, DC: National Academies Press.

13. Goodman, E. (1998, January 15). No easy fix for child care. *San Francisco Chronicle,* p. A23.

14. Minkler, M. (1999). Personal responsibility for health? A review of the arguments and the evidence at century's end. *Health Education and Behavior, 26,* 121–140.

15. Morse, D. (2000, February 11). If you can't smoke in the office, snuff can be a secret vice. *Wall Street Journal,* p. A1.

16. Stein, J., Deputy Director of the National Organization for Victim Assistance, quoted in J. Shiver, Jr. (1997, August 25). Home violence underreported, U.S. study says. *Los Angeles Times,* p. A1.

17. McLoughlin, E., & Fennell, J. (n.d.). Channeling grief into policy change: Survivor advocacy for injury prevention. *Injury Prevention Newsletter,* Vol. 13. San Francisco, CA: The Trauma Foundation.

Community Connections

Hughes, K., & Dorfman, L. (1993). Dangerous promises: The role of alcohol advertising in violence against women. Paper presented at the annual meeting of the American Public Health Association, San Francisco.

Woodruff, K. (1996). Alcohol advertising and violence against women: A media advocacy case study. *Health Education Quarterly, 23,* 330–345.

ADDITIONAL RESOURCES

Print

Chapman, S., & Lupton, D. (1994). *The fight for public health: Principles and practice of media advocacy*. London: BMJ Publishing Group.

Cutting, H., & Themba-Nixon, M. (2006). *Talking the walk: A communications guide for racial justice*. Oakland, CA: AK Press.

Dean, R. (2006, October). *Issue 16: Moving from head to heart: Using media advocacy to talk about affordable housing*. Available: http://www.bmsg.org/pub-issues.php.

DeJong, W. (1996). MADD Massachusetts versus Senator Burke: A media advocacy case study. *Health Education Quarterly, 23,* 318–329.

Dorfman, L., & Wallack, L. (1993). Advertising health: The case for counter-ads. *Public Health Reports, 108,* 716–726.

Jernigan, D., & Wright, P. (Eds.). (1994). *Making news, changing policy: Case studies of media advocacy on alcohol and tobacco issues*. Washington, DC: Center for Substance Abuse Prevention.

Ryan, C. (1991). *Prime time activism*. Boston: South End Press.

Seevak, A. (1997, December). *Issue 3: Oakland shows the way*. Berkeley Media Studies Group. Available: http://www.bmsg.org/pub-issues.php.

Shaw, R. (1999). *Reclaiming America: Nike, clean air, and the new national activism*. Berkeley, CA: University of California Press.

Internet

Action Media. Available: http://www.actionmedia.org/.

Alliance for Justice. Available: http://www.allianceforjustice.org.

Berkeley Media Studies Group. Available: http://www.bmsg.org.

Community Media Workshop. Available: http://www.cmw.org.

FrameWorks Institute. Available: http://www.frameworksinstitute.org/.

The Praxis Project. Available: http://www.thepraxisproject.org.

The Spin Project. Available: http://www.spinworks.org.

INDEX